Critical Limb Ischemia

Critical Limb Ischemia

Edited by

Marc Bosiers
AZ St-Blasius
Dendermonde, Belgium

Peter A. Schneider
Hawaii Permanente Medical Group
Honolulu, Hawaii, USA

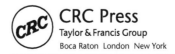

CRC Press
Taylor & Francis Group
Boca Raton London New York

CRC Press is an imprint of the
Taylor & Francis Group, an **informa** business

CRC Press
Taylor & Francis Group
6000 Broken Sound Parkway NW, Suite 300
Boca Raton, FL 33487-2742

First issued in paperback 2019

ISBN-13: 978-1-4200-8189-3 (hbk)
ISBN-13: 978-0-367-38551-4 (pbk)

This book contains information obtained from authentic and highly regarded sources. Reasonable efforts have been made to publish reliable data and information, but the author and publisher cannot assume responsibility for the validity of all materials or the consequences of their use. The authors and publishers have attempted to trace the copyright holders of all material reproduced in this publication and apologize to copyright holders if permission to publish in this form has not been obtained. If any copyright material has not been acknowledged please write and let us know so we may rectify in any future reprint.

Library of Congress Cataloging-in-Publication Data

Critical limb ischemia / edited by Marc Bosiers, Peter A. Schneider.
    p. ; cm.
  Includes bibliographical references.
  ISBN-13: 978-1-4200-8189-3 (hardcover : alk. paper)
  ISBN-10: 1-4200-8189-6 (hardcover : alk. paper) 1. Extremities
(Anatomy)—Blood—vessels—Diseases. 2. Ischemia. I. Bosiers, Marc.
II. Schneider, Peter A.
  [DNLM: 1. Extremities—blood supply. 2. Ischemia—diagnosis. 3.
Ischemia—therapy. 4. Vascular Surgical Procedures—methods. WG 500
C934 2009]
  RC951.C753 2009
  616.7′2—dc22

                                        2009013935

Visit the Taylor & Francis Web site at
http://www.taylorandfrancis.com

and the CRC Press Web site at
http://www.crcpress.com

Preface

Critical limb ischemia (CLI) has emerged as a major international public health challenge that has so far only partially been met. CLI remains an undertreated condition with highly morbid outcomes. Fortunately, the management of CLI has recently improved significantly as new treatment options have been developed and the disease process has become the focus of renewed interest and attention on the part of the medical community and society at large. The management of CLI will likely mature significantly in the next few years, and this will be to the great advantage of current and future vascular patients who face the potential of disability, amputation, and death that has traditionally been associated with CLI.

The area of CLI diagnosis and treatment is experiencing an explosion in interest by multiple specialties. New techniques have come on line, new medications are available, and new information about how bad this problem really is has surfaced. However, an optimal overall approach to CLI has not yet crystallized. Most published material on CLI is available only on a specialty-by-specialty basis, and approaches vary substantially. There is minimal cross-pollination between specialties and continents, and there is no one book that collates all available treatments in an effort to derive a multidisciplinary approach. Because many questions remain unanswered in this endeavor, we have gathered and summarized the knowledge that has accumulated to date by various specialties involved in CLI detection, evaluation, and management by all means. It is the aim of the book to provide a practical and multidisciplinary guide to CLI. We invited a broad array of international opinion leaders and respected experts from a variety of disciplines including cardiology, radiology, vascular medicine, and vascular surgery. This book provides comprehensive and latest available information in a field that is growing rapidly. Diverse aspects of CLI are covered, including demographic and public health issues, diagnosis, bedside evaluation, risk factor management, diagnostic evaluation, medical treatment, endovascular and open surgical management, amputation, and long-term follow-up and management.

We believe that the management of CLI, while having made great strides recently, is poised for dramatic near-term progress. Many diverse areas of knowledge will be put into day-to-day practice. By offering a practical guide for a multidisciplinary approach to CLI, we hope to contribute to this process.

Marc Bosiers
Peter A. Schneider

Contents

Contributors

Enrico Ascher Department of Surgery, Maimonides Medical Center, New York, New York, U.S.A.

Marc Bosiers Department of Vascular Surgery, AZ St-Blasius, Dendermonde, Belgium

Piergiorgio Cao Division of Vascular and Endovascular Surgery, University of Perugia, Ospedale S. Maria della Misericordia, Perugia, Italy

Neal S. Cayne Department of Surgery, New York University Medical Center, New York, New York, U.S.A.

Charlie C. Cheng Department of Surgery, The University of Texas Medical Branch, Galveston, Texas, U.S.A.

Gianmarco de Donato Unit of Vascular and Endovascular Surgery, Policlinico Le Scotte, University of Sienna, Sienna, Italy

Paola De Rango Division of Vascular and Endovascular Surgery, University of Perugia, Ospedale S. Maria della Misericordia, Perugia, Italy

Koen Deloose Department of Vascular Surgery, AZ St-Blasius, Dendermonde, Belgium

Nicholas J. Gargiulo III Department of Surgery, Montefiore Medical Center, New York, New York, U.S.A.

Amelia C. M. Giampietro Service of Interventional Radiology, Ospedale Regionale di Lugano, sede Civico, Lugano, Switzerland

Donald L. Jacobs Department of Surgery, Saint Louis University, Saint Louis, Missouri, U.S.A.

Traci A. Kimball University of Colorado Denver, Anschutz Medical Campus, Section of Vascular Surgery, Department of Surgery, Aurora, Colorado, U.S.A.

Massimo Lenti Division of Vascular and Endovascular Surgery, University of Perugia, Ospedale S. Maria della Misericordia, Perugia, Italy

Christos Lioupis Department of Vascular Surgery, AZ St-Blasius, Dendermonde, Belgium

Evan C. Lipsitz   Department of Surgery, Montefiore Medical Center, New York, New York, U.S.A.

Robyn A. Macsata   Washington DC VA Medical Center, Washington, D.C., U.S.A.

George H. Meier   Division of Vascular Surgery, University of Cincinnati College of Medicine, Cincinnati, Ohio, U.S.A.

Frans L. Moll   Department of Vascular Surgery, University Medical Center Utrecht, Utrecht, The Netherlands

Raghunandan Motaganahalli   Department of Surgery, Saint Louis University, Saint Louis, Missouri, U.S.A.

Mark R. Nehler   University of Colorado Denver, Anschutz Medical Campus, Section of Vascular Surgery, Department of Surgery, Aurora, Colorado, U.S.A.

Nicolas Nelken   Division of Vascular Therapy, Hawaii Permanente Medical Group, Honolulu, Hawaii, U.S.A.

Patrick Peeters   Department of Cardiovascular and Thoracic Surgery, Imelda Hospital, Bonheiden, Belgium

Peter A. Schneider   Division of Vascular Therapy, Hawaii Permanente Medical Group, Honolulu, Hawaii, U.S.A.

Carlo Setacci   Unit of Vascular and Endovascular Surgery, Policlinico Le Scotte, University of Sienna, Sienna, Italy

Anton N. Sidawy   Washington DC VA Medical Center, and Georgetown and George Washington Universities, Washington, D.C., U.S.A.

Michael B. Silva, Jr.   Department of Surgery, The University of Texas Medical Branch, Galveston, Texas, U.S.A.

Niten Singh   Vascular Surgery Service, Madigan Army Medical Center, Tacoma, Washington, U.S.A.

Ralf W. Sprengers   Departments of Vascular Surgery and Nefrology and Hypertension, University Medical Center Utrecht, Utrecht, The Netherlands

Kristien Van Acker   Department of Endocrinology, St. Jozef Hospital, Bornem, Belgium

Jos C. van den Berg   Service of Interventional Radiology, Ospedale Regionale di Lugano, sede Civico, Lugano, Switzerland

Frank J. Veith   Department of Surgery, Cleveland Clinic Foundation, Cleveland, Ohio, and Department of Surgery, New York University Medical Center, New York, New York, U.S.A.

Jürgen Verbist Department of Cardiovascular and Thoracic Surgery, Imelda Hospital, Bonheiden, Belgium

Marianne C. Verhaar Departments of Nefrology and Hypertension, University Medical Center Utrecht, Utrecht, The Netherlands

Roger Walcott Georgetown University Hospital, Washington Hospital Center, and Washington DC VA Medical Center, Washington, D.C., U.S.A.

Willem Willaert Department of Cardiovascular and Thoracic Surgery, Imelda Hospital, Bonheiden, Belgium

Dean T. Williams School of Medical Sciences, Bangor University, and Department of Vascular Surgery, Ysbyty Gwynedd Hospital, Bangor, Wales, U.K.

1 Bedside Evaluation of Lower Extremity Ischemia for Critical Limb Ischemia: A Multidisciplinary Practical Guide

Niten Singh
Vascular Surgery Service, Madigan Army Medical Center, Tacoma, Washington, U.S.A.

Peter A. Schneider
Division of Vascular Therapy, Hawaii Permanente Medical Group, Honolulu, Hawaii, U.S.A.

INTRODUCTION

The results of lower extremity vascular therapy rely on early and accurate diagnosis, intervention that is customized to the patient's needs, and long-term follow-up to ensure the integrity of the treatment. Understanding and performing a thorough history and physical examination facilitate these tasks and remain an essential component of managing lower extremity ischemia.

Much emphasis has been placed on the development and adoption of minimally invasive therapeutic options for vascular disease. However, the results of these procedures, and all therapeutic options, are likely to be poor if there is misunderstanding about the degree of ischemia, the course of the ischemic process, the quality of the tissues, the damage to vital structures, and the levels of disease involved. Understanding key phrases in the history and specific physical findings help to classify which patients warrant further diagnostic and therapeutic evaluation and how rapidly it should be carried out. As Rutherford states, "There are few areas in medicine in which the conditions encountered lend themselves so readily to diagnosis solely on the basis of thoughtful history and careful physical examination as do vascular diseases" (1). Much about the treatment plan can be gleaned by the history and physical examination of a vascular patient. In the following chapter, we review important aspects of the history and physical examination of vascular patients with lower extremity ischemia.

EDUCATING PHYSICIANS ABOUT LOWER EXTREMITY ISCHEMIA

Although medical school training programs strive for uniformity in their educational processes, bedside evaluation of the vascular system does not appear to be a universally strong point. Medical students and residents may not know how to perform a standard physical examination of the vasculature. Endean et al. used a structured clinical examination to evaluate the performance and interpretation of the vascular physical examination by interns and medical students. The test consisted of the ability to identify a pulse and interpret the findings. All groups performed poorly, with the medical students scoring 43% correct, Postgraduate year 1 residents (PGY1) 39%, and PGY2 62% (2). Many unnecessary delays, useless diagnostic tests, and limb loss events may be prevented by a reasonable level of understanding during the initial evaluation. Numerous efforts have been initiated in several countries to increase the awareness of peripheral arterial disease (PAD) among healthcare providers and the general population. The finding that a reduced ankle-brachial index is a marker for cardiac and vascular death and disability has raised the profile of PAD awareness. In addition, it is not uncommon to see advertisements in print and on television regarding PAD, and in the United States more screening programs have been initiated.

PRESENTATION OF LOWER EXTREMITY ISCHEMIA

In the evaluation of lower extremity ischemia, there are two forms of presentation: acute and chronic. Chronic ischemia is almost always due to progressively worsening atherosclerosis. Occasionally, other entities such as popliteal aneurysms may cause occlusion of tibial vessel runoff. Most patients with chronic ischemia have well-developed collateral flow and usually do not have a limb that requires urgent revascularization. Patients present with symptoms of claudication, which may or may not be lifestyle limiting or critical limb ischemia, which is manifested by rest pain or tissue loss. A thorough evaluation can usually be performed on an elective basis. Because chronic ischemia develops gradually, patients may present with profound levels of ischemia and have relatively mild symptoms. Claudication may progress to rest pain and then to gangrene, usually over a course of months to years. Diabetic patients with critical limb ischemia may present initially with tissue loss as repetitive trauma and rest pain may not be noticed secondary to a sensory neuropathy.

Patients with acute ischemia do not have the luxury of an elective workup. Acute ischemia is generally due to an embolic, thrombotic, or traumatic event. These groups can generally be separated on the basis of presentation. Patients with an embolic event will have minimal reserve to compensate for the lack of blood flow and have more profound and possibly permanent ischemia if not revascularized in a timely fashion. Those with an acute thrombosis of an area of stenosis will likely have some collateral flow to allow for limb viability (3). In general, these patients require urgent treatment and evaluation. Often a quick history is taken, and guided by the physical examination findings a decision is made to evaluate the arterial tree.

HISTORY
Chronic Ischemia

The history of a patient with chronic lower extremity ischemia involves identifying the factors that are modifiable and those that require intervention. As such, specific questions regarding the patients' impression of their problem are extremely important. For example, the pain in the lower extremity may bother patients with claudication during activity, but they may have other comorbidities that preclude this symptom from interfering with their lifestyle. As such, a thorough review of past medical history such as coronary artery disease, chronic obstructive pulmonary disease (COPD), diabetes mellitus, and smoking is imperative to managing these patients. It is important to know if someone has well-controlled diabetes as this will impact interventions. In addition, a patient who is still smoking should be counseled on cessation as this may alleviate the progression of claudication symptoms.

Claudication is a relatively reproducible finding and does not occur at rest. It occurs in the lower extremity muscle group one level below the arterial disease. For example, superficial femoral artery (SFA) disease classically results in calf claudication. In general patients with claudication, eliciting the walking distance at which symptoms occur is important as symptoms occur at a predictable distance and worsen with uphill walking or a faster pace.

Differentiating vascular claudication from spinal compression, which can cause similar symptoms, can be confusing for the nonvascular specialist. If lumbar spine compression is causing the problem, symptoms are less with flexion of the spine, and activities such as walking uphill, upstairs, and leaning forward (i.e., while pushing a grocery cart) relieve these symptoms (4). Other entities such as degenerative joint disease of the hip, knees, and ankle can cause pain in the lower extremity but are focal with movement and not consistent with vascular causes of claudication.

In the interview of a patient with lower extremity claudication, numerous questions are pertinent, such as the following:

- Which specific symptom brought the patient for consultation?
- Does the patient have claudication?
- How far can the patient walk?
- Does it improve quickly with rest?
- Is it reproducible?
- Is it worse when walking uphill or upstairs?
- Does the pain interfere with the patient's lifestyle?
- Has the patient ever tried an exercise regimen?
- Has the patient been prescribed any medications for the pain?

Patients with aortoiliac occlusive disease may experience buttock and thigh claudication in addition to calf claudication. Men may experience impotence, as this finding, along with previously mentioned symptoms, is the classic Leriche's triad for aortoiliac occlusive disease.

Women may present with chronic ischemia differently than men as some studies on the basis of objective data have shown that women have a higher prevalence of intermittent claudication and severe ischemia; however, they may not report their symptoms as readily as men (5). Furthermore, women may experience claudication differently than men or may have a lower activity level that does not allow them to experience it as men do (6,7).

In other presentations such as critical limb ischemia, manifesting with rest pain or tissue loss, the above-mentioned past history is extremely important, as these patients will likely have multilevel arterial disease and during the history a treatment plan can be formulated. Rest pain occurs in most distal place aspect of the extremity, the foot, dorsum of the foot, and toes. Patients will complain of pain at night while in the supine position that improves upon placing the extremity in the dependent position. Typically these patients will attempt to maintain their extremity in a dependent position and often will describe sleeping in a reclining chair and avoid elevation of the leg. Patients with rest pain usually have a history of progressive and worsening claudication unless the foot is insensate, such as in patients with neuropathy (8).

In patients with tissue loss, any evidence of acute or chronic infection should be sought as these patients may require a course of antibiotic therapy. In these patients, a history of the length of time they have had the ulceration is important, as is the ambulatory status of the patient as this impacts treatment options. In these situations, ischemia is not the culprit in tissue loss, but it is the main factor that prevents healing.

Diabetic Patients

Diabetic patients present a challenge as they often present with advanced disease secondary to their neuropathy, as mentioned above. Injuries will go unnoticed, and with the blunted inflammatory response seen in diabetic patients, ulceration in the foot will likely proceed in the absence of palpable pedal pulses. The misconception is that diabetics have "microvascular occlusive disease," when in reality they have microvascular dysfunction that does not rule them out for endovascular or open revascularization procedures (9). In this group of patients, a history of good glucose control and adherence to their medications is important prior to embarking on an intervention. Also, understanding that a diabetic patient will likely have tibial vessel occlusive disease with sparing of the pedal vessels, which may preclude an endovascular option, is important as the rate-limiting step in this patient will be conduit for a bypass; therefore, a history of prior cardiac surgery or vascular procedure requiring use of the greater saphenous vein should be elicited.

Rule of "Threes"

A useful method for evaluating lower extremity ischemia is an algorithmic technique that involves the presenting cause, workup, and treatment options. This technique has not been found in published series, but we will give credit to Anton Sidawy, who has taught it to his trainees. It is as follows:

1. Presenting cause:
   A. Lifestyle-limiting claudication
   B. Rest pain
   C. Tissue loss
2. Method to work up patients:
   A. History and physical examination
   B. Noninvasive studies
   C. Invasive studies
3. Treatment options:
   A. Conservative/medical management
   B. Endovascular options
   C. Open operative repair
4. If bypass is considered, three considerations:
   A. Inflow
   B. Outflow
   C. Conduit
5. If bypass is contemplated, three ways to configure the greater saphenous vein:
   A. Reversed
   B. Translocated
   C. In situ

By employing this algorithm for patients seen in the clinic with lower extremity ischemia, the majority of treatment plans can be employed. Obviously, it is generalized but allows one to teach medical students and residents the basic tenets of diagnosis and treatment of patients with lower extremity ischemia.

Acute Ischemia

The history of patients with acute ischemia is fairly straightforward, and the main detail to elicit in these patients is the time from the onset of the symptom. Most patients can pinpoint the exact time their symptoms started. The classic "five Ps," pain, pallor, pulselessness, paresthesias, and paralysis, may or may not be present. It is the goal to place the patient in one of the three Rutherford's criteria, which are the following: class 1, the limb is viable and remains so even without therapeutic intervention; class 2, the limbs are threatened and require revascularization for salvage; and class 3, limbs are irreversibly ischemic and salvage is not possible (10). As mentioned above, most patients with acute ischemia have either an embolic event or an acute thrombosis of a stenotic lesion. Patients with an embolic event may not manifest with a history of chronic symptoms, and a history of cardiac arrhythmias such as atrial fibrillation should be sought. In addition, any familial history of hypercoagulable disorders should be elicited. Subjective questioning of sensory and motor function is important, as this will decide the type of therapy that will be pursued. In patients with a history of chronic symptoms, identifying the level of disease can be helpful in considering treatment options as these patients may tolerate a longer period of ischemia, and options such as thrombolysis can be considered.

PHYSICAL EXAMINATION FOR PATIENTS WITH CHRONIC AND ACUTE LOWER EXTREMITY ISCHEMIA

In most vascular patients, the need and level of intervention can be gleaned from the physical examination after being directed by the appropriate history. We will review the physical examination of patients with lower extremity ischemia in this section.

General Appearance

In patients with claudication, there is no reliable "first impression" in that these patients will generally be sitting quite comfortably without any telltale signs of ischemia. Patients with rest pain may be sitting comfortably, as maintaining their leg in the dependent position relieves pain. This is in contrast to patients with tissue loss, who will usually have a visible wound or dressing in place.

The skin of patients of ischemia has several important findings. Loss of hair of the legs may be the first subtle sign of ischemia. The temperature of the skin is cooler in patients with critical limb ischemia. Capillary refill time can be obtained by pressing the nail bed and noting the time for color to return. Normal capillary refill time is less than two seconds, but in many patients with chronic ischemia, it may be greater than five seconds (11). Often patients with chronic ischemia and those with renal failure will have thickening of the nails, making capillary refill difficult to examine.

In patients with severe ischemia, it can be noted that while sitting, there is erythema over their leg (dependent rubor; Fig. 1). If the leg is elevated, it will appear pale (elevation pallor; Fig. 2). This is a very significant finding of severe ischemia as the patients are depending on gravity and collateral supply for blood to reach their foot. The patients with chronic ischemia may have muscle atrophy of the calf region as well. Patients with rest pain will often have toes that are tender to the touch. Also, other subtle signs of poor perfusion may be minor scrapes and cuts on the skin that do not appear to be healing. Finally, tissue loss will manifest as distal ulcers (i.e., over the toes or dorsum of the foot).

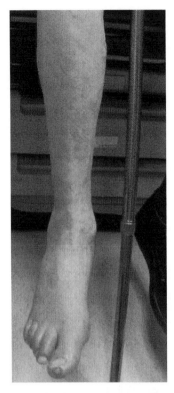

FIGURE 1 Dependent rubor.

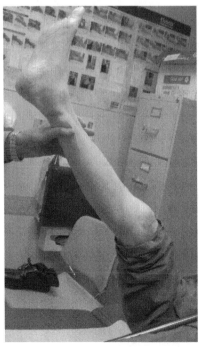

FIGURE 2 Elevation pallor.

TABLE 1 Characteristics of Lower Extremity Ulcers

Ulcer type	Location	Painful
Arterial	Dorsum of the foot and toes	Yes
Venous	Behind medial malleolus (gaiter distribution)	Variable
Neuropathic	Pressure points of foot (i.e., under metatarsal head)	No

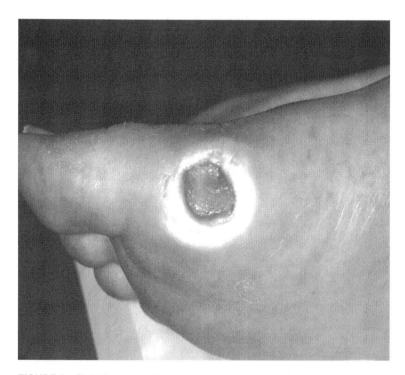

FIGURE 3 Diabetic neuropathic ulcer.

Ulceration may occur without ischemia particularly in diabetic patients, but the ischemic ones are particularly painful and are in random locations—usually from trauma (Table 1). Diabetic neuropathic ulcers (Fig. 3) and venous ulcers (Fig. 4) are usually painless. As gangrene progresses, the nerves in the dead tissue are insensate, and it is usually less painful. In patients with gangrene and pain, it is usually because of live but severely ischemic tissue, like in the forefoot or heel. When dry gangrene occurs (Fig. 5), the body has been able to demarcate the process, and it usually does not progress very rapidly (days, weeks, or even months, instead of hours) as the ischemia may limit the extent of spread. However, wet gangrene (Fig. 6) can progress rapidly, and it is usually due to infection and enough viability of tissue to maintain infection. Often in patients with dry gangrene, there is not enough blood supply to manifest an infection, but after these patients have been revascularized, their dry gangrene may convert to wet

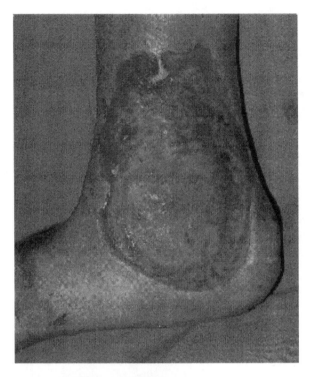

FIGURE 4 Venous ulcer.

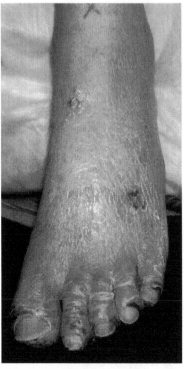

FIGURE 5 Dry gangrene of the forefoot.

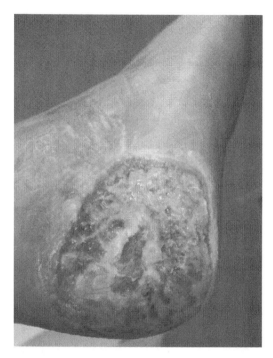

FIGURE 6 Wet gangrene of the heel.

gangrene. Blood is the best antibiotic known to human, and when it is decreased, infection may advance unchecked. If there is persistent infection in the foot after revascularization or when there is good perfusion, one must think of retained foreign body or osteomyelitis.

In patients with tissue loss, the extent of soft tissue loss must be weighed against benefits of reestablishing blood flow. For example, a patient with a significant heel ulcer and exposed bone may not be able to heal the area even with restored blood flow as calcanectomy or other procedures may not allow for tissue coverage of the area and the foot may remain functionless. Exposed tendons and other vital structures may necessitate amputation, even if adequate blood flow is present in face of tissue loss.

Pulse Examination

Pulses are graded as follows: 0, absent; 1, diminished; 2, normal; 3, increased; and 4, bounding. Starting with the abdominal examination, the aorta is palpated. In obese individuals, this may not be possible. The aorta generally bifurcates at the level of the umbilicus, and if the patient is extremely thin, as in many patients with aortoiliac occlusive disease, the calcified aorta or iliac vessels can be palpated. Often using a stethoscope here may reveal a bruit, which may be the first sign of an iliac stenosis.

The femoral pulses can be palpated by identifying them in the groin. To identify the area of the common femoral artery in patients who are obese or do not have palpable pulses, first identify the anterior superior iliac spine and the

pubic tubercle; a line drawn from these two areas represents the inguinal ligament, which may not correspond with the skin fold particularly in obese individuals. Approximately one-third of the way medially will identify the femoral
artery. In patients without a palpable pulse, a firm (calcified) artery may be felt
especially if the patient is thin. In this scenario, pulses may be palpated distally
but not proximally; this usually indicates a calcified femoral artery. Again,
auscultation with a stethoscope in this area may reveal a bruit signifying iliac or
femoral stenosis. The SFA can be palpated throughout its course under the
sartorius muscle as it enters the adductor canal in thin individuals. A 3+ or
greater bounding pulse may signify a stenosis distal to the artery, and auscul-
tating with a stethoscope throughout the artery may reveal a bruit.

The popliteal artery is often difficult to palpate unless properly performed.
The patient should be supine and the knee slightly flexed. Both thumbs of the
examiner should be placed on either side of the patella and the fingers in the
popliteal fossa. The concept should be closing the space between the fingers and
the thumbs (Figs. 7 and 8). Both hands should compress the area, and the
pulsation will be felt between the fingers. Once again, unless the patient is
extremely thin, a bounding pulse in this area may represent a popliteal aneurysm or a significant stenosis of the below-knee segment and a bruit may confirm
this finding. If a popliteal aneurysm is suspected, then an ultrasound should be
planned to further evaluate this area.

The doralis pedis (DP) is the extension of the anterior tibial (AT) artery and
is located over the dorsum of the foot and can be found by palpating just lateral

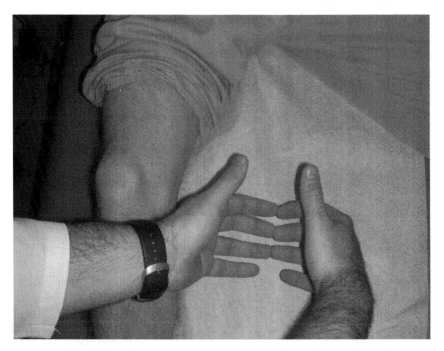

FIGURE 7 Popliteal artery palpation—position of hands with fingertips touching and thumbs on
either side of patella.

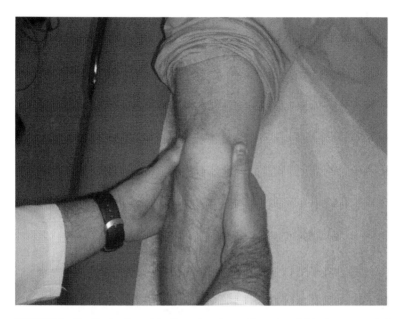

FIGURE 8 Popliteal artery palpation—hands positioned and "closing space between fingers and thumbs."

to the extensor hallucis tendon. To locate this area, the great toe can be dorsi-flexed, and lateral to the tendon is the location where the DP lies. The posterior tibial (PT) artery can be felt by palpating just posterior to the medial malleolus. If neither of these arteries is palpable, then the terminal branch of the peroneal artery, the lateral tibial artery, may be palpable over the medial aspect of the fibula at the ankle.

Oftentimes in patients with ischemia, maneuvers to elicit a suspected area of stenosis can be performed at the bedside. For example, if an SFA lesion is suspected, having the patients exercise by performing plantar and dorsiflexion of the foot may reveal a bruit in the suspected area. Listen for bruits before and after exercise: if a bruit is noted it should be traced proximally and distally to see where it is the loudest. For example, if there is a femoral artery bruit one should auscultate the iliac arteries as well as the length of the SFA in the medial thigh and popliteal artery behind the knee. These concepts are simple but usually overlooked aspects of the bedside examination.

Acute Ischemia

Patients with acute ischemia will generally have severe pain in the lower extremity. On examination, the calf muscles, which are dependent on the inline flow of the SFA, may be tender. In this scenario, there may not be edema as this often occurs after reperfusion, but as the ischemia advances, neurological deficits are apparent. Sensory function will be lost first, followed by motor function. In this situation, the presence of Doppler signals does not mean the limb is not threatened, especially if the patient has palpable pulses on the contralateral leg and may be suffering from myonecrosis at this point. In this case, after discerning a timeline as to when this has occurred and from the physical examination, the treatment is generally straightforward. Patients presenting early in the course may undergo anticoagulation, arteriography, and thrombolysis as needed. Those with a neurological deficit, especially motor, should be taken to the operating room and the muscle inspected before attempting thrombectomy/ embolectomy as the reperfusion of dead muscle could be deadly to these patients.

If acute ischemia has progressed past this point, patients may present with blistering of the skin and edema if the leg is kept in a dependent position, indicating very advanced ischemia. Once again, the history and physical examination are the essential components in the management of these patients.

BEDSIDE EXAM WITH THE HANDHELD DOPPLER

Oftentimes, patients with lower extremity ischemia will not lend themselves to a simple examination. In the case of an experienced examiner, palpation is straightforward, but to those less experienced, confirming a palpable pulse with a Doppler is useful. In this case, a handheld Doppler should be employed to further interrogate the pulses. It is simply done by placing it over the above-mentioned area and listening for the Doppler signal. Generally, it is classified as triphasic (normal), biphasic (likely diseased), and monophasic (severely diseased).

In patients without palpable pulses, the Doppler can be used to provide additional information. In patients with strongly palpable femoral pulses but no palpable pulses, distally Doppler signals in the foot can be indicative of SFA or popliteal artery disease. In a patient without palpable pedal pulses, obtaining a Doppler signal at one of the pedal vessels may indicate tibial vessel disease as well. Another finding when suspecting tibial vessel disease in the presence of pedal Doppler signals is to occlude either the DP or the PT distally and place the Doppler probe on the other pedal artery. If the signal is no longer present in the other pedal artery, then the original signal was only retrograde filling via the arch vessels of the foot and the tibial vessel (PT or AT) is likely stenotic or occluded proximally. Patients with multilevel disease may have weak signals, and venous signals may be hard to discern from monophasic signals. In this instance, placing the Doppler probe over either the DP or the PT and squeezing the foot to increase venous emptying may augment the arterial signal, allowing it to be differentiated.

In addition to identifying flow, the Doppler and a blood pressure cuff can be used to calculate the ankle-brachial index (ABI) (Fig. 9). This index is obtained by placing a pneumatic cuff around the leg above the malleolus and using the Doppler to obtain pressures at the DP and PT arteries. These pressures are then divided by the highest brachial artery pressure and the normal ratio is 1.0. Patients with claudication may have an ABI of 0.4 to 0.8. Ankle-brachial indices at rest and after exercise are useful in patients with suspected claudication, especially if the resting ABI is only mildly diminished. After exercise, the ABI will drop from its resting level as peripheral vasodilation is maximized. Those with more severe ischemia may have an index 0.1 to 0.4, or it may even be undetectable (Table 2). Patients with diabetes will often have calcified vessels; therefore, their ABI will be falsely elevated.

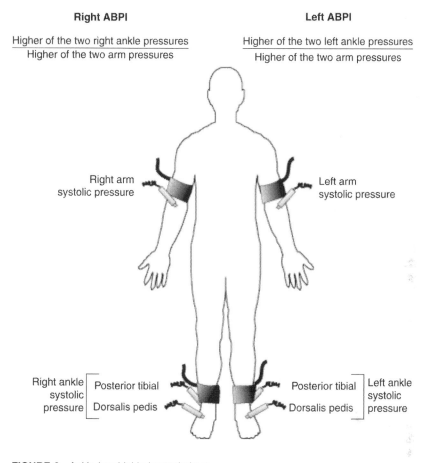

FIGURE 9   Ankle-brachial index technique.

TABLE 2   Ankle-Brachial Index Values and Clinical Presentation

Clinical presentation	Ankle brachial index
Normal	0.95–1.0
Claudication	0.40–0.80
Rest pain	0.20–0.40
Ulceration	0.10–0.40
Acute ischemia	<0.15

CONCLUSIONS

Performing a thorough history and examination of the vascular patient can allow for a diagnosis and treatment plan to be initiated without the need for invasive diagnostic studies. As advancements are made in vascular imaging, we must not forget this important concept.

REFERENCES

1. Rutherford RB. Basic consideration for clinical evaluation. In: Rutherford RB, ed. Vascular Surgery. 6th ed. Philadelphia: WB Saunders, 2005.
2. Endean ED, Sloan DA, Veldenz HC, et al. Performance of the vascular physical examination by residents and medical students. J Vasc Surg 1994; 19:149–156.
3. Ouriel K, Veith FJ, Sashara AA. A comparison of urokinase with vascular surgery as initial treatment for acute arterial occlusion of the legs. Thrombolysis or peripheral arterial surgery (TOPAS) investigators. N Engl J Med 1998; 338:1105–1111.
4. Dormandy JA, Ruhterford RB. TASC Working group: management of peripheral arterial disease. J Vasc Surg 2000; 31(1 pt 2):S1–S296.
5. Sigvant B, Wiberg-Hedman K, Berggvist D, et al. A population-based study of peripheral arterial disease prevalence with special focus on critical limb ischemia and sex differences. J Vasc Surg 2007; 45:1185–1191.
6. Higgins JP, Higgins JA. Epidemiology of peripheral arterial disease in women. J Epidemiol 2003; 13:1–14.
7. McDermott MM, Greenland P, Liu K, et al. The ankle brachial index associated with leg function and physical activity: the Walking and Leg Circulation Study. Ann Intern Med 2002; 136:873–883.
8. Andersen CA, Roukis TS. The diabetic foot. Surg Clin North Am 2007; 87:1149–1177.
9. Akbari CM, LoGerfo FW. Diabetes and peripheral vascular disease. J Vasc Surg 1999; 30: 373–384.
10. Rutherford RB, Baker JD, Ernst C, et al. Recommended standards for reports dealing with lower extremity ischemia: revised version. J Vasc Surg 1997; 26:517–538.
11. McGee SR, Boyko EJ. Lower extremity ischemia: a critical review. Arch Intern Med 1998; 158:1357–1364.

2 Clinical Presentation of Critical Limb Ischemia

Piergiorgio Cao, Paola De Rango, and Massimo Lenti
Division of Vascular and Endovascular Surgery, University of Perugia, Ospedale S. Maria della Misericordia, Perugia, Italy

INTRODUCTION

Critical limb ischemia (CLI) is a *clinical* definition involving a spectrum of clinical features to describe chronic and severe compromise in limb perfusion that results in failure to meet the basal metabolic needs. It is ordinarily manifested by the presence of rest pain, with or without trophic skin changes or tissue loss, including ischemic ulceration and/or ischemic gangrene with appropriate documentation of circulatory impairment. Typically, narcotic medications are required for analgesia.

Contemporary care of CLI consists in attempts at aggressive limb savage. It is fundamentally important for the clinician to recognize early the symptoms of CLI and to determine the time course of development of the ischemia. When the clinical history and physical examination suggest relatively rapid progression, then early or "urgent" revascularization may be required to prevent further deterioration and irreversible tissue loss. Although data confirm that some patients with CLI and intermittent rest pain may improve noticeably during periods of presumed improved cardiac hemodynamics and have small ulcerations that heal with protective dressing alone, these represent a minority of the CLI population. There is general belief that patients with chronic ischemic rest pain or tissue necrosis inevitably progress to limb loss without prompt revascularization. On the basis of this information, vascular specialists recognize the need for early evaluation and treatment of patients with CLI. It is only through control of risk factors, successful revascularization, and aggressive medical therapy that such patients will survive maintaining their ability to deambulate. Despite this belief, data indicate that many CLI patients have delayed treatment with onset of symptoms weeks or months before vascular referral.

The management of patients with CLI is difficult. A number of patients can precipitate to early amputation because of misinterpretation of their symptoms. Indeed, there are patients presenting a variety of lower extremity symptoms other than claudication, not currently considered typical for CLI. Furthermore, the extensive comorbid conditions that accompany CLI (diabetes, coronary artery disease, chronic pulmonary disease) may restrict their activities sufficiently to preclude any claudication before CLI onset. All these data suggest that, despite the systemic nature of atherosclerosis, progression and manifestations of this disease process are not uniform. However, patients who develop rest pain, ulcers, or gangrene have an overall worse prognosis than those who do not. The development of these symptoms may indicate both a limited ability to compensate for the chronic occlusion of major arteries and a greater risk for major amputation and death.

It is important to note that the knowledge of antecedent natural history of patients with CLI is still largely deficient with minimal ability to identify at-risk patients and prevent disease progression. Data suggest that there is not a continuous spectrum of lower extremity ischemia, in which a patient passes from mild claudication to rest pain, ischemic ulcers, and then ischemic gangrene. Although many clinicians assume that CLI evolves through progressive stages of severity in a stepwise manner, multiple natural history studies reveal that in very few patients does claudication progress to CLI, and only 4% are at risk of limb loss (1,2). In a systematic review of 13 population studies, Hooi et al. noted only a small percentage of patients with intermittent claudication that progressed to CLI (2). On the contrary, subsequent failure of the endovascular or bypass graft puts the patient at increased risk for development of CLI. Thus in most patients CLI can progress directly from the first to the last and most severe stages of ischemia.

The majority of studies attempting to address CLI natural history are limited by the inclusion of patients with various degrees of limb ischemia, including pre-CLI stages (before rest pain or foot lesion development). This prevents a clear understanding of the natural history of CLI. CLI populations are difficult to study because large numbers of patients are lost to follow-up or die in longitudinal studies. Indeed, representing the end stage of peripheral arterial occlusive disease, CLI is associated with both a significantly reduced life expectancy and an elevated risk of major amputation of the involved extremity when improvement in arterial flow is not established. Most patients with CLI have a tremendous disease burden with poor baseline function, including loss of ability to deambulate and ability to live independently in an abbreviated survival. Even though revascularization may prevent limb loss, this outcome does not universally result in ambulation of functional independence.

CLINICAL MANIFESTATIONS

According to the TransAtlantic Inter-Society Consensus recommendation 16: "The term critical limb ischemia should be used for all patients with chronic ischemic rest pain, ulcers or gangrene attributable to objectively proven arterial occlusive disease." Therefore, the clinical manifestation of CLI includes typical chronic rest pain or patients with ischemic lesions, ulcers, or gangrene. *The Consensus also stated that the term CLI implies chronicity and therefore applies to patients with presence of these symptoms for more than two weeks.*

PAIN

Ischemic rest pain, the main feature of patients with CLI, is typically described as burning, dysesthetic pain, usually worse in the distal foot and in the toes and usually most severe at night. Rest pain is generally intolerably severe, aggravated by elevation, and relieved with dependency, presumably resulting from the increase in arterial pressure from gravity in a limb with a nonfunctioning venoarteriolar reflex due to ischemia. The pain occurs or worsens with reduction of perfusion pressure: leg elevation with loss of the supplemental effects of gravity on blood flow.

Because of the intolerable, persisting pain, sleep becomes impossible for most of the patients, causing a further decline of their general physical and psychologic conditions. Indeed, rest pain usually occurs at night when the limb is no longer in a dependent position, wakes the patients and forces them to get up or take a short walk to obtain partial relief from the dependent position.

Patients with ischemic pain often sleep in sitting position or with their ischemic leg dangling over the side of the bed. As a consequence of the need for prolonged dependent position of the ischemic leg, ankle and foot edema develop, aggravating foot pain and ischemic lesions.

In diabetic patients the superficial pain sensation may be altered and they may experience only deep ischemic pain such as calf claudication and ischemic rest pain. In the most severe cases of CLI, rest pain is continuous, with episodes lasting minutes to hours but with constant diffuse pain remaining in between. Often the pain cannot be adequately relieved from foot dependency and responds only to opiates.

According to the TASC II (3), ischemic pain needs to be differentiated from other common causes of foot pain to allow early recognition and treatment of ischemic patients.

The pain in CLI is caused by a combination of ischemia, area of tissue loss, and ischemic neuropathy. In the latter, pain needs to be differentiated from neuropathic nonischemic pain, frequently present in diabetic patients. Ischemic neuropathy results in severe, sharp, shooting pain that does not necessarily follow the anatomic distribution of peripheral nerves but is usually most pronounced at the distal part of the extremities. Diabetic neuropathy usually results in a decrease in sensation, but in some patients, it results in severe, seriously disabling pain that has the same characteristics of neuropathic ischemic pain. Indeed it may appear as a burning sensation worsening at night when there is less distraction. However, contrary to ischemic rest pain, diabetic neuropathy shows a symmetrical distribution in both legs and failure to relieve by dependency of the foot. Furthermore, it is often associated with cutaneous hypersensivity and decreased vibratory sensation and reflexes.

Peripheral neuropathy other than that caused by diabetic neuropathy may be caused also by vitamin B_{12} deficiency, syringomyelia, alcohol excess, toxins, and commonly used drugs, such as cancer chemotherapy agents. Any condition producing isolated sensory neuropathy can generate foot pain similar to ischemic pain.

Patients may have foot pain caused by "complex regional pain syndrome," previously defined as "causalgia" or "reflex sympathetic dystrophy." This pain can be easily distinguished from ischemic pain because the circulation is adequate in these patients. However, these complex regional syndromes may be the consequence of delayed revascularization leading to inadvertent ischemic damage to peripheral nerves.

A common cause of continuous foot pain is nerve root compression from different underlying conditions. In these cases, the pain is typically associated with backache, and pain distribution follows lumbosacral dermatomes.

Other very common and harmless, although difficult to diagnose, causes of foot pain are "night cramps" that usually involve the calf, very rarely the foot alone. These may be associated with muscle spasm and chronic venous insufficiency.

Buerger's disease may also present with rest pain in the feet, usually in younger smokers. Although the pathophysiology is distal limb ischemia, this is caused by an occlusive, inflammatory vascular process involving both arteries and veins.

Similarly, pain may be caused by a number of other systemic inflammatory diseases such as gout and rheumatoid arthritis. Finally, local causes of foot pain such as tarsal nerve compression, plantar fasciitis, and digital neuroma should be excluded.

ULCERS AND GANGRENE

Further progression of tissue hypoxia ultimately leads to tissue ulceration and gangrene. However, in many patients, particularly diabetic patients with diabetic neuropathy, CLI does not progress from rest pain to tissue loss but the initial presentation is with a neuroischemic ulcer or gangrene. On the basis of literature, there are significant differences at this stage of CLI between patients with or without diabetes. The former have been recognized and distinguished in a separate subcategory of CLI in the TASC (3): "diabetic foot ulcers."

Nondiabetic gangrene and ulcers usually affect the digits or the pressure points (the heel in bedridden patients) and may extend to the distal parts of the foot. Gangrene is usually caused by a minor local trauma, local pressure (fitting shoes), or use of local heat. Gangrenous tissue can shrink and form a scar leading to mummification and spontaneous amputation. However, necrotic tissue may also be infected with spreading of tissue loss.

The majority of lower leg ulcers above the ankle (especially medial) have a venous origin, whereas ulcers in the foot are most likely due to arterial insufficiency. Malleolar ulcers could also be due to mixed arterial/venous origin or to skin infarct from systemic disease/embolism. Characteristics of ulcers are detailed as follows:

- Arterial ulcers are commonly caused by atherosclerotic disease of *the large arteries* but may also be due to atheroembolism or thromboangiitis obliterans (Buerger's disease). In other cases, the disease of the arterial bed is located in the microcirculatory *system*, as in diabetic microangiopathy or vasculitis and collagen vascular diseases. Arterial ulcers are characterized by severe pain, various shapes with pale, dry base and are located on the toes, foot, or ankle.
- Venous ulcers, a consequence of venous insufficiency, are typically associated with mild pain and are located in the malleolar area. The appearance is irregular with pink, moist base.
- Mixed venous/arterial ulcers due to a combination of the previous two are similar to venous ulcers. These are located at the malleolar area and show mild pain and irregular shape with pink base. However, if nonhealing, revascularization may be required.
- Neuropathic ulcers are all those caused by neuropathy, including diabetes, vitamin B_{12} deficiency, etc. These ulcers are typically painless, deep with a surrounding callus, and can often become infected. The location is characteristic. These affect the plantar surface of the foot (weight/bearing) and are often associated with foot deformation.
- Neuroischemic ulcers, due to a combination of neuropathic and ischemic, are similar to arterial ulcers for characteristics and prognosis but can be located on both the toe and the plantar surface of the foot. However, because of nerve damage, pain is reduced.
- Skin infarct ulcers are due to a variety of systemic hematologic diseases, leading to obstruction of small vessels or microembolism: sickle cell anemia, polycithaemia, leukemia, thalassemia, thrombocytosis, etc. These infarcts are small, multiple, severely painful ischemic areas located on the malleolar site or in the lower third of the leg.

- Drug injection, artifactual or factitious, is another cause of lower limb ulcers.
- Other more rare ulcers are commonly caused by thrombophilia in malignancy (squamous cell carcinoma, Kaposi's sarcoma, metastasis, lymphosarcoma) or by gout, pyoderma gangrenosus, and necrobiosis lipoidica.
- Infectious ulcers are known to be caused by leprosy or mycotic diseases.

Diabetic Foot

It has been estimated that about 15% of people with diabetes will develop foot ulcers during their lifetime and about 14% to 24% will require amputation. Diabetic foot complications are the most common cause of nontraumatic lower extremity amputations in the world, but also the most preventable when detected early and treated appropriately. Early identification of the patient at risk and preventive foot care could prevent up to 85% of diabetic amputations (4).

The most common pathway associated with the development of diabetic ulcers includes peripheral neuropathy; approximately 30% of diabetics have mild to severe forms of nerve damage. Loss of protective sensation leads to insensate foot more vulnerable to pressure points and repetitive activity (5). Motor nerve defects and limited joint mobility can cause structural foot deformities with pressure points further predisposing the patient to foot lesions. Because of autonomic neuropathy, loss of sweating, dry fissured skin, and increased arteriovenous shunting occur. Healing requires a greater increase in perfusion than needed to maintain intact skin.

Although the majority of diabetic ulcers are neuropathic, the TASC (3) classifies diabetic foot ulcerations in three broad categories, which are

- ischemic,
- neuroischemic, and
- neuropathic.

Neuropathic ulcers are typically painless with regular margins and punched out in appearance, located on the plantar surface of foot. The foot typically appears as a dry, warm foot, red in appearance with dilated veins and increased blood flow (Arterio-Venous shunt). Other features are the presence of normal pulses, calluses, bone deformity, and loss of sensation, reflex, and vibration.

Ischemic ulcers typically occur in the absence of distal pulses. These ulcers are severely painful, with irregular margins, and are commonly located on toes. The foot is cold, pale, or cyanotic and shows decreased blood flow with collapsed veins and without bone deformity or sensory degeneration.

The differentiation of these ulcerations might be difficult in diabetic patients, but ischemia has to be excluded in all ulcers, given its major impact on outcome. Some patients have clear signs of CLI (toe pressure <30 mmHg), while in others blood flow is impaired to a lesser degree (toe pressure 30–70 mmHg), but they are still unable to heal foot lesions. Furthermore, increased arteriovenous shunt blood flow, due to autonomic neuropathy, can result in a relatively warm foot, falsely reassuring the clinician. The relative incompressibility of calcified distal arteries in diabetic patients with an apparent ankle-brachial index (ABI) within normal limits should be taken into account in the evaluation of diabetic foot.

The most commonly used classification systems for diabetic foot ulcers are the Wagner and the University of Texas classification, both providing description of ulcers to varying degrees and are useful to plan treatment and assess prognosis (6). The Wagner system assesses ulcer depth and the presence of osteomyelitis or gangrene according to the following grades:

Grade 0: pre- or post-ulcerative lesions
Grade 1: partial/full thickness ulcer
Grade 2: penetrating tendon or capsule
Grade 3: deep osteitis
Grade 4: partial foot gangrene
Grade 5: whole foot gangrene

The University of Texas System is based on ulcer depth and presence of wound infection and of clinical signs of CLI. The classification includes three grades and four stages. The grades of this system are the following:

Grade 0: pre- or post-ulcerative lesions
Grade 1: superficial wound, not involving tendon, capsule, or bone
Grade 2: wound penetrating bone or joint

Within each wound grade, there are four stages, which are as follows:

Stage A: clean wound
Stage B: nonischemic, infected wound
Stage C: ischemic noninfected wound
Stage D: ischemic infected wounds

Both classifications have been largely employed and useful in predicting outcome. However, besides the type of classification used, there is no doubt that the presence of ischemia significantly worsens the prognosis of foot ulcerations (7). It has been recognized that diabetic patients with CLI benefit from early revascularization. Nevertheless multiple revascularization procedures may be required and close surveillance is mandatory since failure rates are high. It has been recognized that the incidence of major amputation in patients with CLI increases markedly with age, smoking, and diabetes. The greatest risk factor for CLI remains diabetes. Major amputation is 10 times more frequent in diabetic patients than in nondiabetics with CLI. Although diabetes affects about 2% to 5% of the Western populations, 40% to 45% of all major amputees are diabetic (2). An aging population with an increasing prevalence of diabetes is developing in Western countries. The associated CLI is thus poised to be a major health concern and potential burden to the health care system. Economically sensible, safe, and successful strategies for management and therapeutic treatments are necessary for successful clinical outcome and require a better definition.

SUBCRITICAL LIMB ISCHEMIA

It has been recently suggested that there is a subgroup of patients with CLI in whom severely reduced circulation to the foot does not manifest as rest pain, ischemic ulceration, or ischemic gangrene. Authors have defined "chronic subcritical limb ischemia (CSLI)." It has been recognized that patients with peripheral arterial disease do not usually go through gradual progression from claudication to advanced stages of CLI because many develop CLI without warning. At least part can be explained by this asymptomatic stage, CSLI, in patients who do not ambulate for various reasons and therefore do not present with claudication or attribute their limited walking ability to other conditions such as arthritis or cardiopulmonary compromise. At this stage foot skin is intact; however, they do not have sufficient perfusion to heal foot wounds, and should they receive minor trauma, the wound would result in nonhealing ischemic lesions and evident CLI with limb threat. These patients need to be discovered before these events precipitate in order to apply (*i*) preventive foot care to avoid foot infection, (*ii*) risk factor control to improve mortality outlook, (*iii*) regular follow-up, and (*iv*) attentive care. However, there is currently no evidence to support that aggressive revascularization at early CSLI can be efficiently managed by medical treatment to prevent progressive disease (8).

CONCLUSIONS

Patients with symptomatic peripheral arterial disease of the lower extremities may present with a spectrum of discomfort ranging from intermittent claudication to limb-threatening ischemia, including rest pain, ischemic ulcerations, and gangrene. The clinical marker of CLI is the presence of constant and intolerable pain requiring pharmacologic assistance to obtain relief.

It is estimated that only 45% of patients with CLI are alive without amputation at one year (2). The fate of survivors is similarly poor. Many who do survive with intact lower limb suffer from chronic pain that requires analgesia. The rate of limb loss in patients with CLI is significant, with approximately 25% who could not have circulation to the leg restored, or who failed revascularization, requiring below- or above-knee amputation within six months of presentation. Several large studies have reported that more than one-third of patients presenting with CLI required major amputation within 12 months of presentation (2).

Early recognition of clinical symptoms is essential to improve unfavorable outcomes.

REFERENCES

1. Dormandy JA, Murray GD. The fate of the claudicant. A prospective study of 1969 claudicants. Eur J Vasc Surg 1991; 5(2):131–133.
2. Hooi JD, Stoffers HE, Knottnerus JA, et al. The prognosis of non-critical limb ischaemia: a systematic review of population-based evidence. Br J Gen Pract 1999; 49(438):49–55.
3. Norgren L, Hiatt WR, Dormandy JA, et al. TASC II Working Group. Inter-society consensus for the management of peripheral arterial disease (TASC II). J Vasc Surg 2007; 45(suppl S):S5–S67.
4. Moulik PK, Mtonga R, Gill GV. Amputation and mortality in new-onset diabetic foot ulcers stratified by etiology. Diabetes Care 2003; 26(2):491–494.
5. Frykberg R. An evidence based approach to diabetic foot infections. Am J Surg 2003; 186:S44–S54.
6. Lipsky B. International Consensus group on diagnosing and treating the infected diabetic foot. A report from the international consensus on diagnosing and treating the infected diabetic foot. Diabetes Metab Res Rev 2004; 20(suppl 1):S68–S77.
7. Oybo SO, Jude EB, Tarawneh I, et al. A comparison of two diabetic foot ulcer classification systems: the Wagner and the University of Texas wound classification systems. Diabetes Care 2001; 24(1):84–88.
8. White JV, Rutherford RB, Ryjewski C. Chronic subcritical limb ischemia: a poorly recognized stage of critical limb ischemia. Semin Vasc Surg 2007; 20(1):62–67.

3 | Classification Systems for CLI

Marc Bosiers, Christos Lioupis, and Koen Deloose
Department of Vascular Surgery, AZ St-Blasius, Dendermonde, Belgium

Jürgen Verbist and Patrick Peeters
Department of Cardiovascular and Thoracic Surgery, Imelda Hospital, Bonheiden, Belgium

The main purpose of defining and grading chronic arterial limb ischemia is to predict outcome and to standardize reporting practices. Many classification systems for grading the severity of chronic arterial occlusive disease have been suggested. In the case of *critical limb ischemia* (CLI), attempts at a precise definition based on clinical grades of classification systems have been problematic. Current CLI definitions have been criticized for being arbitrary, unclear, and not able to predict outcome accurately.

A number of terms require definition before analyzing the criteria for classifying chronic arterial limb ischemia and defining CLI. The term *ischemic rest pain* has been well characterized as a severe pain that is localized to the forefoot and toes or to the vicinity of focal ischemic lesions (1). It is brought on or worsened by elevation and relieved by dependency, and it is intolerably severe—not readily controlled by analgesics. Diffuse pedal ischemia with ischemic rest pain is commonly associated with ankle pressures lower than 40 mmHg and toe pressures lower than 30 mmHg (2). The term *ischemic ulcer* implies that there is insufficient arterial perfusion to support the healing process of the ulcer in distal parts of the extremity. Ulcers may be entirely ischemic in etiology or may initially have other causes (such as traumatic or neuropathic) but cannot heal because of the severity of the underlying peripheral arterial disease (PAD). Associated with ulcers, there is usually ischemic rest pain and objective evidence of diffuse pedal ischemia, such as critical reductions in the ankle or toe pressures: an ankle pressure upper limit of 60 mmHg is recommended for this category and a toe pressure of 40 mmHg (2). The ankle and toe pressure levels needed for healing are, therefore, higher than the pressures found in ischemic rest pain, implying the additional perfusion that is required to heal an ulcer, especially if secondary infection is present. *Gangrene* may be focal, affecting the digits or, in a bedridden patient, the heel, but in severe cases it may involve the distal parts of the forefoot. Focal gangrene may be caused by focal arterial thrombosis or atherothrombotic microembolism and therefore not be associated with diffuse pedal ischemia and ischemic rest pain. Gangrene associated with diffuse pedal ischemia extended is almost invariably associated with typical ischemic rest pain. For patients with gangrene, the presence of CLI is suggested by an ankle pressure less than 70 mmHg or a toe systolic pressure less than 50 mmHg (3). It is important to understand that there is not complete consensus regarding the vascular hemodynamic parameters required to make the diagnosis of CLI, and no single level can cleanly separate categories, but they do have a rational basis (2,3).

The first classification system for CLI was introduced by Fontaine et al. in 1954. Patients with ischemic rest pain but no skin lesions categorized as belonging to stage III PAD and patients who had skin lesions as stage IV PAD. Chronic CLI is used simply as a collective term (Fontaine III and IV) (4). The problem with this simple definition of CLI is that it includes a whole spectrum of patients, from those with mild, easily controlled rest pain to patients with extensive gangrene of the foot, in whom there is no alternative to an early major amputation.

In 1981, an ad hoc working party developed a definition of *critical ischemia* (5). The authors included an ankle systolic pressure of less than 40 mmHg in patients with chronic ischemic rest pain and an ankle systolic pressure less than 60 mmHg in patients with ulcers or gangrene. Patients with diabetes were excluded from the definition and no other report was applied to such patients. The definition was based on the concept of *limb-threatening ischemia*, a term used to describe ischemia of such severity that in the absence of a successful revascularization the leg will require a major amputation. The term *limb salvage* was added to describe this indication for surgery. The definition of CLI aimed at defining this indication for limb salvage surgery.

Recommendation for clinical categories of chronic limb ischemia was also made in 1986, by a committee reporting standards of the Society for Vascular Surgery (SVS) and the North American Chapter of the International Society of Cardiovascular Surgery (ISCVS). This had the same resting ankle pressure limit but added the possibility of measuring the toe pressure, which had to be below 30 or 40 mmHg for patients with ulcers or gangrene or "a barely pulsatile ankle or metatarsal plethysmographic tracing" (6). Another definition of chronic CLI was developed in a European Consensus Document that selected a common pressure level (50 mmHg ankle and 30 mmHg toe pressure) to define a group of patients who would inevitably require amputation in the absence of successful revascularization (7). However, using the same criteria both for those with rest pain and for those with tissue loss, though may be simpler it does not recognize the difference between the level of perfusion pressure required to preserve intact tissue and ward off ischemic rest pain and the additional perfusion for healing ischemic foot lesions (8).

CLI is also equivalent to the grades II and III, which includes categories 4, 5, and 6 of the North American recommendations for reporting standards (2). According to these recommendations, symptomatic chronic arterial occlusive disease is stratified into six categories to provide the greater breadth required for many clinical research studies. Gangrene is divided into two levels according to its extent and the possibility of salvaging a functional foot remnant. Simpler broader gradations, based on Fontaine's original clinical staging, are offered in parallel in Table 1. A particular subgroup of patients with PAD does not fall within the definitions of either claudication or chronic CLI. These patients are completely asymptomatic because they are sedentary and therefore do not claudicate. If they manage to avoid trauma, they may not have ulcers or gangrene, though they may have low perfusion pressures and low ankle systolic pressures. They are nevertheless very vulnerable, and they may easily proceed to CLI. Because such patients may benefit from preventive measures and close follow-up to detect and deal with the development of manifestations of CLI, there is a need to identify and characterize this group of asymptomatic patients with very low perfusion pressures and therefore high risk (9).

All these post-Fontaine definitions are limited in that they cannot identify a group of patients who will inevitably require a major amputation in the absence of

TABLE 1 Clinical Categories of Chronic Limb Ischemia

Grade	Category	Clinical description	Objective criteria
0	0	Asymptomatic—no hemodynamically significant occlusive disease	Normal treadmill or reactive hyperemia test
	1	Mild claudication	Completes treadmill exercise[a]; AP after exercise >50 mmHg but at least 20 mmHg lower than resting value
I	2	Moderate claudication	Between categories 1 and 3
	3	Severe claudication	Cannot complete standard treadmill exercise[a]; AP after exercise <50 mmHg
II[b]	4	Ischemic rest pain	Resting AP <40 mmHg, flat or barely pulsatile ankle or metatarsal PVR; TP <30 mmHg
III[b]	5	Minor tissue loss—nonhealing ulcer, focal gangrene with diffuse pedal ischemia	Resting AP <60 mmHg, ankle or metatarsal PVR flat or barely pulsatile; TP <40 mmHg
	6	Major tissue loss—extending above transmetatarsal level, functional foot no longer salvageable	Same as category 5

[a]Five minutes at 2 mph on a 12% incline.
[b]Grades II and III and categories 4, 5, and 6 are embraced by the term chronic critical ischemia.
Abbreviations: AP, ankle pressure; PVR, pulse volume recording; TP, toe pressure.

successful revascularization. It is simply not known what would happen to a patient with severe leg ischemia in the absence of treatment. Furthermore, the division between subgroups has been made using arbitrary pressure limits, excluding occasionally patients with rest pain or possibly even ulcers, and therefore they may be of little utility in the management of individual patients.

More recently, Wolfe and Wyatt analyzed the literature and suggested that a "low-risk" and a "high-risk" group should be identified within patients with severe leg ischemia (8). The term *chronic subcritical ischemia* was suggested for a particular subgroup that falls between the definitions of claudication and chronic CLI. The low-risk group contained only patients with rest pain alone and an ankle pressure above 40 mmHg (subcritical ischemia). The high-risk group contained patients with rest pain and either tissue loss or an ankle pressure below 40 mmHg (critical ischemia). For patients with subcritical ischemia, 100% cumulative patency is equivalent to 64% resolution of symptoms at one year as the rest pain in some (9%) may have improved without treatment. For patients with critical ischemia, 100% cumulative patency is equivalent to 93% limb salvage at one year. The authors concluded that "reconstructive surgery" should be viewed from the following more realistic perspective, which means that for the group of patients with critical ischemia, a surgical/radiological intervention appears to be virtually imperative to save the limb, while for the less severely affected group with subcritical ischemia, limb loss does not appear to be inevitable and pharmacotherapy and medical treatment may buy sufficient time for the crisis to pass. They also recommended that future reports should identify these two groups separately. However, their analysis may be unreliable, because most of the literature on which the conclusions were based showed methodological flaws and contradictions (did not quote Doppler pressure, many included patients with intermittent claudication, and many were postoperative series) (9). Confusion may also arise by the alternative use of the term *subcritical ischemia* as defined in this report and as more recently suggested by the SVS/ISCVS document, referring to asymptomatic, sedentary patients with low perfusion pressures and low ankle systolic pressures (2).

The TransAtlantic Inter-Society Consensus (TASC) II for the management of peripheral arterial disease, published in 2007, included a definition of CLI (3). According to this, CLI is a manifestation of PAD that describes patients with typical chronic ischemic rest pain or patients with ischemic skin lesions, either ulcers or gangrene. Chronic ischemic disease was defined as the presence of symptoms for more than two weeks. Ischemic rest pain should be considered at an ankle pressure below of 50 mmHg or a toe pressure less than 30 mmHg, while other causes of pain at rest should be considered in a patient with an ankle pressure above 50 mmHg, although CLI could be the cause. The authors noticed that a subgroup of PAD patients fall outside the definition of either claudication or CLI. These patients have severe PAD with low perfusion pressures and low ankle systolic pressures, but are asymptomatic. They are usually sedentary and, therefore, do not claudicate, or they may have diabetes with neuropathy and reduced pain perception. The natural history of this subgroup of severe PAD is not well characterized. These patients are presumed vulnerable to develop clinical CLI and outcomes of excess mortality, and amputation would be expected. The term *chronic subclinical ischemia* has been ascribed to this subgroup (3).

Overall, the term critical limb ischemia should be used for all patients with chronic ischemic rest pain, ulcers, or gangrene attributable to objectively proven arterial occlusive disease. The term critical limb ischemia implies chronicity and is to be distinguished from acute limb ischemia. In general, the prognosis is ominous and very much worse than that of patients with intermittent claudication; however, it is impossible to describe the natural history of these patients. Most available information looks at patients treated conservatively, but they are clearly a selected subgroup in no way representative of all patients with rest pain, ulcers, or gangrene. Large numbers of patients are also lost to follow-up or dying in longitudinal studies, leading to incomplete data sets. There is, however, information on what happens to an unselected group of patients newly diagnosed with CLI and receiving the currently available standard therapy. In general, such information suggests that a year after the onset of CLI, only about half the patients will be alive without a major amputation, although some of these may still have rest pain, gangrene, or ulcers. Approximately 25% will have died, and 25% will have required a major amputation (9). Hence the increased focus on developing new surgical, endovascular, and pharmacological approaches to the management of this small, but very seriously ill, group of patients. The current classification systems of CLI and ankle/toe systolic pressure levels cannot identify these subgroups of patients who will be benefited by conservative treatment or primary amputation and this should be probably an area for future research.

REFERENCES

1. Cranley JJ. Ischemic rest pain. Arch Surg 1969; 98(2):187–188.
2. Rutherford RB, Baker JD, Ernst C, et al. Recommended standards for reports dealing with lower extremity ischemia: revised version. J Vasc Surg 1997; 26(3):517–538.

3. Norgren L, Hiatt WR, Dormandy JA, et al. Inter-society consensus for the management of peripheral arterial disease (TASC II). Eur J Vasc Endovasc Surg 2007; 33(suppl 1): S1–S75.
4. Fontaine R, Kim M, Kieny R. [Surgical treatment of peripheral circulation disorders.] Helv Chir Acta 1954; 21(5–6):499–533.
5. Jamieson C. The definition of critical ischaemia of a limb. Br J Surg 1982; 69(suppl): S1.
6. Suggested standards for reports dealing with lower extremity ischemia. Prepared by the Ad Hoc Committee on Reporting Standards, Society for Vascular Surgery/North American Chapter, International Society for Cardiovascular Surgery. J Vasc Surg 1986; 4(1):80–94.
7. Second European Consensus document on chronic critical leg ischemia. Eur J Vasc Surg 1992; 6(suppl A):1–32.
8. Wolfe JH, Wyatt MG. Critical and subcritical ischaemia. Eur J Vasc Endovasc Surg 1997; 13(6):578–582.
9. Anonymous. D1 Definition and nomenclature for chronic critical limb ischemia. J Vasc Surg 2000; 31(suppl):S168–S175.

4 The Physiological Evaluation of Critical Lower Limb Ischemia

Dean T. Williams
School of Medical Sciences, Bangor University, and Department of Vascular Surgery, Ysbyty Gwynedd Hospital, Bangor, Wales, U.K.

INTRODUCTION

It is the aim of all vascular clinicians, where possible, to maintain the integrity and improve the function of ischemic lower limbs by increasing perfusion via the least perilous process. This risk/benefit balance is often a delicate one in individuals with multiple or severe comorbidities.

The clinical evaluation remains the cornerstone of the assessment in critical lower limb ischemia. The addition of noninvasive testing can underpin or contradict the initial diagnosis of limb ischemia, particularly where the clinical evaluation is confounded by coexisting morbidities. Only after the diagnosis of limb ischemia has been made and therapeutic intervention considered a viable proposition should we proceed to demonstrate the anatomical distribution of arterial disease.

It has, for many years, been accepted as good practice that noninvasive, laboratory tests should be performed in individuals who have, or are suspected to have, significant peripheral arterial occlusive disease (PAOD) (1). Noninvasive tests of lower limb perfusion are now widely used both in hospitals and the community. Increasingly, algorithms for managing various lower limb diseases include noninvasive tests to provide a measure of perfusion and exclude the presence of physiologically significant PAOD.

A vascular laboratory can augment the management of critical limb ischemia (CLI) by clarifying the diagnosis, establishing the level of disease, quantifying severity, and indicating prognosis (2). Noninvasive tests, by avoiding contrast media, are inherently safe compared with other imaging modalities (Table 1).

Noninvasive tests are also employed to measure the efficacy of interventions aimed at improving limb perfusion.

Clinically, CLI is defined by the TransAtlantic Inter-Society Consensus (TASC) II document (3) as severe disease (chronic ischemic rest pain for greater than two weeks or tissue loss) *attributable to objectively proven* PAOD. The inherent difficulty with this definition is that the clinical picture may be a result of multiple influences not solely attributable to identified PAOD. This is potentially further confounded by only employing invasive methods to diagnose PAOD. Invasive tests can clearly demonstrate occlusive disease, but are poor at reflecting the physiological changes that result. Objective, noninvasive tests can accurately reflect hemodynamic changes resulting from occlusive disease and indicate distal perfusion. They are therefore an essential addition to the criteria employed in defining chronic critical lower limb ischemia.

TABLE 1 Summary of Advantages and Disadvantages for Noninvasive Assessments

Laboratory	Radiology
Advantages	
General	
Relatively low cost	
Can reduce requirement of contrast imaging	
Ease of availability	Generally limited availability
No radiation	Radiation exposure (CT, DSA)
Low risk, noninvasive	Higher risk (intravenous/arterial puncture)
Nontoxic/No contrast	Potential toxicity related to contrast
Potential quantitative severity measurement	Generally qualitative measurement
Post-intervention testing and monitoring	Hazardous and restricted use
Close patient contact	Patient can be isolated
Small probes and equipment	Confined space—claustrophobia risk
Color Duplex imaging	
Reflect severity of hemodynamic change	Reflect anatomical change mainly
Image vessel wall and surrounding tissue	Only MR+/− CT image tissues
Doppler waveform analysis	
Reflect severity of hemodynamic change	Reflect anatomical change mainly
Relatively easy to perform	Complex procedures
Distal perfusion indicators	
Indicate perfusion close to point of interest	No measurement of perfusion
Continuous monitoring possible	Restricted—generally brief
Disadvantages	
General	
Results very operator dependent	Minimal operator dependency
Generally no therapeutic action (except ultrasound-guided intervention)	Potential therapeutic intervention (DSA/angioplasty/stenting)
Color Duplex imaging	
Interpretation of stored images difficult	Images easily inspected after test
Patient obesity—potential reduced efficacy	Obesity has less influence
Doppler waveform analysis	
Vessel calcification can compromise tests	Calcification less problematic
Arterial anatomical detail limited	Good arterial anatomical detail
Segmental pulse and pressure tests	
Vessel calcification can compromise tests	Calcification less problematic
Arterial anatomical detail limited	Good arterial anatomical detail
Practical issues regarding cuff application	No similar restriction (lower limb edema, cellulitis, ulceration)
Cutaneous sensors sensitive to environment (potential for variation in readings)	No similar sensitivity issues
Cutaneous perfusion indicators	
Restricted use in clinical setting	No similar concerns
Small study area (vulnerable to local variations in perfusion)	No similar concerns
Cutaneous sensors sensitive to environment (potential for wide variation in readings)	No similar environment issues
Cutaneous perfusion tests generally slow	Tests performed relatively quickly

Abbreviations: MR, magnetic resonance imaging; CT, computerized tomography; DSA, digital subtraction angiography.

AN OBJECTIVE ASSESSMENT: THE VASCULAR LABORATORY

When a patient presents with ulceration or necrosis, an absence of lower limb pulses together with the typical features of lower limb PAOD directs the clinical evaluation toward the diagnosis of critical ischemia due to arterial insufficiency. However, subjective information can be unreliable. The classical symptoms and signs of critical ischemia in some individuals can be absent. In particular, individuals with diabetes mellitus represent a diagnostic and therapeutic challenge in this respect. Typically in diabetes mellitus, individuals, possibly resulting from the presence of impaired sensation due to peripheral neuropathy, may not perceive pain normally associated with ischemia, chronic ulceration, or necrosis. Arterial calcification associated with diabetes can render vessels rigid and palpation of distal pulses impossible. Therefore a diagnosis of critical lower limb ischemia is best confirmed or established by objective, noninvasive testing. When a patient presents with the classical picture of limb (and life)-threatening critical ischemia due to arterial insufficiency with tissue loss, the management is aimed at improving arterial inflow as quickly as possible, wherever possible. This requires the attainment of optimum images of the arterial tree to plan and perform intervention, usually by employing an invasive test that requires injection of a contrast medium to demarcate arteries from surrounding tissues. The three main modalities are magnetic resonance angiography (MRA), computerized tomographic angiography (CTA), and digital subtraction angiography (DSA). Generally, because of the associated risks, DSA is only performed if a therapeutic procedure is being considered.

Frequently however, individuals present with more complex clinical pictures, requiring additional objective diagnostic information and alternative therapeutic strategies. Laboratory tests offer safe diagnostic verification and can provide valuable data on which to base a therapeutic strategy. Color duplex imaging (CDI), by using ultrasound and Doppler assessments, can be used as the sole anatomical assessment tool on which to plan therapeutic intervention. The relative merits of duplex versus other modalities in defining disease distribution are constantly debated. The technologies involved with duplex imaging, magnetic resonance, and computerized tomography continue to evolve. Studies often reflect the enthusiasm of the researchers for one modality over another (4,5). In practice, the availability of both the imaging modality and appropriately trained staff will influence the decision regarding which modality is employed.

The clinical utility or usefulness of all invasive and noninvasive tests can be influenced by patient comorbidities. Diabetes in particular not only complicates clinical assessment but also influences the efficacy of noninvasive tests, and this must be considered when interpreting results.

THE MEASUREMENT OF LOWER LIMB PERFUSION

All methods of assessing lower limb perfusion have their advantages and limitations. An ability to judge the relative merits of noninvasive testing and to understand the limitations of the various modalities requires an appreciation of circulatory physiology.

Potentially, the most accurate evaluation of blood flow and tissue perfusion requires invasive measurement and sampling. Practically, in the assessment of lower limb perfusion, technological improvements provide us with ever increasing levels of equipment sophistication. It, however, remains that an understanding of circulatory physiology and the characteristics of noninvasive perfusion indicators in health allow us to identify and interpret abnormalities associated with disease.

The following text will discuss applied circulatory physiology, focusing on its clinical relevance and influence on the assessment methods.

PERIPHERAL ARTERIAL BLOOD FLOW

Maintenance of blood flow at the capillary level facilitates adequate and continuous tissue oxygenation, delivery of nutrients, and removal of waste products. Flow provides the energy needed to create a capillary pressure fundamental to the fluid dynamics that occur at the capillary basement membrane, "Starling forces."

At a basic mechanistic level, the effective supply of blood is dependent on an effective pump, an efficient network of pipes that carry and deliver blood with minimal loss of energy, and the ability to modify flow to requirements. The distal end organ circulation is integral to the dynamics of blood flow. An assessment of cardiac function is an integral part of the evaluation of limb perfusion.

Blood flow can be measured directly or indirectly using many techniques. Doppler analysis indirectly measures blood flow by detecting frequency changes to the reflected signal caused by red blood cells moving toward or away from the source. This frequency shift is converted to velocity in meter or centimeter/second.

Flow in a vessel is dependent on

1. pressure difference between the two ends, the pressure gradient, and
2. vascular resistance.

The flow through a vessel is summarized by Ohm's law, where

$$\text{flow } (Q) = \frac{\text{pressure gradient}}{\text{resistance}}, \quad \text{measured in milliliters or liters/minute.}$$

Conductance is a measure of blood flow at a given pressure gradient and is the reciprocal of resistance. Equations describing fluid flow characteristics through vessels reflect steady state situations where flow and diameter are constant. The steady flow through smooth constant diameter vessel leads to streamline laminar flow with a parabolic profile. Blood flow in arteries is pulsatile and the diameter variable. Calculations therefore represent approximations for minimal energy losses and cannot be strictly applied.

Flow reduction (and therefore energy loss) is inversely proportional to the fourth power of the radius (Poiseuille's law). This formula is

$$Q = \frac{\pi \Delta P r^4}{8 \eta L}$$

where Q is the flow, ΔP the pressure difference across vessel, r the radius, η the viscosity, and L the length.

This reflects that in cross section, proportionally far less blood is influenced by friction at the blood/vessel wall interface in larger vessels when compared with that in smaller vessels. This effect is intimately related to fluid viscosity and the shear forces created between moving layers that are in contact. Viscosity is a measure of energy dissipation. Whole blood has viscoelasticity, with an elastic, energy-storing capacity due to transient red cell deformity during changes in blood flow in systole and diastole. Viscous energy losses are due to more permanent cell deformity and cell movement in plasma. Plasma also has varying degrees of viscosity and is elevated in individuals who smoke cigarettes. Blood with a high hematocrit has higher viscosity. This causes a greater resistance to moving forces resulting in greater energy loss and reduced flow. Blood in small vessels has relatively fewer red cells and as a result the reduced viscosity offsets the reduction in vessel radius seen in arterioles and capillaries.

Increased arterial pressure during systole improves flow by increasing not only the pressure gradient but also the diameter of distensible vessels, so reducing resistance to flow. In stenotic disease, nonlinear, turbulent flow adjacent to an area of vessel surface irregularity and immediately post-stenosis results in further energy loss and reduced flow. Distensability, which is related to compliance, dampens peak pressure in larger arteries during systole and by elastic recoil helps provide continued flow through the microvascular bed during diastole. Poorly distensible vessels will give higher systolic blood pressure readings but this may not reflect the cardiac output. Pressure pulse transmission through the major vessels is much quicker than the blood flow in the lumen and very much quicker in less-compliant walls. The ability of atherosclerotic, less-compliant vessels to maintain capillary bed flow during diastole is impaired.

Narrowing of arteries due to atherosclerosis, therefore, influences flow distally through many processes. The resulting loss of energy and reduction in flow is greater than would be expected by simple assumption that percentage reduction in diameter is directly proportional to the percentage loss of flow distally. Typically, blood flow at a pressure of 50 mmHg may be less than one-fourth of that seen at 100 mmHg.

At a tissue level, many variables interact to influence blood flow and tissue perfusion (Table 2).

It is apparent that because of the detrimental effects of many other physiological anomalies, for individuals with equivalent degrees of PAOD, those who smoke cigarettes and have diabetes are more likely to suffer critical lower limb ischemia.

TABLE 2 Influences on Tissue Perfusion

General
    Cardiac output
    Distance and elevation relative to heart
    Blood viscosity, hematocrit, rheological variation, and plasma viscosity

Local
    Peripheral arterial occlusive disease
    Arteriolar reactivity: deinnervation, vasospastic disorders
    Capillary wall function: thickness, porosity
    Interstitial fluid and plasma osmolarity
    Tissue pressures: excessive interstitial fluid (edema), extrinsic pressures
    Venous and lymphatic drainage

Arterial Insufficiency and Compensatory Mechanisms

Ischemia occurs when there is insufficient perfusion to meet the requirements of tissue, resulting in cellular dysfunction and death. There is a continuous interaction between the variable metabolic demands of tissue and the provision of an adequate blood supply. This relationship is dynamic. Local tissue ischemia due to initial increased metabolic demands stimulates rapid physiological responses that result in increased tissue perfusion designed to meet the new requirements. These responses are typically seen during muscular activity and following tissue injury. In health, therefore, transient focal ischemia is intimately related to normal lower limb circulatory dynamics. Any disease that impedes on this vascular physiological reserve may cause cellular dysfunction and ultimately tissue loss. In chronic lower limb ischemia due to impaired large vessel blood flow, circulatory dynamics are compromised and increased metabolic demands may result in prolonged ischemia. This effect may be augmented by a dysfunctional or impaired microcirculatory perfusion at a tissue level, as in diabetes (6). Severe atherosclerosis, by causing a reduction in luminal cross-sectional area can result in a dampening of the circulatory response to elevated tissue demands, resulting in symptoms and signs of arterial insufficiency. CLI, typically due to multilevel stenoses or occlusions and frequently confounded by reduced cardiac output, results in lower limb perfusion insufficient to support even basal tissue metabolism, leading to symptoms and signs of limb ischemia at rest (Fig. 1).

There are two main compensatory mechanisms to a significant reduction in lower limb inflow due to PAOD. Initially, there is a reduction in vascular peripheral resistance associated with a downregulated sympathetic innervation. The resulting arteriolar dilatation increases the overall diameter of the vascular bed, thus reducing resistance to flow. Then over a longer period there is a development of collateral arterial branches, arteriogenesis.

Noninvasive, physiological testing has an advantage over a qualitative angiographic evaluation in that it has the potential to quantitatively measure the influence of these mechanisms on limb perfusion.

THE DIAGNOSIS OF CRITICAL LIMB ISCHEMIA

There have been efforts to define CLI using quantitative measurement. Systolic blood pressure measurements at the ankle or the hallux should be included in the assessment of the lower limb to support the clinical diagnosis (3). An ankle pressure of less than 50 mmHg or a toe pressure less than 30 mmHg at rest indicate that there is insufficient perfusion distal to the point of the tourniquet to facilitate healing, and chronic pain may be due to ischemia. The TASC II document also forwarded transcutaneous oxygen tension ($TcPO_2$) as a confirmatory test. These tests have inherent weaknesses that can confound the diagnosis of CLI. These issues will be discussed later in the text.

LIMITATIONS OF NONINVASIVE TESTING

The expectations generated by the introduction of many of the noninvasive tests have been tempered universally by failings when applied to clinical practice.

The efficacy of noninvasive tests is influenced by many factors both technical and biological. Noninvasive tests are generally dynamic and the interpretation of

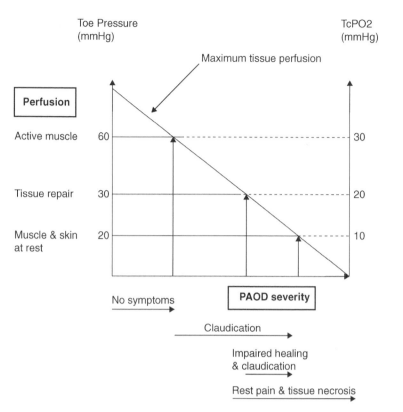

FIGURE 1 Lower limb perfusion and clinical presentation. *Note*: A representation of metabolic demands versus compromised lower limb perfusion due to varying severities of PAOD. Estimated toe pressures and TcPO$_2$ values. *Abbreviations*: PAOD, peripheral arterial occlusive disease; TcPO$_2$, trancutaneous oxygen tension. *Source*: From Refs. 23, 31, and 43.

results more operator dependent than the "snapshot" mechanistic invasive tests that provide processed data that is easier to interpret by all. Laboratory tests can be technical, relying on focused application and interpretation, as well as operator ability.

A further potential limitation to physiological tests is that there is a range of values in health and disease that can overlap. In health, macro- and microvascular physiology varies between individuals and varies continually in response to stimuli. This can hinder the ability of a test to provide definitive answers regarding the presence (or absence) and the severity of disease. The setting of threshold values to indicate significant disease, although attractive, is therefore inherently flawed.

Noninvasive tests, particularly those that employ cutaneous perfusion detectors, are vulnerable to environmental variation, particularly changes in room temperature. Ideally, tests should be performed in a controlled laboratory setting. Performing noninvasive tests outside the laboratory in a clinical setting introduces potential environmental variation that can profoundly influence results.

THE ASSESSMENT OF THE EFFICACY OF TESTS: HOW DEPENDABLE IS THE RESULT?

There are various noninvasive modalities that reflect lower limb perfusion. Understanding the methods and their limitations allows for better interpretation and provides for their more effective integration into the management of individuals with suspected or diagnosed CLI.

Obtaining a Result

Accuracy defines how close a measured value reflects the actual (true) value. *Precision* is defined as the ability of a device to produce the same value or result, given the same input conditions and operating in the same environment. A device may be precise, but not reflect the true value, so losing accuracy.

Reliability is the ability of a person or system to perform and maintain its functions in routine circumstances, as well as hostile or unexpected circumstances. Laboratory tests are vulnerable to variation in the ability of operators and their familiarity with equipment, called intra-operator variation. The operator and the environment in which a test is performed may therefore influence precision, accuracy, and reliability.

Reproducibility is one of the main principles of the scientific method and refers to the ability of a test or experiment to be accurately reproduced, or replicated, by someone else working independently.

Noninvasive tests vary in technical difficulty, but all are vulnerable to poor reproducibility, or inter-operator variation. Reproducibility is particularly vulnerable where a test requires greater operator skills and interpretation. Further, precision and/or accuracy may be compromised where tests that are sensitive to environmental conditions are employed toward the limits of their operative range.

Ideally, the same trusted, competent operator should perform all tests under the same conditions using the same machine. This would reduce the likelihood of operator error in performing and interpreting findings and reduce the influence of the environment on results and negate worries regarding reproducibility (7). Frequently, where limb perfusion is severely reduced, the limitations of all imaging modalities become exaggerated. Paradoxically, accuracy can therefore be compromised in the very situation where good information is that much more valuable.

It is prudent to acclimatize patients in a controlled environment, particularly when the outside temperatures are low. Generally, tests reflecting macrovascular physiology, such as CDI, Doppler waveform, or segmental systolic blood pressure measurement, are less vulnerable to environmental influences. Unfortunately, tests that employ infrared detectors for pressure measurement and tests of local perfusion are particularly vulnerable to the environmental conditions. This is a particular problem where limb perfusion is severely compromised, as in CLI, because readings are low, and variations due to environmental factors can have a proportionately greater effect on the result.

Interpreting the Result

Ideally, a test should perfectly reflect the presence of health or disease. However, as demonstrated in arterial disease, there are varying degrees of severity, the detection of which is of great importance in clinical practice. In the assessment of the effects of PAOD on lower limb perfusion, variations in severity should ideally be reflected by a proportionate range of values. In the context of this chapter, effective detection or exclusion of critical ischemia is particularly important. However, there are limitations for each noninvasive method of assessment, both in their application and interpretation.

Quantitative and Qualitative Analysis

Tests measuring a variable should have a range of values to which can be assigned parameters for health and disease. These are quantitative tests. However, some tests are vulnerable to large variation when applied in a clinical setting and are potentially unusable. Such tests however can be valuable when used in a qualitative manner and not assigned numerical value.

Test Validation

When compared with a criterion standard, how good was a test at detecting the presence of disease? This represents its *sensitivity*. The *specificity* reflects how good a test was at excluding disease in its absence. Accuracy here represents the percentage of the total number of results that correctly identified the presence or absence of disease.

A good test will be highly sensitive. However, when presented with a positive result, the next question that needs to be answered is the likelihood that disease is present. This is its *positive predictor value* (PPV). Conversely, if the test is negative, the likelihood that there is no disease is the *negative predictor value* (NPV). Ideally, a good vascular screening test would be highly sensitive but also have a high predictor value so that the chance of a false-positive (test positive but no underlying disease) or false-negative (test negative but underlying disease) result would be small.

In a vascular evaluation, it is not just the presence of disease but also the impact of the disease on limb perfusion that needs quantifying. It is worth noting that the criterion standard for lower limb arterial assessment has been DSA. This is the criterion standard in terms of anatomical distribution of disease, but not in terms of the hemodynamic effects of atherosclerosis and the assessment of distal limb perfusion. In the evaluation of limb perfusion, other tests have the potential to afford better efficacy. Further, it is worth remembering that anatomical detail is not necessary if noninvasive tests indicate that limb perfusion is adequate and vascular intervention not required.

Analysis and validation will be discussed for each modality.

METHODS OF NONINVASIVE ASSESSMENT

Vascular clinics employ noninvasive tests at the patient's first attendance, thus providing subjective and objective data in determining a diagnosis and planning management. The type of initial noninvasive testing employed will depend on the availability of trained technical staff and equipment. Some clinics employ CDI. Many clinics use segmental pressures, typically ankle and toe pressures, and Doppler waveform analysis as first-line objective tests.

Vascular laboratories should contain equipment suited to both the vascular clinician and technician (Fig. 2). The different methods of noninvasive testing for limb ischemia can broadly be separated into those that reflect larger vessel dynamics and those that reflect tissue perfusion. The more commonly used modalities are discussed in more detail below.

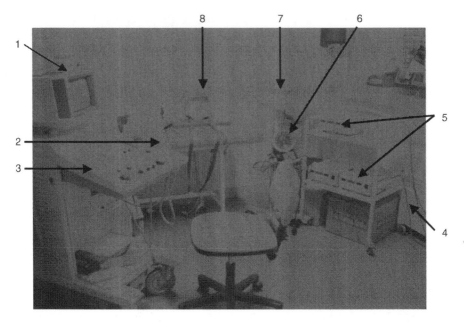

FIGURE 2 A vascular laboratory. List of contents: 1. skin thermometer, 2. linear array Doppler probe, 3. color Doppler imaging processor and monitor, 4. thermostatically controlled room heater, 5. transcutaneous oxygen and carbon dioxide measurement equipment, 6. blood pressure measurement equipment, 7. handheld Doppler waveform measuring equipment, and 8. examination couch and basic exercise cycle ergometer.

COLOR DUPLEX IMAGING

This modality is the mainstay of many vascular laboratories. A successive reduction in the size of new models means that this modality is becoming increasingly portable. It remains very operator dependent and is expensive to purchase. It is however a very useful and versatile tool in the assessment of lower limb vasculature.

This technique combines brightness mode (B-mode) ultrasound with pulsed Doppler spectral waveform analysis and color flow imaging. It facilitates the noninvasive assessment of the vessel location, its wall, and a detailed analysis of blood flow characteristics at various points within the lumen at contiguous multiple levels.

Typically, a 5- to 7.5-MHz linear array (flat) transducer probe is used. This has multiple piezoelectric crystals that emit a single constant signal due to electrically induced deformity. The array also detects the reflected signals. Curvilinear, lower frequency probes are employed for imaging deeper vessels, particularly the aortoiliac segment. More obese patients may require lower frequency probes to analyze vessels normally studied using linear probes. There is a loss of acuity when employing curvilinear probes that can compromise the assessment. Spectral waveform analysis can display details of the waveform patterns at selected points within the lumen. Typically, the waveform has a well-defined outline (band width) in normal vessels with laminar blood flow (Fig. 3). Stenoses cause an increased velocity of blood locally. Turbulent post-stenotic

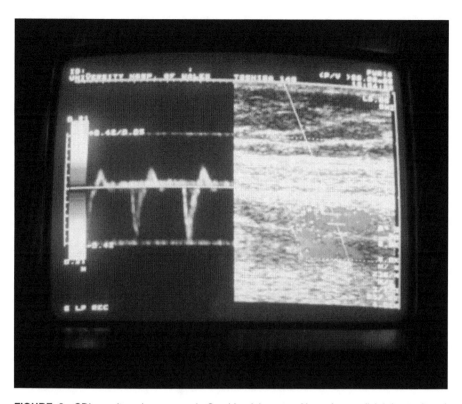

FIGURE 3 CDI monitor view—normal. Combined images. Normal superficial femoral and profunda femoris arteries. Smooth vessel wall and homogenous filling of lumen (in color on-screen) suggesting laminar flow (*right*). Note the oblique dotted line with two parallel bars that allow the operator to select a point of interest for waveform analysis. Doppler analysis of selected point of flow in lumen (between two parallel lines) (*left*). *Note*: Doppler probe was held pointing away from heart, therefore, the triphasic profile appears upside down.

flow causes a widening of the waveform outline due to the wider range of velocities, termed "spectral broadening." Color flow imaging displays the blood flow in the entire lumen within the section being studied. It allows geometric measurement of a stenosis by comparing the relative thickness of the wall with the section with visualized flow. Homogenous color depicts normal laminar blood flow, bright and granular color patterns indicate turbulent flow, termed "aliasing." This type of picture typically occurs where stenotic lesions cause a less than 50% reduction in the internal diameter, equivalent to a 75% reduction in cross-sectional area of the lumen (Fig. 4). Doppler analysis of selected central parts of the luminal blood flow, applying appropriate probe angulation for measurement, can give an accurate measurement of blood velocity. Velocities within a 50% stenosis would typically be doubled to approach 200 cm/sec. Comparison of elevated peak velocities within a stenotic lesion with proximal velocities during systole is used to grade hemodynamic severity, usually presented as a percentage loss of cross-sectional area.

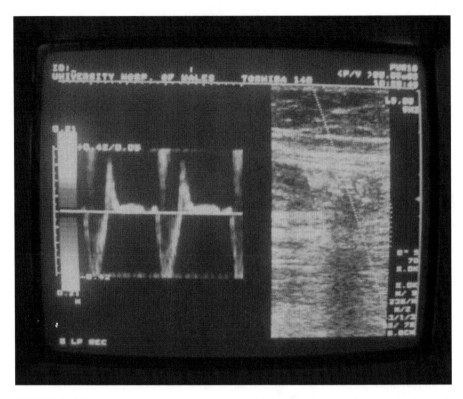

FIGURE 4 CDI monitor view—abnormal. Image of irregular stenosis of superficial femoral artery (*right*). Doppler analysis of flow within stenosis shows high peak velocities, the highest velocities disappearing from the bottom of the screen and reappearing at the top (*left*).

It is the measurement of peak red cell velocities (centimeter/second or meter/second), rather than a calculation of total blood flow through the luminal area (liter/minute), that is used to help estimate the severity of a stenotic lesion. CDI can precisely and reliably identify and grade arterial disease. It can therefore replace invasive techniques in localizing and grading arterial disease. CDI can also prevent patients with less severe or inoperable disease being unnecessarily exposed to invasive procedures (8–11). Higher frequency probes have also demonstrated accurate visualization of distal vessels (12). CDI is employed in the surveillance of arterial bypass grafts and is increasingly being used as a first-line investigation for patients presenting to vascular clinics.

Arterial calcification can interfere with CDI. Medial sclerosis, frequently seen in the iliofemoral and infrageniculate arteries in diabetes, typically has a uniformly high signal on B-mode ultrasound, but generally permits flow analysis. Calcification of atherosclerotic plaques, a particular feature of patients with chronic kidney disease secondary to diabetes, can reflect ultrasound signals, preventing flow analysis within the lumen. However, waveform analysis proximal and distal to these areas can indicate whether significant disease is present. Dampened waveforms with reduced peak velocity indicate the presence of significant stenotic disease proximal to the point of analysis. Further, there is the potential to fail to localize significant arterial disease proximally, particularly in obese individuals and to miss distal disease in small vessels so preventing accurate anatomical mapping. Obese individuals with type 2 diabetes are potentially a challenge for this modality. CDI, in common with invasive tests, does not reflect tissue perfusion. The efficacy of this technique remains intimately bound to the skills of the operator and the enthusiasm of the vascular clinician. The reproducibility and validity of this modality is summarized in Table 1.

SEGMENTAL PLETHYSMOGRAPHY AND PULSE VOLUME RECORDING

Pulse volume recording (PVR) is a long-established oscillometric technique that uses a pneumatic cuff insufflated to approximately 65 mmHg to allow quantitative measurement of waveform amplitude. Measurements can be taken at multiple sites from the thigh to the toe. Many of the early vascular laboratories used this type of plethysmography as the mainstay of their investigation. Plethysmography is the measurement of volume change due to changes in the amount of blood contained in the tissues. A local pressure of 65 mmHg allows good skin contact and optimum sensitivity. Pulse plethysmography measures volume change during the cardiac cycle. As limb length remains fixed, volume change is reflected by variation in circumference, and this can be measured to reflect limb perfusion. Decreasing amplitude and loss of normal waveform are indicators of PAOD. Together with segmental lower limb pressure measurement, these tests facilitate the evaluation of both the level and severity of PAOD (2). In the presence of critical PAOD, cuff insufflation to 65 mmHg may approach systolic blood pressures, making pulse volume changes slight or absent. The presence of critical ischemia would then therefore be established using measurement of systolic pressure. Comparing waveform profiles before and after exercise or changing limb dependency can enhance the diagnostic utility of these tests. Again tests indicating the patency of large vessels proximal to the ankle may not reflect more distal PAOD or perfusion.

Toe plethysmography requires a more sensitive mercury strain gauge oscillatory measurement, but increasingly infrared detectors are used to quantitatively assess the wave profile or contour. Using photosensors, as used in pulse oximetry, is not strictly plethysmography, as they do not measure volume change, but generate a wave profile that reflects changes in blood flow in the tissue bed. At a local level, tissue perfusion can be indicated by detecting changes in the amount of blood in the cutaneous microvasculature during the cardiac cycle, *photoplethysmography* (PPG). A quantitative measurement of the pulse pressure can be performed, with decreased amplitude associated with disease. A qualitative assessment of the contour can also be performed. The presence of a dichrotic notch in early diastole due to superimposed reflected pressure waves is lost in significant PAOD (Fig. 5). This is discussed further under waveform analysis.

Digital studies have the potential to improve the sensitivity of these tests in detecting more distal disease and reflect tissue perfusion. Arterial calcification, particularly associated with diabetes, reduces distensibility and may influence any technique measuring volume change during the cardiac cycle. PPG has the potential advantage of not relying on this phenomenon. However, quantitative

Severity of PAOD

normal   mild   moderate   severe/critical

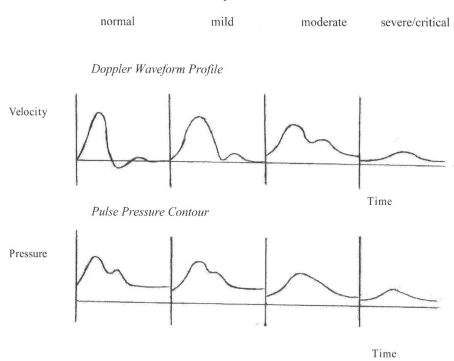

FIGURE 5 Doppler and plethysmographic waveform profiles. *Note*: Comparative changes in waveforms during the cardiac cycle in the presence of peripheral arterial occlusive disease of increasing severity.

measurement of digital photoplethysmographic profiles is prone to error, particularly in the presence of poor perfusion, and its efficacy is limited (13,14). Combining PPG with other modalities may marginally improve its sensitivity, but the accuracy of many noninvasive tests begins to fall toward the extreme of disease, and combining pressure and plethysmographic modalities may have little benefit (15).

Segmental oscillometry provides limited anatomical detail regarding disease distribution in larger vessels. It is now much less frequently used because of the increasing availability and improving reliability of other methods of noninvasive assessment (16). Issues surrounding the reliability and reproducibility of methods employing compression and infrared measurement are discussed later in the chapter.

LOWER LIMB SYSTOLIC BLOOD PRESSURE MEASUREMENT
Ankle Pressure and Ankle-Brachial Pressure Index
This widely used method compares the synchronous measurement of upper and lower limb systolic blood pressures. The higher of the upper limb systolic pressures is used in calculating the ankle-brachial pressure index (ABPI). This

represents a ratio of the brachial pressure compared with the pressure at the ankle. In health, all limb pressures should be similar, and the ratio near 1. Multiple segmental pressure measurements are now generally not performed and have been restricted to a single measurement at the ankle that provides comparable information and is much simpler to perform (17).

Brachial blood pressure is commonly measured by auscultation with a stethoscope. The lower limb segmental pressure at the ankle cannot be measured by this technique. One of the commonest methods of measuring ankle pressure is by handheld Doppler. This is a single-crystal probe that emits and detects a continuous signal. During the ankle pressure analysis, the return of blood flow in the vessel selected during pressure cuff deflation is detected by the Doppler probe. The flow is relayed audibly to the operator via a speaker on the handset. The audible signal also relays information on blood flow characteristics when not employed as a detector of reperfusion. The Doppler probe is able to detect blood flow in limbs that are pulseless because of low flow or hard incompressible artery walls. More elaborate Doppler devices are available, which both display and analyze the blood flow characteristics detected using a single-crystal probe (Figs. 2 and 6). Infrared detectors can also be used to detect reperfusion and measure systolic pressure demonstrating comparable accuracy when used in a controlled environment (18).

The posterior tibial artery is anatomically the most consistent artery at the ankle, while the dorsalis pedis on the foot dorsum is the most convenient artery in which to detect Doppler signals. These two vessels are the most commonly used to measure ankle pressures. The lateral tibial artery, a terminal branch of the peroneal artery, although the least consistent anatomically, is frequently less affected by atherosclerotic disease than tibial vessels and should be used in assessing ankle pressures. Systolic pressures are recorded at each vessel and the highest value generally used to calculate the ABPI.

The calculation of indices facilitates the evaluation of limb perfusion without the need to refer to brachial pressures when quoting ankle or toe pressures. However, indices can be misleading where brachial pressures are low because of upper limb arterial stenotic disease or cardiac failure. An ABPI of 0.5, for example, may suggest moderate PAOD, but a critically low ankle pressure of 45 mmHg would be present if the brachial systolic pressure were 90 mmHg. Where low brachial systolic pressures are encountered or ankle pressures approach critical values, absolute values should be quoted and ratios avoided. An ankle pressure that is less than 50 mmHg, irrespective of the brachial value, supports the diagnosis of chronic CLI due to PAOD.

Validation
The ABPI value in the absence of hemodynamically significant PAOD should be 1. A value less than this indicates PAOD. Initial work in individuals with no PAOD found a range of values, the great majority between 0.9 and 1, with only an occasional value less than 0.9. The values below 0.9 may have been due to occult PAOD. The lower limit should therefore be no lower than 0.9. ABPI values are well known to be vulnerable to the influence of arterial calcification, particularly in diabetes. Its sensitivity is compromised in stiff vessels where the external cuff pressures required to collapse the artery are greatly in excess of the systolic pressure and reflect more the vessel wall rigidity. Various attempts have been made to define an upper limit to the normal range above which ABPI

measurement is inaccurate. It has become clear however that varying degrees of vessel rigidity not only result in grossly elevated values but also falsely elevate results across the range of pressures (18). The sensitivity and predictor values of ankle pressure measurement are therefore prone to being compromised, particularly in diabetes. Generally, in the absence of diabetes, ABPI measurement is accurate. In diabetes, the PPV is high, a low ABPI being very likely to reflect the presence of significant PAOD. Unfortunately, the sensitivity and NPVs are relatively poor. A value that is normal or demonstrates moderate, noncritical PAOD may hide significant PAOD. An alternative test may then be required, particularly where there is a clinical suspicion of critical disease (18,19).

Reliability and Reproducibility

Although a relatively simple test, Doppler methodology is open to variation in technical ability and relies on the detection of an audible signal by the operator. The reliability of the method is vulnerable as several aspects of the method are dependent on the operator. Compression cuffs must be correctly sized and placed relative to the limb being analyzed. Suboptimal probe positioning when detecting arterial flow, insufficient or poor quality ultrasound gel, and movement of the probe during measurement can all influence the quality of the audible signal. The reproducibility of the technique is also vulnerable as demonstrated in our vascular clinics where, not infrequently, values are markedly different to those taken elsewhere. A good and constant technician will provide reliable results. The use of photosensors placed on the skin of the foot or at the toe would potentially reduce dependence on the reliability of the operator in detecting reperfusion, making the test more reproducible, but photosensors are vulnerable to variation in cutaneous perfusion due to the environment and may therefore be less reliable than the Doppler method.

The *toe pole test* is an alternative method of determining lower limb pressures, particularly where ankle pressures are grossly elevated. Commonly, a handheld Doppler is used to detect the loss of signal at the ankle as the limb is elevated. The pressure can be calculated by measuring the vertical height from the bed. Pressure at the toe can also be measured using infrared or laser flow detectors by the same technique. The measurements are lower in practice than methods employing pressure cuffs and the accuracy of this technique in critical ischemia is not proven (20,21).

Toe Pressure and Toe-Brachial Pressure Index

Toe-brachial pressure index (TBPI) is the most distal segmental pressure. The toe pressure is usually obtained at the hallux. A small toe tourniquet is used to occlude arterial flow. There are several techniques employed to detect reperfusion when measuring toe pressures, including handheld Doppler, laser Doppler, strain gauge, and infrared photosensors. The digital arteries are generally too small to facilitate handheld Doppler analysis (22). Infrared sensors, reflective or transmitted, are probably the most commonly used reperfusion detectors, but rely on the presence of toes able to accommodate tourniquet and sensor. The range of normal values for this test is not universally agreed and like ABPI, there are a range of values in health and disease. There is loss of energy by the time blood reaches the digital arteries and normal systolic pressures are reduced by 10% to 20% compared with the ankle and brachial measurements (23). Generally,

TBPI values more than 0.75 suggest the absence of hemodynamically significant PAOD (18). A toe pressure of less than 30 mmHg supports the diagnosis of critical ischemia. As for ABPI, absolute measurements should be quoted where brachial pressures are low or toe pressures approach critical values.

This measurement has the potential to indicate the perfusion at the point of interest and reflect the sum effects of all arterial disease, whether focal, multisegmental, or diffuse. Further, it has the potential to detect disease in the lower leg and foot, distal to the pressure cuff used for ABPI measurement. In particular, the test has attracted much interest as it has the potential to offer a more effective objective assessment of PAOD than ABPI in diabetes. More distal disease affecting the lower leg and foot is a particular feature of PAOD in diabetes. The arterial calcification frequently encountered in the lower limb arteries of patients with diabetes appears to be less severe in digital arteries. Thus the potential for artificially raised systolic pressures as caused by calcified, poorly compliant arteries at the ankle is reduced (24). This test may then reveal arterial insufficiency, otherwise hidden by a normal or elevated ABPI (25).

It has been suggested that where an ABPI is more than 1.15, TBPI should be calculated (26). In the presence of diabetic peripheral neuropathy, arterial calcification is more likely, and the accuracy of ABPI must then be in doubt (27). However, as described earlier, a low ABPI is highly indicative of significant PAOD with a very high PPV, regardless of the presence of diabetes (18).

Validation
Concerns regarding this technique are similar to those surrounding ABPI, particularly in relation to diabetes. Studies have demonstrated reduced toe pressures in patients with neuropathy and recurrent ulceration or a history of foot infection, but no significant reduction of toe pressures in the absence of foot disease (28,29). It has been suggested that toe measurements may also be influenced by autonomic neuropathy, paradoxically reducing pressures due to a reduced peripheral resistance (30). Other researchers have found that, paradoxically, toe pressure measurement using infrared detectors was better at excluding than detecting PAOD (22).

However, many of these studies failed to use a criterion standard vascular assessment and are likely to have failed to detect significant arterial disease. TBPI has been demonstrated to more accurately reflect critical and noncritical PAOD than ABPI and some recommend its routine use in clinical practice (31,32). The test is more sensitive than ABPI in detecting PAOD in diabetes, although its PPV is reduced (18).

Reproducibility and Reliability
An important limitation of this technique is that it is not only susceptible to conditions that influence the cutaneous circulation when employing infrared or laser Doppler detectors but also anatomical variation. Absent or variable toe length and width and variation in cuff width all influence its usefulness (33).

DOPPLER WAVEFORM ANALYSIS
Doppler waveform analysis of blood flow can be used in isolation without the need to combine it with a more complex ultrasound and array of transducers. A single-crystal Doppler probe produces and receives a continuous signal. The

profile produced by the reflected signal is displayed on-screen. The Doppler probe is identical to that used in detecting audible signals during Doppler blood pressure measurement. However, the characteristics of the flow are not judged by interpreting audible changes, but by analysis of the displayed waveform. Higher ultrasonic frequencies are employed where possible, typically 5 to 8 MHz. The Doppler signal is not pulsed as with the CDI and is not able to selectively analyze parts of the flow in its cross section. The test is relatively easy to perform and does not require the use of a tourniquet.

Doppler waveforms can be interpreted qualitatively or quantitatively. Qualitative analysis is based on visual interpretation of the shape of the wave profile. The waveform throughout the lower limb arteries is normally triphasic with preservation of reverse flow (Fig. 5). As described for CDI, a significant stenosis causes an increase in waveform amplitude locally, signifying the presence of a lesion. Reverse flow during early diastole is the result of the summation of waves reflected from decreasing luminal diameters and multiple perpendicular surfaces at vessel bifurcations as the initial systolic blood volume travels distally. These reflected waves cause a transient reverse in red cell velocities, which in health briefly overcome forward velocities. In the presence of reduced blood flow, vasodilatation increases the overall luminal cross-sectional area, reducing both the impedance to flow and reflected waves. Waveforms then demonstrate a reduction in peak velocities with loss of reverse flow, with two forward, or if severe, only a single forward phase (Fig. 5). This change in the waveform profile to a bi- or monophasic pattern, with forward flow only, is diagnostic of hemodynamically significant PAOD (Fig. 6). Waveform changes may also occur proximal to a significant lesion.

The audible Doppler signal can relay useful information to the experienced operator. A clearly triphasic signal is indicative of a normal flow, but less well-defined signals must be interpreted with caution and not used as a basis for diagnosing the presence or absence of arterial disease. Qualitative analysis, by current definitions, is not recommended for supporting the diagnosis of critical ischemia. However, in the presence of symptoms and/or signs of critical lower limb ischemia, demonstrating a monophasic, severely damped or absent Doppler signal in all vessels at the ankle is highly suggestive of critical disease.

Quantitative analysis of the waveform amplitude and velocity during the cardiac cycle facilitates comparative analysis and estimation of disease severity (Fig. 6). Commonly employed measurements based on these parameters include pulsatility index (PI), resistance index (RI), and spectral broadening index (SBI).

Validation

Quantitative waveform analysis has demonstrated good correlation with angiographic findings in evaluating occlusive arterial disease (34). There have been concerns that in diabetes, autonomic neuropathy, by reducing the sympathetic innervation to the cutaneous vasculature, can potentially reduce peripheral vascular resistance, altering the waveform in the absence of significant atherosclerosis (35). It has been demonstrated subsequently that it is likely that these studies failed to detect PAOD in individuals who had peripheral neuropathy and that qualitative waveform analysis is sensitive and accurate in individuals both with and without diabetes (18). Quantitative analysis can potentially be misleading in situations of low flow or poor signal quality, as demonstrated in Figure 6, where analysis of qualitatively abnormal monophasic waveforms has resulted in relatively normal indices.

Reproducibility and Reliability

The method requires familiarity with the use of a Doppler probe and more complex equipment than employed using handheld Doppler. However, the absence of both pressure cuff usage and the need to interpret an audible Doppler signal reduces the number of operator-dependent steps. The method therefore has the potential to be more robust and create reproducible results. The method does not employ cutaneous perfusion detectors and so is more reliable in a changeable clinical setting.

CUTANEOUS PERFUSION INDICATORS

Accurate and reliable information on perfusion at a local level has the potential to be invaluable in managing patients with chronic lower limb disease. Therapeutic intervention would be guided by such data and be able to predict outcomes (36). Critical ischemia would be diagnosed, treatment options explored, and outcomes measured. Invasive measurement of perfusion is not feasible. There are several methods available that indicate tissue perfusion. However, tests that reflect local perfusion are prone to weaknesses in their reproducibility and reliability. Their application in routine clinical practice remains limited. The main modalities are discussed below.

Infrared Photosensors

Infrared light can be detected either by a sensor placed opposite the source, after passing through tissue, or be reflected back to a sensor in the same housing as the emitter. The relative amounts of oxy- and deoxyhemoglobin alter the absorbance of the light, and this is detected by the sensor. Near-infrared sensors are commonly employed in bedside tests for peripheral hemoglobin oxygen saturation monitoring. Blood pressure can also be accurately measured using infrared sensors (37). These sensors are not generally used as indicators of tissue oxygenation as the hematocrit is influenced by many factors and hemoglobin saturation does not correlate linearly with tissue perfusion. Near-infrared sensors can be used to detect cutaneous and muscular perfusion and reperfusion by measuring degrees of desaturation of hemoglobin. Many of these tests are dynamic, comparing oxygen values before and after exercise or temporary occlusion of arterial inflow and measuring saturation recovery times. Differences have been demonstrated between patients with PAOD and controls, but wide variation in results exists and assessing the severity of PAOD with this modality is unproven (38–40).

PPG is the detection of the waveform reflected from the cutaneous vascular bed using infrared light. The amount of blood contained within the vasculature relative to the total tissue volume changes during the cardiac cycle. Normally biphasic with a dicrotic notch at the toe, the waveform may be dampened in the presence of arterial disease. Infrared sensors are small and may detect local perfusion changes that may not reflect the perfusion of surrounding tissues. Influences from a local focus of infection or proximity to a wound edge are examples of this.

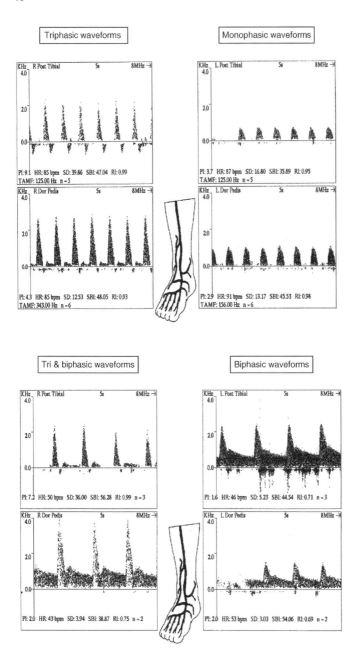

FIGURE 6 Selection of printouts of continuous Doppler waveforms at ankle. *Note*: Waveforms detected at the dorsalis pedis and posterior tibial vessels. Note qualitative changes in profiles and quantitative analyzes for each study. Indices calculated include PI, pulsatility index, SBI, spectral broadening index, and RI, resistance index. The indices describe differing aspects of waveform displacement at varied points during the cardiac cycle (Dopplex Assist, Huntleigh Healthcare, Cardiff, U.K.).

Reliability

Tests that use infrared absorbance are sensitive to environment change, and their reliability in a clinical setting is vulnerable. These devices are prone to reflect influences on cutaneous perfusion other than arterial disease alone. Changes in perfusion due to variation in room temperature, poor cardiac perfusion, vasoactive medications, and dehydration all have the potential to affect the measurement. Again, this modality can indicate perfusion but is prone to the same confounding influences that affect the reliability of infrared measurements.

Temperature (Thermography) and Color Measurement

Both temperature and color are indicators of perfusion and can be measured, mainly employing infrared detectors. As with many perfusion indicators, their results may be confounded by many factors, particularly infection, neuropathy, medication, and the environment (41). Although these tests are attractive in their simplicity, they are limited by their vulnerability to these multiple influences, and guarded interpretation is required, particularly when not performed in controlled conditions. They may be of greater use in the follow-up of individual patients, rather than a general screening tool.

The reliability of cutaneous perfusion indicators is discussed further in the section on transcutaneous oxygen measurement.

Transcutaneous Oxygen Tension and Carbon Dioxide

$TcPO_2$ technique is used in clinical practice and as a research tool. The device applied to the skin consists of a small heating element and Clarke's silver electrode sensor. The area under the sensor is then typically heated to 44°C, for 10 to 15 minutes, thus "arterializing" the skin microcirculation. Although there is potential to cause a skin burn, in practice there is no discomfort and the residual red mark disappears after an hour or so. The test is rather slow and requires a synchronous comparative measurement typically from the anterior chest wall to allow for variations in general cutaneous perfusion between individuals due to factors such as medication and cardiac output. Calculation of a regional perfusion index (RPI) can be performed, much like the ABPI, using the chest measurement as the baseline comparison. Numerous studies of non-invasive lower limb perfusion have identified that a $TcPO_2$ of less than 30 mmHg is consistent with poor healing in both lower limb amputation and ulcer healing (42,43). Values in patients with diabetes, particularly with peripheral neuropathy (and no macrovascular disease), are often lower than that in nondiabetic controls because of a decreased cutaneous microcirculatory response to local heating (6). $TcPO_2$ has been widely used in diabetes in an effort to predict healing of amputation sites and intransigent foot ulceration in patients with distal PAOD, frequently not amenable to intervention (44,45).

Validity

$TcPO_2$ is a well-established indicator of arterial oxygen tension used widely in neonatal medicine. It is quantifiable and accurately reflects cutaneous perfusion. Accurate results require considered application as it is affected by several factors. Less is known about carbon dioxide measurement and its relevance to perfusion assessment.

Reproducibility and Reliability
Potential confounding influences to measurement include respiratory disease, incorrect sensor placement, local infection, skin thickness, edema, limb position, and environmental changes (room temperature and atmospheric pressure). Only in a strictly controlled environment is the method reproducible. In a less-controlled clinical environment it is unfortunately very easy for this test to produce hugely variable and unreliable results that are greatly at variance with the true values. These factors generally limit its use to inpatient assessment and research.

The following methods are employed less frequently clinically to assess lower limb perfusion.

Laser Applications
Laser Doppler Flowmetry
This method measures skin perfusion (flux) over small areas by detecting the light reflected off moving red cells. Used extensively as a clinical research tool with some clinical applications, the technique is generally employed to measure cutaneous perfusion change, such as reactive hyperemia after transient arterial occlusion or the reaction of the cutaneous vasculature to various stimuli. Laser flow measurements are expressed generally as degrees of change of readings following a stimulus and are not afforded units, although measurements are sometimes afforded units of perfusion or flux (46).

Toe Pressure Measurements Using Laser Doppler
Toe pressure measurements using laser Doppler, as a detector of reperfusion, may have an advantage over infrared detectors at lower pressures (47).

Skin Perfusion Pressure
Skin perfusion pressure, an alternative to toe pressure measurement, employs laser to measure perfusion changes in response to controlled application of pressure. The technique is limited by its inability to assess larger areas quickly and variations in baseline values when commencing analyzes affecting its precision. Environmental variation may also influence reliability (48).

Laser Doppler Imaging
Laser Doppler imaging (LDI) is an adaptation of this technique, which affords a wider imaging area. The depth of laser penetrance into the skin can also be varied, thus altering the type of microvasculature being studied.

Capillaroscopy (Videomicroscopy)
This method directly images the cutaneous capillary bed, thus facilitating the assessment of their density and function. Red cell velocities can be measured when combined with laser Doppler.

This technique is again limited because of the small area of analysis and potential failure to reflect larger areas of limb perfusion. It is used largely as a research tool (49). Both laser Doppler and capillaroscopy have limited application to current clinical practice.

SUMMARY

Noninvasive tests, by indicating changes in circulatory physiology, provide a safe and effective means for detecting and measuring arterial insufficiency. Each method has advantages and disadvantages that influence their efficacy. Appropriate application and skilled interpretation provide for the most effective use of these tests. The combination of clinical evaluation and noninvasive testing is fundamental to achieving a thorough vascular assessment and optimizing the management of individuals with CLI.

REFERENCES

1. Raines JK, Darling RC, Buth J, et al. Vascular laboratory criteria for the management of peripheral vascular disease of the lower extremities. Surgery 1976; 79(1):21–29.
2. Nicholas GG, Myers JL, DeMuth WE Jr. The role of vascular laboratory criteria in the selection of patients for lower extremity amputation. Ann Surg 1982; 195(4):469–473.
3. Norgren L, Hiatt WR, Dormandy JA, et al., for the TASC II working group. Inter-Society Consensus for the Management of Peripheral Arterial Disease (TASC II). J Vasc Surg 2007; 45(1):S5–S67.
4. Ouwendijk R, de Vries M, Stijnen T, et al. Multicenter randomized controlled trial of the costs and effects of noninvasive diagnostic imaging in patients with peripheral arterial disease: the DIPAD trial. AJR Am J Roentgenol 2008; 190(5):1349–1357.
5. Collins R, Cranny G, Burch J, et al. A systematic review of duplex ultrasound, magnetic resonance angiography and computed tomography angiography for the diagnosis and assessment of symptomatic, lower limb peripheral arterial disease. Health Technol Assess 2007; 11(20):1–184.
6. Williams DT, Price P, Harding KG. The influence of diabetes and lower limb arterial disease on cutaneous foot perfusion. J Vasc Surg 2006; 44(4):770–775.
7. de Graaff JC, Ubbink DT, Legemate DA, et al. Interobserver and intraobserver reproducibility of peripheral blood and oxygen pressure measurements in the assessment of lower extremity arterial disease. J Vasc Surg 2001; 33(5):1033–1040.
8. Aly S, Sommerville K, Adiseshiah M, et al. Comparison of duplex imaging and arteriography in the evaluation of lower limb arteries. Br J Surg 1998; 85(8):1099–1102.
9. Ascher E, Mazzariol F, Hingorani A, et al. The use of duplex ultrasound arterial mapping as an alternative to conventional arteriography for primary and secondary infrapopliteal bypasses. Am J Surg 1999; 178(2):162–165.
10. Ascher E, Hingorani A, Markevich N, et al. Lower extremity revascularization without preoperative contrast arteriography: experience with duplex ultrasound arterial mapping in 485 cases. Ann Vasc Surg 2002; 16(1):108–114.
11. Mandolfino T, Canciglia A, D'Alfonso M, et al. Infrainguinal revascularization based on duplex ultrasound arterial mapping. Int Angiol 2006; 25(3):256–260.
12. Hofmann WJ, Walter J, Ugurluoglu A, et al. Preoperative high-frequency duplex scanning of potential pedal target vessels. J Vasc Surg 2004; 39(1):169–175.
13. Parameswaran GI, Brand K, Dolan J. Pulse oximetry as a potential screening tool for lower extremity arterial disease in asymptomatic patients with diabetes mellitus. Arch Intern Med 2005; 165(4):442–446.
14. Alnaeb ME, Crabtree VP, Boutin A, et al. Prospective assessment of lower-extremity peripheral arterial disease in diabetic patients using a novel automated optical device. Angiology 2007; 58(5):579–585.
15. Carter SA, Tate RB. Value of toe pulse waves in addition to systolic pressures in the assessment of the severity of peripheral arterial disease and critical limb ischemia. J Vasc Surg 1996; 24(2):258–265.
16. Jonsson B, Lindberg LG, Skau T, et al. Is oscillometric ankle pressure reliable in leg vascular disease? Clin Physiol 2001; 21(2):155–163.
17. Gale SS, Scissons RP, Salles-Cunha SX, et al. Lower extremity arterial evaluation: are segmental arterial blood pressures worthwhile? J Vasc Surg 1998; 27(5):831–838.

18. Williams DT, Harding KG, Price P. An evaluation of the efficacy of methods used in screening for lower-limb arterial disease in diabetes. Diabetes Care 2005; 28(9): 2206–2210.
19. Khattak M, Abdulnabi K, Williams DT. Abstracts of papers, 5th International Symposium on the Diabetic Foot, Noordwijkerhout, The Netherlands, May 9–12, 2007.
20. Pâhlsson HI, Wahlberg E, Olofsson P, et al. The toe pole test for evaluation of arterial insufficiency in diabetic patients. Eur J Vasc Endovasc Surg 1999; 18(2):133–117.
21. Smith FC, Shearman CP, Simms MH, et al. Falsely elevated ankle pressures in severe leg ischaemia: the pole test—an alternative approach. Eur J Vasc Surg 1994; 8(4):408–412.
22. Kröger K, Stewen C, Santosa F, et al. Toe pressure measurements compared to ankle artery pressure measurements. Angiology 2003; 54(1):39–44.
23. Carter SA, Lezack JD. Digital systolic pressures in the lower limb in arterial disease. Circulation 1971; 43(6):905–914.
24. Vincent DG, Salles-Cunha SX, Bernhard VM, et al. Noninvasive assessment of toe systolic pressures with special reference to diabetes mellitus. J Cardiovasc Surg (Torino) 1983; 24(1):22–28.
25. Johansson KE, Marklund BR, Fowelin JH. Evaluation of a new screening method for detecting peripheral arterial disease in a primary healthcare population of patients with diabetes mellitus. Diabet Med 2002; 19(4):307–310.
26. Schaper NC, Apelqvist J, Bakker K. The international consensus and practical guidelines on the management and prevention of the diabetic foot. Curr Diab Rep 2003; 3(6):475–479.
27. Edmonds ME, Roberts VC, Watkins PJ. Blood flow in the diabetic neuropathic foot. Diabetologia 1982; 22(1):9–15.
28. Chew JT, Tan SB, Sivathasan C, et al. Vascular assessment in the neuropathic diabetic foot. Clin Orthop Relat Res 1995; (320):95–100.
29. Stevens MJ, Goss DE, Foster AV, et al. Abnormal digital pressure measurements in diabetic neuropathic foot ulceration. Diabet Med 1993; 10(10):909–915.
30. Uccioli L, Monticone G, Durola L, et al. Autonomic neuropathy influences great toe blood pressure. Diabetes Care 1994; 17(4):284–287.
31. Ramsey DE, Manke DA, Sumner DS. Toe blood pressure-a valuable adjunct to ankle pressure measurement for assessing peripheral arterial disease. J Cardiovasc Surg (Torino) 1983; 24(1):43–48.
32. Ubbink DT, Tulevski II, den Hartog D, et al. The value of non-invasive techniques for the assessment of critical limb ischaemia. Eur J Vasc Endovasc Surg 1997; 13(3):296–300.
33. Pâhlsson HI, Jörneskog G, Wahlberg E. The cuff width influences the toe blood pressure value. Vasa 2004; 33(4):215–218.
34. Bagi P, Sillesen H, Bitsch K, et al. Doppler waveform analysis in evaluation of occlusive arterial disease in the lower limb: comparison with distal blood pressure measurement and arteriography. Eur J Vasc Surg 1990; 4(3):305–311.
35. Corbin DO, Young RJ, Morrison DC, et al. Blood flow in the foot, polyneuropathy and foot ulceration in diabetes mellitus. Diabetologia 1987; 30(7):468–473.
36. Ubbink DT, Spincemaille GH, Reneman RS, et al. Prediction of imminent amputation in patients with non-reconstructible leg ischemia by means of microcirculatory investigations. J Vasc Surg 1999; 30(1):114–121.
37. Sadiq S, Chithriki M. Arterial pressure measurements using infrared photosensors: comparison with CW Doppler. Clin Physiol 2001; 21(1):129–132.
38. McCully KK, Landsberg L, Suarez M, et al. Identification of peripheral vascular disease in elderly subjects using optical spectroscopy. J Gerontol A Biol Sci Med Sci 1997; 52(3):B159–B165.
39. Komiyama T, Shigematsu H, Yasuhara H, et al. Near-infrared spectroscopy grades the severity of intermittent claudication in diabetics more accurately than ankle pressure measurement. Br J Surg 2000; 87(4):459–466.
40. Jawahar D, Rachamalla HR, Rafalowski A, et al. Pulse oximetry in the evaluation of peripheral vascular disease. Angiology 1997; 48(8):721–724.
41. Boyko EJ, Ahroni JH, Stensel VL. Skin temperature in the neuropathic diabetic foot. J Diabetes Complications 2001; 15(5):260–264.

42. Takolander R, Rauwerda JA. The use of non-invasive vascular assessment in diabetic patients with foot lesions. Diabet Med 1996; 13(suppl 1):S39–S42.
43. Kalani M, Brismar K, Fagrell B, et al. Transcutaneous oxygen tension and toe blood pressure as predictors for outcome of diabetic foot ulcers. Diabetes Care 1999; 22(1): 147–151.
44. Christensen KS, Klarke M. Transcutaneous oxygen measurement in peripheral occlusive disease. An indicator of wound healing in leg amputation. J Bone Joint Surg Br 1986; 68(3):423–426.
45. Ballard JL, Eke CC, Bunt TJ, et al. A prospective evaluation of transcutaneous oxygen measurements in the management of diabetic foot problems. J Vasc Surg 1995; 22(4): 485–492.
46. Leahy MJ, de Mul FF, Nilsson GE, et al. Principles and practice of the laser-Doppler perfusion technique. Technol Health Care 1999; 7(2–3):143–162.
47. de Graaff JC, Ubbink DT, Legemate DA, et al. The usefulness of a laser Doppler in the measurement of toe blood pressures. J Vasc Surg 2000; 32(6):1172–1179.
48. Yamada T, Ohta T, Ishibashi H, et al. Clinical reliability and utility of skin perfusion pressure measurement in ischemic limbs–comparison with other noninvasive diagnostic methods. J Vasc Surg 2008; 47(2):318–323.
49. Jorneskog G, Brismar K, Fagrell B. Skin capillary circulation is more impaired in the toes of diabetic than non-diabetic patients with peripheral vascular disease. Diabet Med 1995; 12(1):36–41.

5 | Imaging and Diagnostic Tools for CLI

Amelia C. M. Giampietro and Jos C. van den Berg
Service of Interventional Radiology, Ospedale Regionale di Lugano, sede Civico, Lugano, Switzerland

INTRODUCTION

Peripheral arterial occlusive disease (PAOD) of the lower extremities is a chronic and progressive disease with an incidence ranging from 4.5% to 8.8% among people older than 55 years. PAOD is an important cause of morbidity and an adverse prognostic indicator in the elderly population, even when it is not a frequent primary cause of mortality (1,2). The initial symptom of PAOD of the lower extremities is normally an intermittent claudication caused by the inability to sufficiently augment blood flow in response to exercise. Only a quarter of the patients deteriorate to a higher Fontaine class (III or IV) or incapacitating symptoms (Fontaine class IIB) and require intervention. The ultimate amputation rate of the patients suffering from intermittent claudication is limited to 1% per year (3).

Although the diagnosis can usually be obtained by clinical examination, including measurement of ankle-brachial index followed by duplex ultrasound evaluation, the selection of the appropriate treatment requires detailed information of the arterial tree. The purpose of additional imaging is to better define the anatomic site, grade of disease severity, status of distal circulation, and to demonstrate the presence of unsuspected lesions. Other indications include confirmation of duplex findings, unreliable or equivocal duplex findings (calcified vessels), nonavailability of duplex, acquisition of additional anatomic information, and procedural planning in complex pathology. Imaging should be performed comprising the aortoiliac territory and feet. Imaging in patients with critical limb ischemia (CLI) has the main purpose of identifying those cases that are amenable to angioplasty (1,4).

Although catheter-based digital subtraction angiography (DSA) preserves its role of gold standard to evaluate the peripheral ischemia, its intrinsic invasiveness and costs, together with the risk of complications, have raised the demand for alternative imaging methodologies to assess number and severity of vascular lesions and to select the correct treatment planning (5–8). For successful evaluation of vascular pathology in general, an imaging study must enable accurate measurements, demonstrate intraluminal abnormalities and mural disease, and depict (patency of) side branches (9).

The current imaging options in patients with clinically suspected CLI are duplex ultrasound, computed tomography angiography (CTA), magnetic resonance angiography (MRA), and DSA (with or without 3D rotational angiography). In this chapter, an overview of the technical aspects of the currently available modalities (except duplex ultrasound) will be given and advantages and disadvantages of each technique will be discussed.

COMPUTED TOMOGRAPHY ANGIOGRAPHY

The first CTA examinations were obtained almost 20 years ago, in the early 1990s. Over the last two decades computed tomography (CT) applications have improved on both efficiency and efficacy, particularly in the field of vascular CT applications.

Using first-generation scanners, acquisition of single images took several minutes. With the introduction of spiral CT in the early 1990s, fundamental and far-reaching improvement of CT imaging was possible, which opened the pathway to entirely new applications, but still a limited area of interest could be examined during a single contrast injection.

Many factors contributed to the rapid CT development. In particular, technological developments in slip-ring gantry design, faster gantry rotation times, and, ultimately, multiple-row detector arrays have paved the way for CTA, rapidly overcoming its major initial limitation, that is, the lack of longitudinal anatomic coverage (10–13). Furthermore, a concurrent increase in computational power allowed for rapid reconstruction of large data sets. Volumetric imaging of larger scan ranges can now be performed in a single breath-hold, avoiding possible artifacts caused by misregistration.

CTA, by combining the luminal information provided by DSA with the cross-sectional view supplied in traditional axial CT, offers the advantages of both those imaging technologies, thereby offering additional visualization of vessel wall and extraluminal processes, and anatomic relationships with adjacent structures. The evaluation of the lower extremity arterial system is probably the most technically demanding clinical application for CTA, given the demand for extensive longitudinal anatomic coverage and high spatial resolution, to visualize small-diameter vessels.

Imaging protocols for CTA may vary from institution to institution and should be tailored to the available hardware, the anatomic coverage needed, and the clinical questions to be answered. There are three basic scan parameters that need to be optimized to obtain the highest possible quality for a study: *longitudinal resolution, scan speed, and luminal contrast enhancement.*

Longitudinal resolution used to be a limiting factor in three-dimensional computed tomography (3D CT); the advent of faster gantry rotation and multiple-row detector arrays has enabled to reduce nominal section thickness from 0.5 to 2.5 mm, with a resulting nearly isotropic voxel acquisition (i.e., imaging with a resolution that is equally high in all directions). Volumetric, near-isotropic data sets allow for 3D reconstruction in any plane with virtually no loss of image quality, thus enhancing the diagnostic possibilities as compared to axial source images.

Shorter scan times, in addition to reducing the likelihood of motion artifacts, have the added benefit of decreasing the volume of contrast medium to be administered. Since the contrast bolus duration for a CTA should be equivalent to the actual scan duration, shorter scan times result in lower contrast doses with positive impacts on patient safety, comfort, as well as cost (14).

Short bolus durations associated with short scan durations, however, require accurate scan time setting: scanning too early can result in incomplete opacification of the arterial system on early images, while waiting too long to start the image acquisition can result in a drop-off of the luminal enhancement on those images acquired toward the end of the scan. Both these circumstances can influence the study effectiveness negatively, resulting in nondiagnostic studies or complicate the selection of 3D rendering thresholds (see reconstruction techniques below). For optimal results, an enhancement of the arterial system of at least 250 HU is needed. To achieve optimal CT angiograms, the available speed hardware must be tuned, taking into careful account all various physiological and morphological characteristics of the patients' cardiovascular system and following a systematic approach.

Three methods for selecting scan delay times are known in literature: (*i*) empiric scan delay, (*ii*) timing bolus technique, and (*iii*) automated bolus detection and scan triggering (15,16).

1. Empiric selection of a scan delay is unlikely to be reliable enough to guarantee consistent results, in a variable population, with unpredictable differences in cardiac output.
2. The timing bolus approach involves injection of a 10 to 15 mL bolus of contrast at a rate of 4 to 5 cc/sec, followed by sequential dynamic scanning at 2-second intervals at a specified level within the target vessel after a set delay time. Serial measurements of region-of-interest attenuation within the target vessel can be graphically plotted against time on dynamic images, thus enabling a precise prediction of the time-to-peak enhancement, which is the delay time after start of contrast injection at which scanning should be initiated. One relatively simple refinement of this technique is to immediately follow the timing bolus with a 15- to 20-cc saline "chaser" bolus to prevent pooling of the contrast bolus within the injector line and peripheral veins.
3. MDCT scanners are usually equipped with bolus tracking software with automated or semi-automated scan triggering. This procedure requires the selection of a region-of-interest within the target vessel on a preliminary, that is, unenhanced image. After intravenous contrast medium administration is started, sequential images (every 3–4 seconds) are obtained at the specified level, and when the attenuation within the selected region-of-interest reaches a user-defined threshold, the CTA acquisition is either automatically or manually triggered. Automated bolus detection with scan triggering enables a higher efficiency and a (theoretical) reduction in the amount of contrast to be used. However, as in the timing bolus approach, an additional radiation dose is imparted to the patient for the acquisition of nondiagnostic images used only for determining contrast arrival. This is however counterbalanced by a reduction of the number of examinations with nondiagnostic outcome due to suboptimal enhancement.

Limitation of both timing bolus and (semi)automated technique is the risk of suffering a significant delay between the arrival of contrast and the real start of the CTA acquisition, caused by the reaction time. This lag time is the sum of interscan time, image reconstruction time, time for the scan operator to review the image and initiate the CT angiographic acquisition, and, finally, the time required for the moving table to reach the start position while giving the breathing instructions.

After acquisition of the raw data (thin axial source images), further elaboration is needed to transform the large number of images (>1500) into a digestible format. CTA image reconstruction begins with the choice of a desired section thickness, which is generally the thinnest possible for a given acquisition, to optimize the final 3D reconstruction and provide the highest degree of details for visualizing small structures or abnormalities.

Various 3D reformatting techniques are currently used in practice to aid in the visualization of vascular structures and their anatomic relationships (17). Among those, the most commonly used ones are multiplanar reconstruction (MPR), curved multiplanar reconstruction (curved MPR), maximum intensity projection (MIP), shaded surface display (SSD), and volume rendering (VR) (18). Since all these techniques rely on contrast differences between the enhanced vascular lumen and surrounding structures, it is important not to give any oral contrast prior to the CT examination, as this will disturb evaluation of the aortoiliac segment.

- *MPR (multiplanar reconstruction)*: Reconstruction of source data into two-dimensional (2D) sections with a thickness of one voxel in any arbitrarily defined plane. It is useful for evaluating structures that do not conform to an axial plane. Fast and easily performed at the CT scanner (Fig. 1).
- *MIP*: A technique that was initially introduced in the MRA literature. A specific projection angle is selected and parallel rays are then cast through the image volume. The resulting 2D image displays the maximum attenuation value encountered along the path of each ray (i.e., the brightest pixel) therefore, the effect of overlapping structures obscuring the vessel of interest is limited to only those structures with attenuation values greater than the enhanced blood (i.e., bone, calcium, and metal). The so-called bone removal technique can be used in conjunction with MIP reconstruction techniques. This technique is susceptible to artifacts, especially in regions where arteries are running close to bony structures (Fig. 2).
- *Curved MPR (curved multiplanar reconstruction)*: Displays a curved plane prescribed along an individual vessel contour, depicting the entire midline of the vessel on a single 2D image. This technique is a single-voxel thick tomogram that is helpful in analyzing individual vessels, especially those heavily calcified. Lack of visualization of the lumen of a vessel by extensive calcification, a major drawback of MIP and VR reconstructions, is less critical with curved MPR, which allows evaluation of the lumen even in the presence of such calcification (Figs. 3 and 4). The major disadvantage of curved MPR is its limited spatial resolution, where inaccurate centerline definition can lead to spurious stenoses and occlusions.
- *SSD*: This method uses a single threshold to choose relevant (high-density) voxels; results in visually appealing 3D renderings of vessels; a virtual light source is used to generate reflections that are represented in a grayscale picture, resulting in lighting effects; because of the threshold, this method is susceptible to artifacts and may fail to demonstrate vascular calcifications. This method is useful in determining the anatomical relationship between site of stenosis and bony structures (19); SSD, which is a useful tool for giving an overall picture of the anatomy and shape of a vessel, should never be used when accurate measurements of luminal dimensions are required.
- *VRT (3D volume rendering techniques)*: Probably the most complex 3D reconstruction technique. Voxels within a data set are assigned with a degree of opacity and a color, as a function of their attenuation values. By changing the function, a user-defined curve where either color or opacity is

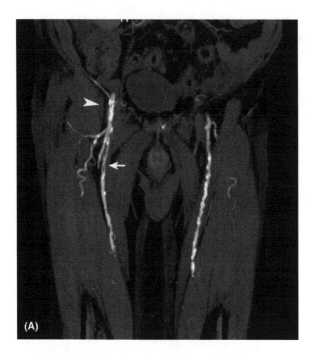

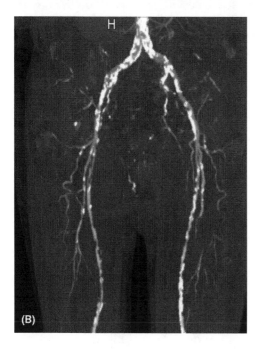

FIGURE 1 MPR of CTA (**A**) demonstrating calcification at the level of the common femoral artery (*arrowhead*) and multiple stenoses of the superficial femoral artery (*arrow*), only a relatively small segment of the artery can be evaluated due to the small thickness of the slice; corresponding MIP image using bone removal software (**B**) offers complete overview of the iliac and femoral arteries; corresponding DSA image (**C**) of multiple stenoses of superficial femoral artery. *Abbreviations*: MPR, multiplanar reconstruction; CTA, computed tomography angiography; MIP, maximum intensity projection; DSA, digital subtraction angiography. (*Continued*)

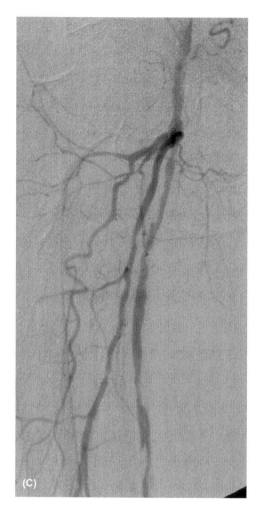

(C)

FIGURE 1 (*Continued*)

plotted against attenuation, structures of different attenuation can either be emphasized or deemphasized (up to the point of invisibility). This feature enables the assessment of the anatomic relationship between vessels, bones, calcium (including calcified plaque), and other structures such as metallic stents (Fig. 3). On the other hand, the arbitrary nature of opacity and color function precludes accurate measurements of vessel diameter (10,20). Reversing window-level transfer function, virtual angioscopic images can be produced (20,21).

Table 1 lists the advantages and disadvantages of the various reconstruction techniques.

When interpreting CTA studies, it must be always taken into consideration that all diagnostic information contained in the study is present in the axial source images, and this is not automatically the case for the various 3D reconstructions. Therefore, it is imperative to carefully review the axial source images in all cases to detect vascular pathology and incidental, nonvascular, abnormalities (22). Calcification of plaque should not be considered a limitation of CTA, although heavily calcified eccentric plaque precludes an adequate MIP and VRT evaluation of CTA, for the reasons indicated above (Fig. 4). Overestimation of stenosis in CTA can occur because of "blooming artifacts." By using a so-called "bone window" setting blooming artifacts can be reduced (Fig. 5). Another technique to avoid measurement error is using an incremental reduction of the volume of a multiplanar volume reconstruction (23). Ring-like calcifications in the arterial wall can mask the patent lumen in MPR images and here evaluation using axial reconstructions is of use (24).

CTA Acquisition Protocols
The CTA should be performed as a single acquisition with coverage from the supraceliac abdominal aorta down the feet (8,11).

The patient should lie supine on the table, feet first with the knees and ankles secured together in a neutral comfortable position to reduce artifact from motion during the scan and to minimize the display field of view. The legs should be as close to the isocenter of the scanner as possible to avoid off-center stair-step artifacts. The feet should not be excessively plantar flexed to avoid artifactual stenosis or even pseudo-occlusion of the dorsalis pedis artery. The

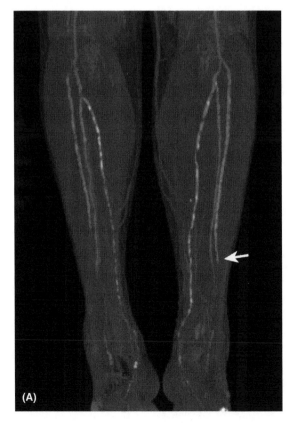

(A)

FIGURE 2   MIP CTA using bone removal software (A) demonstrating interruption of the anterior tibial artery in the distal segment (*arrow*); careful evaluation of the original axial slices (B) demonstrated patency of the distal anterior tibial artery (*arrowhead*); findings were confirmed at DSA (C) during an endovascular procedure of the ipsilateral superficial femoral artery with patency of distal anterior tibial artery (*arrow*). *Abbreviations*: MIP, maximum intensity projection; CTA, computed tomography angiography; DSA, digital subtraction angiography. (*Continued*)

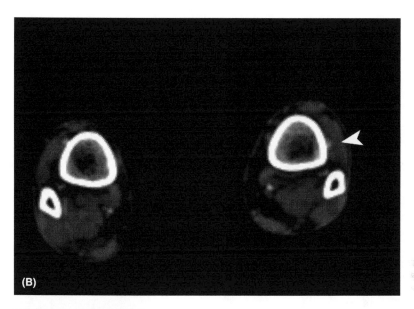

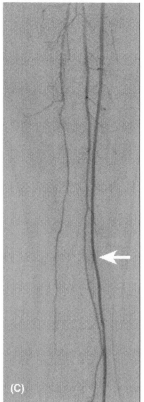

FIGURE 2 (*Continued*)

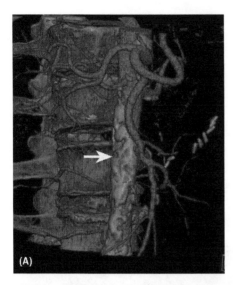

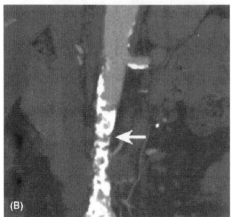

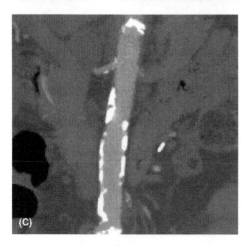

FIGURE 3 VRT reconstruction of CTA (**A**) demonstrating heavily calcified infrarenal abdominal aorta (*arrow*), no luminal information can be obtained; the corresponding sequential MPR images (**B** and **C**) demonstrate the calcification to be located only in the vessel wall (*arrow*), without lumen reduction. *Abbreviations*: VRT, volume rendering techniques; CTA, computed tomography angiography; MPR, multiplanar reconstruction; DSA, digital subtraction angiography.

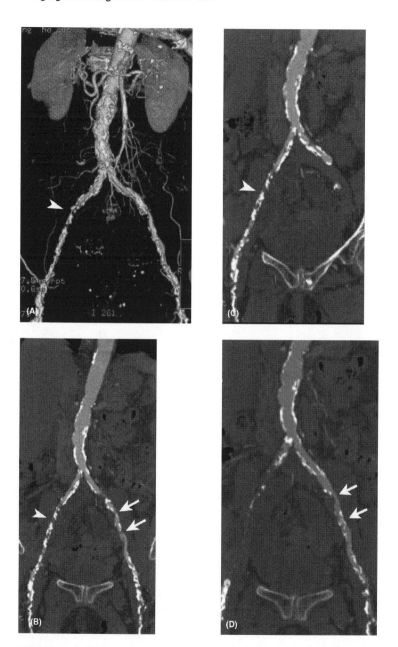

FIGURE 4 VRT reconstruction of CTA (**A**) showing heavily calcified aortoiliac segment, with suspicion of occlusion the right distal common iliac artery (*arrowhead*), right external iliac artery, and left iliac axis appear patent; MPR (*in bone window*) of CTA (**B**) and curved MPR of the right (**C**) and left (**D**) iliac axis allows for better visualization of the lumen, occlusion of the right external iliac artery (*arrowhead*), and a hemodynamically significant stenosis of the left external iliac artery (*arrows*); findings confirmed by CE MRA (**E**). *Abbreviations*: VRT, volume rendering techniques; MPR, multiplanar reconstruction; CTA, computed tomography angiography; CE MRA, contrast-enhanced magnetic resonance angiography. (*Continued*)

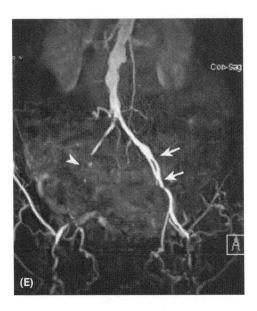

FIGURE 4 (*Continued*)

TABLE 1 Characteristics of Reconstruction Techniques

	Luminal and vessel wall information	Vascular contour	Visualization adjacent structures	Diagnostic accuracy
Axial images	+++	+	+++	++
MPR	+++	+	+++	++
Curved MPR	+++	++	++	+++
MIP	+	++	+	++
SSD	+	+++	+	+
VR	++	+++	++	+
Bone removal	+	++	+	+++

Abbreviations: MPR, multiplanar reconstruction; MIP, maximum intensity projection; SSD, shaded surface display; VR, volume rendering.
Source: Adapted from Ref. 10.

full study consists of a digital radiograph (the "scout" image, needed for planning), an optional unenhanced acquisition, a series for bolus testing or triggering, the angiographic acquisition, and an optional late-phase acquisition.

A scout image, or topogram, should first be acquired to identify the area of coverage. Anatomic coverage usually extends from just cranial to the origins of the renal arteries through the feet with an average scan length of around 120 cm. If the distal vessels are not well opacified (e.g., in cases of femoropopliteal aneurysm or slow circulation in the setting of cardiac failure), a second acquisition may be necessary. This optional late-phase scanning of the popliteal and infrapopliteal vasculature should be initiated only on demand by the technologist upon seeing poor opacification on first-pass imaging (Fig. 6).

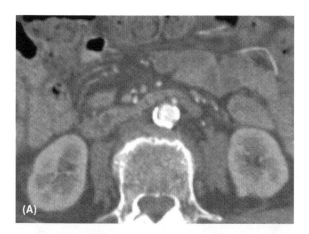

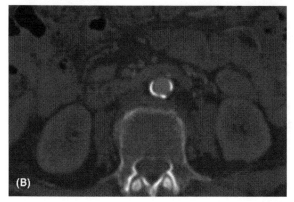

FIGURE 5 Axial CT image at the level of the infrarenal abdominal aorta, using standard abdominal window setting (**A**), and bone window setting (**B**); it can be clearly seen that luminal evaluation is less disturbed by blooming artifact caused by the calcified arterial wall.

The proper administration of nonionic contrast material is key to sufficient opacification of the arteries of the lower extremities. The objective is to image these vessels while enhancing them homogenously without venous or tissue enhancement.

An 18G to 22G canula is placed into a superficial vein within the antecubital fossa, forearm, or dorsum of the hand. A total volume of 100 to 160 mL of contrast material may be needed to opacify all the arteries of the lower extremities sufficiently. In general, about 0.5 to 0.7 g of iodine/kg of body weight is necessary. When using an iodine concentration of 300 to 370 mg/mL and an injection rate of 3.5 to 5.0 mL/sec, sufficient opacification of the abdominal aorta and peripheral arteries is obtained. The total volume of contrast material may be reduced if a higher concentration of iodine (e.g., 370 mg/mL) is used. Monophasic injections during which contrast material is injected at a single rate yield a short-lived peak on curves that track arterial attenuation over time. Biphasic injections, during which the rate is high initially, followed by a different lower rate, may enhance the arteries more consistently (25). After the contrast medium has been injected, flushing with saline pushes the residual material from the venous system into arterial circulation (26,27). Typically, 30 to 50 mL of saline is administered via a dual-chamber injector device. If a

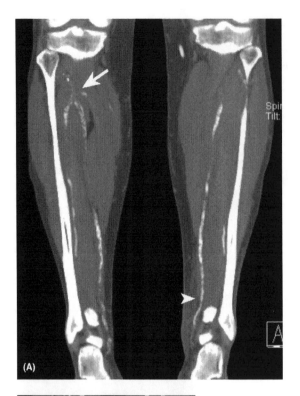

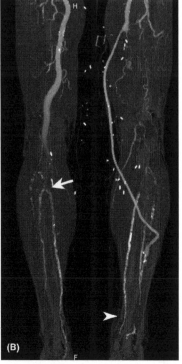

FIGURE 6 MPR of CTA (**A**) and corresponding MIP using bone removal software (**B**) in
early phase in a patient after left popliteal-crural
bypass demonstrating good enhancement of
the left posterior tibial artery (*arrowhead*) and
absence of filling of the right trifurcation; corresponding images obtained with a second pass of
the lower leg (**C** and **D**) show good filling of crural
vessels on the right side as well (*arrowhead*).
Abbreviations: MPR, multiplanar reconstruction;
CTA, computed tomography angiography; MIP,
maximum intensity projection. (*Continued*)

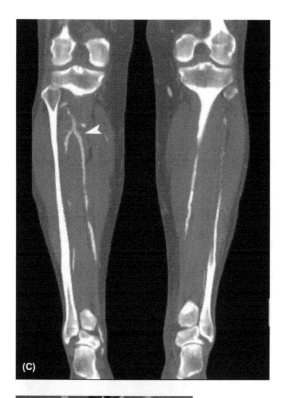

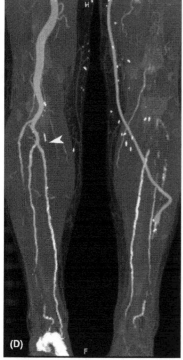

FIGURE 6 (*Continued*)

TABLE 2   Technical Parameters for MDCTA Using Different Scanners

Parameters	4–8 Slice scanners	10–16 Slice scanners	32–64 Slice scanners
Tube voltage (kV)	120	120	120
Tube current time product (mAs)	110	120	170
Collimation (mm)	2.5	0.75	0.6
Pitch	0.375	0.25	0.2
Reconstructed slice thickness (mm)	3.0	1.0	0.6
Convolution kernel	Standard	Standard	Standard

Abbreviation: MDCTA, multidetector computed tomography angiography.

TABLE 3   Injection Protocols for MDCTA Using Different Scanners

	4–8 Slice scanners	10–16 Slice scanners	32–64 Slice scanners
Concentration (mg iodine/mL)	350–400	350–400	350–400
Mono/biphasic	Biphasic	Biphasic	Monophasic
Volume (mL)	150	120	100
Injection rate (mL/sec)	4.0/2.5	4.0/2.5	5.0
Saline chaser (mL; mL/sec)	30; 2.5	30; 2.5	60; 5
Delay (sec)	Test bolus	Test bolus/bolus tracking	Test bolus/bolus tracking

Abbreviation: MDCTA, multidetector computed tomography angiography.

dual-chamber injector is unavailable, the saline may be after-loaded in a single-chamber injector (12).

Depending on the scanner characteristics (number of detector rows), the CTA examination may be carried out with different technical protocols (collimation, gantry rotation time, table speed). Tables 2 and 3 list the technical parameters for multidetector computed tomography angiography (MDCTA) and injection protocols.

MDCTA has many advantages over other modalities commonly used to image the lower extremities, including ultrasonography and DSA. Unlike ultrasonography, CTA of the lower limb is relatively investigator-independent and can be performed easily, even in patients with calcified native arteries or patients who have recently undergone bypass surgery (and still have healing wounds or surgical dressing). When compared with conventional catheter angiography, CTA is less invasive, less expensive, and exposes the patient to less radiation (17). CTA also assesses aspects external to the lumen of the vessel that DSA cannot, including mural thrombus, atheroma, inflammation, and periarterial tissues (Fig. 7). The diagnostic performance of MDCT in detecting arterial atherosclerotic steno-occlusive disease relative to DSA is good, as reported in a systematic review of several studies (28). Pooled sensitivity and specificity for all studies reported in this review were 92% (95% confidence interval 89–95%) and 93% (95% confidence interval 91–95%), respectively.

CTA represents a noninvasive study with high diagnostic yield, convenience, and speed at a substantial cost savings when compared with conventional DSA [that usually requires a (short) hospital stay] (29,30).

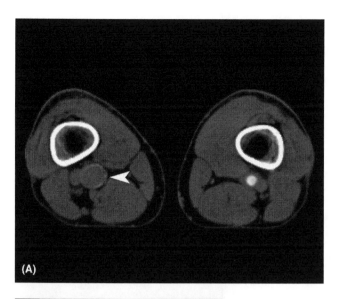

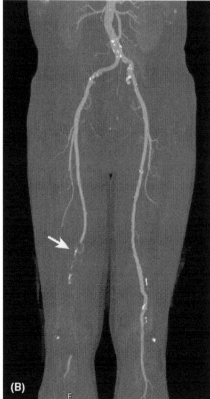

FIGURE 7 MIP CT angiography using bone removal software (**A**) demonstrating occlusion of the distal superficial femoral artery and popliteal artery (*arrow*); evaluation of MPR images (**B**) and axial source images (**C**) reveals presence of a thrombosed popliteal aneurysm. *Abbreviations*: MIP, maximum intensity projection; MPR, multiplanar reconstruction. (*Continued*)

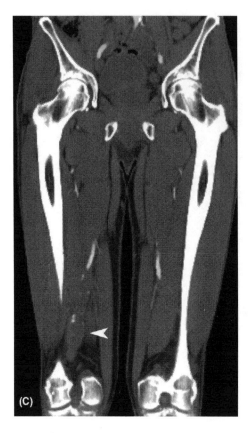

(C)

FIGURE 7   (*Continued*)

MAGNETIC RESONANCE ANGIOGRAPHY

Contrast in magnetic resonance (MR) images depends principally on static tissue parameters: longitudinal relaxation time T1, transverse relaxation time T2, and proton density. In addition, the MR signal is sensitive to flow and movement, which frequently leads to artifacts in MR imaging. MR angiographic sequences, however, use flow-induced signal variations to depict blood vessels or even to obtain quantitative information about blood flow in terms of velocity and direction. Unenhanced MRA comprises those MR techniques that rely solely on flow effects. Unlike contrast-enhanced MRA (CE MRA) and DSA, which depict the vessel lumen filled with contrast agent, it is just the movement of blood that is seen in the unenhanced MR angiogram.

Unenhanced MRA differs from DSA and other angiographic techniques in the fact that blood vessels are depicted noninvasively and without the need for contrast agent injection. Unenhanced MR techniques allow the acquisition of 3D data sets or stacks of 2D images ("source images") covering all vessels in a selected volume of interest. Starting from source images, the postprocessing algorithm (MIP algorithm) is capable of reconstructing a projectional angiographic display of the vessel and enables, without the need for additional measurements, the generation of angiogram-like images from any desired view angle (31,32).

Another main advantage of MRA versus DSA is the fact that with MRA extravascular tissue is shown together with the vessels, thereby permitting the correlation of blood flow abnormalities with associated soft tissue pathologies.

Typically, MRA techniques are designed to make the flowing blood producing hyperintense signal over a background signal from stationary tissue largely suppressed ("bright-blood" angiography). An alternative is to make flowing spins to appear hypointense compared with the stationary background ("black-blood" angiography).

To perform "bright-blood" MRA, two approaches are available, time of flight (TOF) and phase contrast (PC).

- *Amplitude effects* (TOF): Blood flowing into or out of a chosen slice has a different longitudinal magnetization, compared with stationary spins, depending on the duration of stay (TOF) in the slice.
- *Phase effects* (PC): Blood flowing along the direction of a magnetic field gradient is subject to changes of its transverse magnetization compared with stationary spins.

Since unenhanced MRA is based on complex flow phenomena, physiological conditions of flow in the vascular territory of interest are a critical factor for the applicability of the method. Brain vessels, where flow is nearly laminar, provide advantageous conditions for unenhanced MRA. In fact, in clinical routine, unenhanced MRA has proven to be a robust and versatile method for noninvasive imaging of brain vessels (circle of Willis, sagittal sinus) and a suitable technique for depicting extracranial carotid arteries and short segments of peripheral vessels (e.g., lower leg) (33). Unenhanced MRA is in fact well performing in high-velocity arterial flow, where acceptable vessel-background contrasts can be achieved in moderate acquisition times. On the other hand, it shows its limitation in areas of turbulent or very slow flow, where some sort of signal loss is possible and may lead, in severe cases, to a misdiagnosis of the pathological condition (stenosis, aneurysm). In addition to this, anatomic coverage is very limited. Another major limitation of TOF and PC angiography is their high sensitivity to motion artifacts, that can either be caused by patient movements, more likely given the need for relatively long acquisition times, or can occur for physiological reasons in areas of very pulsatile flow (e.g., carotids, aorta, and peripheral arteries) or in regions affected by breathing and heart actions (e.g., thoracic and abdominal).

For all these reasons, another approach to MRA, CE MRA, is nowadays more frequently used. Over the past decade, CE MRA technologies have significantly improved image quality, acquisition speed, reliability, and ease of use. CE MRA performed adopting traditional extracellular gadolinium (Gd)-chelate contrast media can now yield angiographic image quality that is comparable, and in some cases even superior, to that achievable with conventional catheter angiography (34,35). CE MRA, besides being noninvasive, shows inherent clinical benefits with respect to DSA and CTA, since it does not require any exposure to ionizing radiation or nephrotoxic iodinated contrast media. Recently, some issues were raised regarding the occurrence of a syndrome of nephrogenic systemic fibrosis, which might limit the applicability of CE MRA in patients with renal insufficiency (36). It is beyond the scope of this chapter to discuss this in detail.

CE MRA techniques rely on the T1 shortening effect of Gd-chelate contrast agent in blood to generate vascular signal, instead of exploiting the inherent motion of blood flow as in the flow-based TOF and PC techniques. Thanks to this different approach, the vascular signal generated with CE MRA is not hampered by the numerous flow-related artifacts that can degrade the flow-based MRA techniques and can often result in the overestimation of stenoses or the mimicking of a vascular occlusion (37,38). In CE MRA, it is the contrast agent that during its vascular transit, as in conventional angiography, enables the generation of "luminograms" that can visualize both arteries and veins: Arteries are visualized if image acquisition is performed during the arterial phase of the bolus whereas veins are shown if imaging is performed later, that is, during the venous or delayed phase of the bolus. The vascular enhancement is a transient and dynamic process, hence the critical element to be set for a CE MRA, as with CTA, is the proper timing for the image acquisition. Ideally, imaging is to be performed during peak enhancement of the target vessel and when overlapping structures and background tissue are not enhanced. For arterial visualization, this means synchronizing the acquisition to the period of preferential arterial enhancement, when arterial Gd concentration is high and no significant venous or background enhancement has occurred (39,40). Early venous filling can be reduced by putting a cuff or tourniquet around the upper leg (Fig. 8), a simple maneuver that reduces flow significantly (41).

Another advantage of CE MRA being performed using 3D MRA pulse sequences is that it yields volumetric data sets, which can also be postprocessed by applying MPR algorithms and various 3D visualization techniques like maximum MIP and VR display (Fig. 9).

In case of multistation CE MRA examinations (i.e., bolus chase CE MRA), another important information to have from the patient in advance is if he has any underlying condition that could prevent him from staying still for even a short time. These examinations, in fact, usually require subtraction of images and patient motion, between pre- and postcontrast data set acquisitions, can result in spatial misregistration and can lead to degraded image quality.

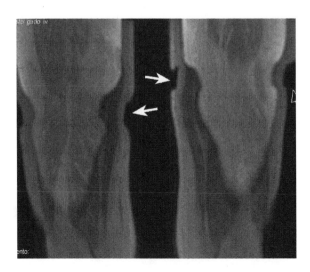

FIGURE 8 T1-weighted MRI of upper leg, clearly depicting a tourniquet (*arrows*) placed to reduce early venous return of contrast. *Abbreviation*: MRI, magnetic resonance image.

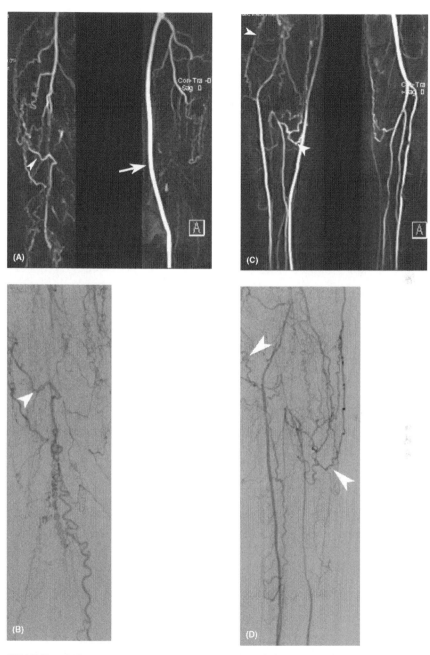

FIGURE 9 MIP image of upper legs (**A**) and lower legs (**B**) demonstrating occlusion of the right superficial femoral artery, and distal enhancement through collaterals (*arrowhead*), note presence of femoropopliteal bypass on the left (*arrow*); corresponding selective DSA of right leg (**C** and **D**) confirming occlusion and demonstrating collaterals (*arrowheads*). *Abbreviations*: MIP, maximum intensity projection; DSA, digital subtraction angiography.

To complete a proper collection of patient's information before the examination, the history of prior interventions, especially vascular or endovascular procedures, should be investigated as well; knowledge of extra-anatomic bypass grafts or stent grafts will ensure proper scan prescription and planning (42).

CE MRA Acquisition Protocols

Ideally, for CE MRA, the intravenous canula is placed in the antecubital fossa and should be sufficiently large (i.e., at least 22 gauge) to support a bolus rate of at least 2 mL/sec. For multistation bolus chase examinations, care must be taken to ensure that the intravenous catheter is stabilized and that the tubing is sufficiently long to allow free movement of the patient and table during the bolus chase table translation. It is advisable to firmly tape the tubing to the patient and to cover potential areas that may snare the tubing. Snaring of the tubing during table translation may not only pull the intravenous catheter out but also stop table translation as some scanners will automatically stop if any resistance or hindrance to table translation is detected.

For most CE MRA examinations, patients are positioned feet first in the supine position in the bore of the magnet. Vascular signal-to-noise ratio (SNR) can be improved by the use of phased array coils and, additionally, by the proper centering of the coil elements about the region(s) of interest.

With the advent of new scanners with higher numbers of reception channels, coverage of the entire body of the patient with multiple coils is now possible, allowing whole body imaging without moving the patient. The use of phased array coils provides the additional benefit of markedly shortening image acquisition times or, with the use of parallel imaging schemes, of acquiring higher spatial resolution image sets in the same time period (35,43,44).

As with CTA, timing is of utmost importance. With traditional extracellular Gd-chelate contrast agents, much of an intravenously administered dose will diffuse rapidly out of the vascular space into adjacent tissues within five minutes, thereby increasing background signal and reducing the vascular contrast-to-noise ratio (CNR). Arteries are best imaged if imaging data are acquired during peak arterial enhancement (i.e., when the concentration of Gd is greatest). The arrival time for the contrast bolus in the region of interest depends on the patient's cardiac output and the status of the vascular segment under investigation (45,46).

Peak contrast enhancement of the abdominal aorta, for example, has been shown to range from 10 to as long as 60 seconds, with the longest delay occurring in a patient with inherently slow flow due to the presence of a large thoracoabdominal aneurysm.

Fundamental to the proper synchronization of arterial CE MRA is the acquisition of imaging data during the period of preferential arterial enhancement prior to the occurrence of significant venous enhancement. Prior to the availability of MR compatible injectors and fast imaging methods, an empiric estimation of the bolus arrival time was used. This technique ("best guess" or "educated guess") used predetermined times (e.g., a 10-second delay for CE MRA of the thoracic aorta and a 12-second delay for renal CE MRA) but generally required higher doses of Gd-chelate (e.g., 40–60 mL or 0.2–0.3 mmol/kg) to ensure sufficiently long arterial phase duration of an adequate Gd concentration. By accurately timing the CE MRA examination, optimized arterial SNR and CNR can frequently be achieved with lower doses of contrast agent, thereby reducing overall examination costs. There are three methods for accurate timing.

The first, and most widely used, method involves performing a test bolus scan to estimate the arrival of contrast in the target vascular bed. This is usually achieved by administering a 1 to 2 mL dose of Gd-chelate contrast agent and measuring its arrival time in the vessel of interest. For optimal results, it is advisable to administer the test bolus in a manner identical to that planned for the full dose during the CE MRA examination. Thus, it should be injected at the same rate and with sufficient saline flush (≥ 30 mL) to ensure that it arrives centrally and does not pool within the tubing set or a peripheral vein. Standardization of injections is easily accomplished using an MR compatible injector. Test bolus imaging should be performed using a fast 2D, T1-weighted, spoiled gradient echo pulse sequence. Imaging parameters (e.g., repetition time, echo time, matrix) should be adjusted to yield a temporal resolution of approximately one image every one to two seconds. The ideal contrast arrival time can be estimated based on the frame with the optimal arterial enhancement.

More recently, two additional methods of real-time triggering for CE MRA have become commercially available. One early technique is referred to as automated bolus detection (e.g., MR SmartPrep, General Electric Medical Systems, Waukesha, Wisconsin, U.S.), in which monitoring for contrast bolus arrival and initiation of the MRA data acquisition are automated and integrated into a single pulse sequence. This monitoring phase of the pulse sequence uses a high temporal resolution (400 milliseconds) fast spin echo pulse sequence to monitor the arrival of contrast into an operator-defined volume of interest, typically a large vessel within the field of view. After a preliminary period (e.g., 10–20 seconds) during which the baseline signal of the monitoring volume is determined, the pulse sequence informs the operator as to when to initiate the contrast administration while continuing its monitoring phase. Once the signal within the monitoring volume exceeds two preset thresholds (typically, 2 standard deviations and 20% rise over baseline signal), the pulse sequence automatically switches to its imaging phase. At the beginning of the imaging phase, the operator can also set a delay period (e.g., 3–5 seconds) prior to the actual 3D MRA data acquisition. The delay period provides an opportunity for the patient to initiate a breath-hold prior to the actual 3D MRA data acquisition.

The second method for real-time CE MRA timing utilizes a fluoroscopic trigger (BolusTrak, Philips Medical Systems, Best, the Netherlands; Care Bolus, Siemens Medical Solutions, Erlangen, Germany; Fluoro Trigger, General Electric Medical Systems, Waukesha, Wisconsin, U.S.). Like the aforementioned automated triggering scheme, the real-time MR fluoroscopic technique also integrates a monitoring phase and an imaging phase into a single pulse sequence. However, with the MR fluoroscopic method, monitoring is performed by the operator visually, using a continuous fast 2D spoiled gradient echo pulse sequence with imaging centered over the vascular bed. With this method, the operator is able to see the arrival of the contrast bolus and to manually initiate the imaging phase. Once again, a delay period can be selected to enable patient breath holding, which is generally preferable for most body applications. Table 4 lists typical scanning parameters for CE 3D MRA at 1.5 T for specific vendors.

Recently, a new Gd contrast agent (gadobenate dimeglumine, Gd-BOPTA, MultiHance; Bracco Imaging SpA, Milan, Italy) has become available in Europe and numerous other countries around the world. Compared with the

TABLE 4 Typical Scanning Parameters for CE 3D MRA at 1.5 T for Specific Vendors

Imaging parameter	General Electric	Philips	Siemens
Pulse sequence	3D FSPGR	3D FFE	3D FLASH
TR (msec)	4–6	4–6	3–5
TE (msec)	1–2	1–2	1–2
Flip angle	45	40	25
FOV	30–40 cm	400 mm	400 mm
Timing	SMARTPREP	BolusTrak	Care bolus

Abbreviations: MRA, magnetic resonance angiography; TR, repetition time; TE, echo time; FOV, field of view.

Gd-chelates traditionally used for CE MRA, this agent has improved T1 relaxivity due to weak interactions of the Gd-BOPTA chelate with serum proteins such as albumin. Several studies have shown that the signal intensity increase with Gd-BOPTA is as much as 50% higher as with conventional Gd contrast agents at the same dose and injection rate, making this agent particularly suitable for CE MRA (47,48). The relative benefits of Gd-BOPTA are more apparent in smaller vessels, which are better visualized using Gd-BOPTA than with traditional extracellular contrast agents (39). However, the use of intravenous low- and high-molecular Gd-chelates for CE MRA is limited by the rapid equilibration of these agents among the intravascular, extravascular, and extracellular compartments. As mentioned in section "CE MRA Acquisition Protocol," imaging during the arterial phase is desirable for strong arterial and minimal confounding background and venous enhancement. But the arterial phase of extracellular contrast material is short because rapid extravasation occurs. Various approaches for prolongation of the arterial phase, such as venous compression for imaging of runoff vessels, have been tested (41).

More recently, a new generation of contrast agents with intravascular distribution, also referred to as blood pool agents (BPAs), has become available. Among the class of contrast agents that provides strong and prolonged vascular enhancement, one preparation, *gadofosveset* (Vasovist®, Bayer Schering Pharma, Berlin, Germany), has been approved for clinical use (49–51). This type of contrast agents offers the same advantages as extracellular contrast agents, with even a stronger T1 relaxation effect, and in addition to this allows for late imaging in the so-called steady state (52). Because scanning times can be longer, higher-resolution images can be obtained with isotropic resolution of 0.6 mm. Overlap of venous structures is therefore not an issue anymore, since all structures can be easily separated from each other (Fig. 10) (51). BPAs are particularly promising in contrasting smaller vessels, vessels with slow flow, and vessels with complex flow (51). Plaque morphology can be depicted in high detail.

DIGITAL SUBTRACTION ANGIOGRAPHY

For many years, DSA has been the only means to visualization of the arterial tree. It involves puncture of the arterial system (usually the common femoral artery), followed by introduction of an angiographic catheter and injection of iodinated contrast medium. Typically, various projections of the different anatomical regions are necessary; for example, for evaluation of the iliac territory consists of an anteroposterior (AP) projection and two oblique projections (with

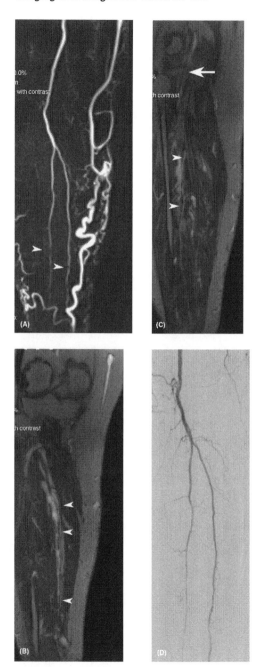

FIGURE 10 First-pass CE MRA (*using gadofosveset*) of right lower leg (**A**) depicting multiple stenosis of the fibular and posterior tibial artery (*arrowheads*); in the steady-state phase, despite venous filling, the posterior tibial artery (*arrowheads*) in (**B**), and the fibular artery and popliteal artery (**C**), (*arrowheads and arrow, respectively*) can be clearly delineated, suggesting absence of stenosis; corresponding DSA (**D**) rules out hemodynamically significant stenoses. *Abbreviations*: CE MRA, contrast-enhanced magnetic resonance angiography; DSA, digital subtraction angiography.

inclination of the X-ray tube of 25°). Evaluation of the iliac bifurcation can be performed on the oblique projection with the image intensifier rotated toward the contralateral side. Evaluation of the femoral bifurcation on the other hand is best performed with an ipsilateral inclination of the C-arm. For evaluation of the superficial femoral and popliteal artery AP projections suffice, while best evaluation of the crural arteries is obtained with slight ipsilateral lateral inclination of the image intensifier (or inward rotation of the leg with the C-arm in AP projection).

In the aorto-iliac segment, the radiation exposure and amount of contrast medium can be reduced significantly using 3D rotational angiography (53). For evaluation of the infra-inguinal arteries there is no place for 3D rotational angiography. DSA is capable of providing dynamic images, information that cannot be obtained with standard CTA and MRA techniques (Fig. 11).

To reduce the amount of iodinated contrast medium used (in patients with renal insufficiency), angiography using CO_2 can be performed. Injection of CO_2 is typically performed by hand injection using a large (50 mL) syringe, which is filled with CO_2 from a plastic bag attached to a CO_2 container. Care should be taken not to mix CO_2 with room air. To facilitate dispersion of CO_2 into the peripheral arteries, it is advisable to place the patient in a Trendelenburg position. Patients usually experience more discomfort during CO_2 injection (54). The diagnostic accuracy of grading stenosis is comparable to angiography with iodinated contrast medium. However, iodine-based vascular opacification remains superior to that with CO_2 in the central and distal arteries. Image quality of crural angiography using CO_2 is generally poor (Fig. 12). Furthermore, the degree of certainty and overall quality score can be found higher for iodine compared with CO_2-based contrast studies (54,55).

When using CO_2 as contrast agent, special software of the angiography system is needed, and some features of angiography systems cannot be used (e.g., road map). Therefore, it will never be possible to completely eliminate use of iodinated contrast medium during a procedure.

As an alternative or as a supplement to CO_2 angiography, Gd has been proposed as contrast medium (up to 50% of lower extremity angiography using CO_2 may yield insufficient results) (56). Gd has the same attenuation characteristics as iodine and therefore no special settings for the X-ray equipment are needed (57). Cases of renal insufficiency at high dose Gd injection have been described but no safety risks are known at low-dosage schemes (<0.4 mmol/kg body weight) (58,59).

COMPARISON OF TECHNIQUES

Martin and colleagues reported that MDCTA (performed with a four-detector scanner) had excellent specificity in revealing severe (>75%) stenoses and arterial occlusions (97% and 98%, respectively) with an acceptable sensitivity (92% and 89%, respectively).

Further progresses in MDCT, with the release of 8-, 16-, and even 64-detector scanners have demonstrated to yield even better results (Table 5).

Conventional angiography will keep a major role in patient care, but mainly in a therapeutic setting. For diagnostic purposes, CTA, especially when performed on multidetector-row CT scanners, has become the preferred imaging test for many clinical situations. MRA can compete with CTA, although,

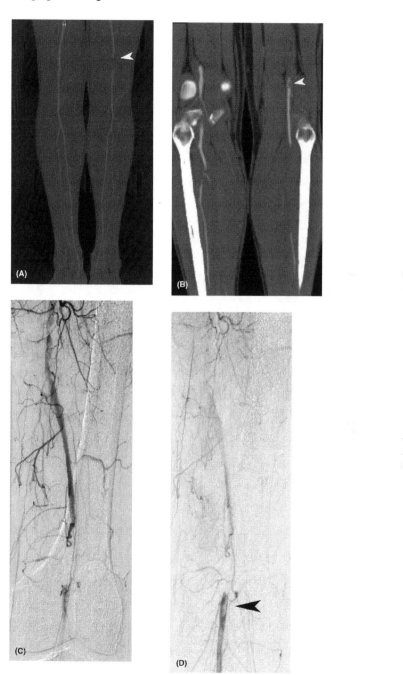

FIGURE 11 MIP CTA using bone removal software (**A**) demonstrating occlusion of the distal superficial femoral artery-proximal popliteal artery due to thromboembolism (*arrowhead*); the corresponding MPR image (**B**) demonstrates the tail of the embolus (*arrowhead*); serial DSA images (**C** and **D**) demonstrate collateral pathways and flow dynamics and show the embolus (*arrowhead*) to advantage; surgical embolectomy was performed uneventfully. *Abbreviations*: MIP, maximum intensity projection; CTA, computed tomography angiography; MPR, multiplanar reconstruction; DSA, digital subtraction angiography.

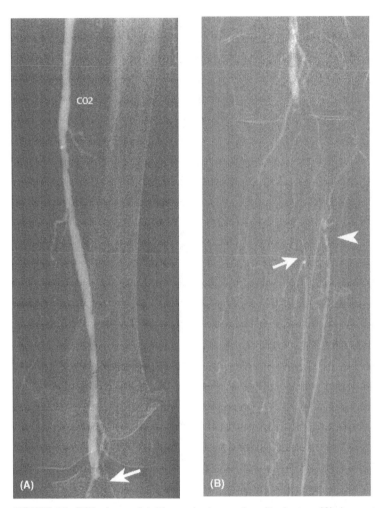

FIGURE 12 DSA of superficial femoral artery and popliteal artery (**A**) demonstrating occlusion of the distal popliteal artery; DSA of the crural segment (**B**) demonstrating flow at the level of the fibular artery (*arrow*) and anterior tibial artery (*arrowhead*); note low resolution compared with DSA using iodinated contrast. *Abbreviation*: DSA, digital subtraction angiography.

with the improved spatial resolution of MDCTA and the easier reformation of the imaging volume, the advantages of MRA have decreased. MRA continues to have a primary role in all cases where radiation exposure can be a concern (especially in young individuals who may need multiple studies over time or when multiphasic imaging is to be performed) or when iodinated contrast is contraindicated (e.g., due to renal dysfunction or allergy) and remains a valuable option in patients with extensive arterial calcification (Fig. 13) (72). MRA on the other hand has contraindications and challenges that do not apply when considering a CTA. The presence of surgical clips or metallic stents can cause artifacts interfering with the interpretation of MRA. Furthermore, patients with pacemakers or cardiac defibrillators cannot undergo MRA, yet many of them

TABLE 5 Results of Recent Studies Comparing MDCT with DSA

Author, year	MDCT rows	Evaluated segment	Sensitivity (%)	Specificity (%)
Puls, 2001 (60)	4	Aorta to ankles	89	86
Ofer, 2003 (61)	4	SMA to pedal arteries	91	92
Heuschmid, 2003 (62)	4	Aorta to ankles	91	90
Martin, 2003 (8)	4	Celiac axis to toes	92	97
Mesurolle, 2004 (63)	2	Celiac axis to 10 cm below trifurcation	91	93
Ota, 2004 (64)	4	L2 to calf	99	99
Catalano, 2004 (1)	4	Diaphragm to feet	96	93
Portugaller, 2004 (65)	4	Aorta to ankles	92	83
Bui, 2005 (66)	4	Celiac axis to toes	90	86
Edwards, 2005 (67)	4	Aorta to ankles	72–79	93
Willmann, 2005 (68)	16	Aorta to ankles	96–97	96–97
Schertler, 2005 (69)	16	Aorta to ankles	96–98	85–89
Fraioli, 2006 (70)	4	Aorta to ankles	91–94	94–96

Abbreviations: DSA, digital subtraction angiography; MDCT, multidetector computed tomography; SMA, superior mesenteric artery.
Source: Adapted from Refs. 28, 30, and 71.

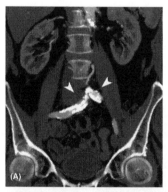

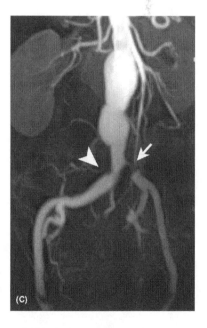

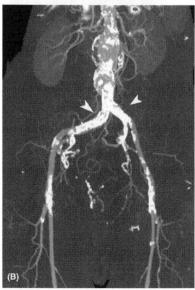

FIGURE 13 MPR (**A**) and MIP (**B**) of CTA demonstrating severe calcification of both common iliac arteries (*arrowheads*), from these images judgment of the residual lumen is difficult; CE MRA (**C**) of the same patient demonstrates absence of significant stenosis on the right side (*arrowhead*), while on the left side a subtotal occlusion is present (*arrow*). *Abbreviations*: MPR, multiplanar reconstruction; MIP, maximum intensity projection; CTA, computed tomography angiography; CE MRA, contrast-enhanced magnetic resonance angiography.

need to be evaluated for stenotic-occlusive arterial disease. Another pitfall that should be mentioned when considering MRA is the evaluation of tortuous arteries that may appear occluded if they are not carefully included in the plane of imaging (Fig. 14). Finally, MRA does not offer visualization of bony landmarks for assisting surgeons in planning operations, a feature that is available with CTA (45,46), and when using high resolution MR imaging (with blood pool contrast agents).

CTA should therefore be considered the first modality to image patients with an initial acute onset of symptoms. CTA can also be performed to supply valuable 3D guides to perform subsequent catheter-based interventions (e.g., evaluation of tortuosity of iliac arteries in planning "crossover" technique, identification of the level of the femoral bifurcation for antegrade puncture). Moreover, with modern CT systems, multiple types of reformatting are now available with a simple click and in just a few seconds. However, the review of all images (including axial source images) in a "movie" fashion on a CT monitor or workstation remains the mainstay of any initial evaluation. In fact, when interpreting CTA studies, attention must always be paid to the extra-arterial structures, since CT is a global examination, and alternative or additional diagnoses may be present.

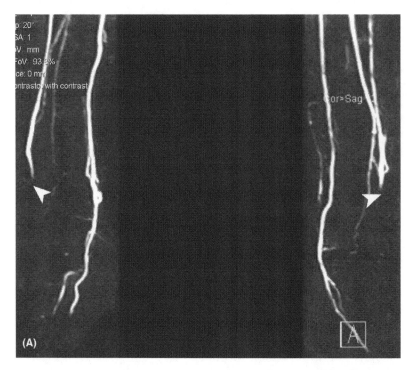

FIGURE 14 CE MRA of feet in AP projection (**A**), showing abrupt ending of the dorsal artery of the foot bilaterally (*arrowheads*); in lateral projection (**B**) it is evident that the forefoot is outside the scanned volume, leading to nonvisualization of the distal arteries (*arrowhead*); similar pitfalls can occur in very tortuous iliac and popliteal arteries. *Abbreviation*: CE MRA, contrast-enhanced magnetic resonance angiography. (*Continued*)

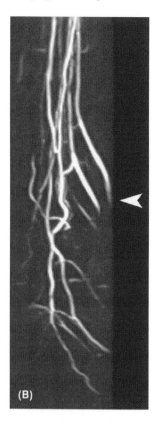

(B)

FIGURE 14 *(Continued)*

CONCLUSION
Clinical examinations and vascular laboratory examinations remain the mainstay for the diagnosis of CLI. Both CTA and MRA performed with state-of-the-art technique can provide information to confirm the diagnosis, to identify the level of arterial obstruction, and to plan an interventional procedure. The role of DSA nowadays is limited to guidance of the interventional procedure itself.

REFERENCES
1. Catalano C, Fraioli F, Laghi A, et al. Infrarenal aortic and lower-extremity arterial disease: diagnostic performance of multi-detector row CT angiography. Radiology 2004; 231(2):555–563.
2. Norgren L, Hiatt WR, Dormandy JA, et al. Inter-society consensus for the management of peripheral arterial disease (TASC II). J Vasc Surg 2007; 45(suppl S):S5–S67.
3. Walsh DB, Gilbertson JJ, Zwolak RM, et al. The natural history of superficial femoral artery stenoses. J Vasc Surg 1991; 14(3):299–304.
4. Rofsky NM, Adelman MA. MR angiography in the evaluation of atherosclerotic peripheral vascular disease. Radiology 2000; 214(2):325–338.
5. Katz DS, Hon M. CT angiography of the lower extremities and aortoiliac system with a multi-detector row helical CT scanner: promise of new opportunities fulfilled. Radiology 2001; 221(1):7–10.
6. Katzen BT. The future of catheter-based angiography: implications for the vascular interventionalist. Radiol Clin North Am 2002; 40(4):689–692.

7. Kreitner KF, Kalden P, Neufang A, et al. Diabetes and peripheral arterial occlusive disease: prospective comparison of contrast-enhanced three-dimensional MR angiography with conventional digital subtraction angiography. AJR Am J Roentgenol 2000; 174(1):171–179.
8. Martin ML, Tay KH, Flak B, et al. Multidetector CT angiography of the aortoiliac system and lower extremities: a prospective comparison with digital subtraction angiography. AJR Am J Roentgenol 2003; 180(4):1085–1091.
9. Lawler LP, Fishman EK. Multi-detector row CT of thoracic disease with emphasis on 3D volume rendering and CT angiography. Radiographics 2001; 21(5):1257–1273.
10. Chow LC, Rubin GD. CT angiography of the arterial system. Radiol Clin North Am 2002; 40(4):729–749.
11. Rubin GD, Shiau MC, Leung AN, et al. Aorta and iliac arteries: single versus multiple detector-row helical CT angiography. Radiology 2000; 215(3):670–676.
12. Rubin GD. Techniques for performing multidetector-row computed tomographic angiography. Tech Vasc Interv Radiol 2001; 4(1):2–14.
13. Rubin GD, Schmidt AJ, Logan LJ, et al. Multi-detector row CT angiography of lower extremity arterial inflow and runoff: initial experience. Radiology 2001; 221(1):146–158.
14. Kock MC, Dijkshoorn ML, Pattynama PM, et al. Multi-detector row computed tomography angiography of peripheral arterial disease. Eur Radiol 2007; 17(12):3208–3222.
15. Yu T, Zhu X, Tang L, et al. Review of CT angiography of aorta. Radiol Clin North Am 2007; 45(3):461–483.
16. Kirchner J, Kickuth R, Laufer U, et al. Optimized enhancement in helical CT: experiences with a real-time bolus tracking system in 628 patients. Clin Radiol 2000; 55(5): 368–373.
17. Siegel MJ. Multiplanar and three-dimensional multi-detector row CT of thoracic vessels and airways in the pediatric population. Radiology 2003; 229(3):641–650.
18. Klucznik RP. Current technology and clinical applications of three-dimensional angiography. Radiol Clin North Am 2002; 40(4):711–728, v.
19. Sameshima T, Futami S, Morita Y et al. Clinical usefulness of and problems with three-dimensional CT angiography for the evaluation of arteriosclerotic stenosis of the carotid artery: comparison with conventional angiography, MRA, and ultrasound sonography. Surg Neurol 1999; 51(3):301–308.
20. Bartolozzi C, Neri E, Caramella D. CT in vascular pathologies. Eur Radiol 1998; 8(5): 679–684.
21. Smith PA, Heath DG, Fishman EK. Virtual angioscopy using spiral CT and real-time interactive volume-rendering techniques. J Comput Assist Tomogr 1998; 22(2):212–214.
22. Flohr TG, Schaller S, Stierstorfer K, et al. Multi-detector row CT systems and image-reconstruction techniques. Radiology 2005; 235(3):756–773.
23. Randoux B, Marro B, Koskas F, et al. Carotid artery stenosis: prospective comparison of CT, three-dimensional gadolinium-enhanced MR, and conventional angiography. Radiology 2001; 220(1):179–185.
24. Silvennoinen HM, Ikonen S, Soinne L, et al. CT angiographic analysis of carotid artery stenosis: comparison of manual assessment, semiautomatic vessel analysis, and digital subtraction angiography. AJNR Am J Neuroradiol 2007; 28(1):97–103.
25. Fleischmann D, Rubin GD, Bankier AA, et al. Improved uniformity of aortic enhancement with customized contrast medium injection protocols at CT angiography. Radiology 2000; 214(2):363–371.
26. Catalano C, Fraioli F, Danti M, et al. MDCT of the abdominal aorta: basics, technical improvements, and clinical applications. Eur Radiol 2003; 13(suppl 3):N53–N58.
27. Cademartiri F, Mollet N, van der LA, et al. Non-invasive 16-row multislice CT coronary angiography: usefulness of saline chaser. Eur Radiol 2004; 14(2):178–183.
28. Heijenbrok-Kal MH, Kock MC, Hunink MG. Lower extremity arterial disease: multidetector CT angiography meta-analysis. Radiology 2007; 245(2):433–439.
29. Schoepf UJ, Becker CR, Hofmann LK, et al. Multislice CT angiography. Eur Radiol 2003; 13(8):1946–1961.
30. Hiatt MD, Fleischmann D, Hellinger JC, et al. Angiographic imaging of the lower extremities with multidetector CT. Radiol Clin North Am 2005; 43(6):1119–1127, ix.

31. Leiner T, Ho KY, Nelemans PJ, et al. Three-dimensional contrast-enhanced moving-bed infusion-tracking (MoBI-track) peripheral MR angiography with flexible choice of imaging parameters for each field of view. J Magn Reson Imaging 2000; 11(4):368–377.
32. Kaufman JA, McCarter D, Geller SC, et al. Two-dimensional time-of-flight MR angiography of the lower extremities: artifacts and pitfalls. AJR Am J Roentgenol 1998; 171(1):129–135.
33. Lell M, Fellner C, Baum U, et al. Evaluation of carotid artery stenosis with multi-section CT and MR imaging: influence of imaging modality and postprocessing. AJNR Am J Neuroradiol 2007; 28(1):104–110.
34. Ho VB, Foo TK, Czum JM, et al. Contrast-enhanced magnetic resonance angiography: technical considerations for optimized clinical implementation. Top Magn Reson Imaging 2001; 12(4):283–299.
35. Meissner OA, Rieger J, Weber C, et al. Critical limb ischemia: hybrid MR angiography compared with DSA. Radiology 2005; 235(1):308–318.
36. Sadowski EA, Bennett LK, Chan MR, et al. Nephrogenic systemic fibrosis: risk factors and incidence estimation. Radiology 2007; 243(1):148–157.
37. Goyen M, Herborn CU, Kroger K, et al. Detection of atherosclerosis: systemic imaging for systemic disease with whole-body three-dimensional MR angiography—initial experience. Radiology 2003; 227(1):277–282.
38. Tatli S, Lipton MJ, Davison BD, et al. From the RSNA refresher courses: MR imaging of aortic and peripheral vascular disease. Radiographics 2003; 23(Spec No):S59–S78.
39. Spinosa DJ, Angle JF, Hartwell GD, et al. Gadolinium-based contrast agents in angiography and interventional radiology. Radiol Clin North Am 2002; 40(4):693–710.
40. Shetty AN, Bis KG, Duerinckx AJ, et al. Lower extremity MR angiography: universal retrofitting of high-field-strength systems with stepping kinematic imaging platforms initial experience. Radiology 2002; 222(1):284–291.
41. Zhang HL, Ho BY, Chao M, et al. Decreased venous contamination on 3D gadolinium-enhanced bolus chase peripheral MR angiography using thigh compression. AJR Am J Roentgenol 2004; 183(4):1041–1047.
42. Ho VB, Corse WR. MR angiography of the abdominal aorta and peripheral vessels. Radiol Clin North Am 2003; 41(1):115–144.
43. Ruehm SG, Hany TF, Pfammatter T, et al. Pelvic and lower extremity arterial imaging: diagnostic performance of three-dimensional contrast-enhanced MR angiography. AJR Am J Roentgenol 2000; 174(4):1127–1135.
44. de Vries M, Ouwendijk R, Flobbe K, et al. Peripheral arterial disease: clinical and cost comparisons between duplex US and contrast-enhanced MR angiography—a multicenter randomized trial. Radiology 2006; 240(2):401–410.
45. Nelemans PJ, Leiner T, de Vet HC, et al. Peripheral arterial disease: meta-analysis of the diagnostic performance of MR angiography. Radiology 2000; 217(1):105–114.
46. Ruehm SG, Goyen M, Barkhausen J, et al. Rapid magnetic resonance angiography for detection of atherosclerosis. Lancet 2001; 357(9262):1086–1091.
47. Knopp MV, Giesel FL, von Tengg-Kobligk H, et al. Contrast-enhanced MR angiography of the run-off vasculature: intraindividual comparison of gadobenate dimeglumine with gadopentetate dimeglumine. J Magn Reson Imaging 2003; 17(6):694–702.
48. Kreitner KF, Kunz RP, Herber S, et al. MR angiography of the pedal arteries with gadobenate dimeglumine, a contrast agent with increased relaxivity, and comparison with selective intraarterial DSA. J Magn Reson Imaging 2008; 27(1):78–85.
49. Collidge TA, Thomson PC, Mark PB, et al. Gadolinium-enhanced MR imaging and nephrogenic systemic fibrosis: retrospective study of a renal replacement therapy cohort. Radiology 2007; 245(1):168–175.
50. Bremerich J, Bilecen D, Reimer P. MR angiography with blood pool contrast agents. Eur Radiol 2007; 17(12):3017–3024.
51. Nikolaou K, Kramer H, Grosse C, et al. High-spatial-resolution multistation MR angiography with parallel imaging and blood pool contrast agent: initial experience. Radiology 2006; 241(3):861–872.
52. Bluemke DA, Stillman AE, Bis KG, et al. Carotid MR angiography: phase II study of safety and efficacy for MS-325. Radiology 2001; 219(1):114–122.

53. Racadio JM, Fricke BL, Jones BV, et al. Three-dimensional rotational angiography of neurovascular lesions in pediatric patients. AJR Am J Roentgenol 2006; 186(1):75–84.
54. Rolland Y, Duvauferrier R, Lucas A, et al. Lower limb angiography: a prospective study comparing carbon dioxide with iodinated contrast material in 30 patients. AJR Am J Roentgenol 1998; 171(2):333–337.
55. Oliva VL, Denbow N, Therasse E, et al. Digital subtraction angiography of the abdominal aorta and lower extremities: carbon dioxide versus iodinated contrast material. J Vasc Interv Radiol 1999; 10(6):723–731.
56. Spinosa DJ, Angle JF, Hagspiel KD, et al. Lower extremity arteriography with use of iodinated contrast material or gadodiamide to supplement CO_2 angiography in patients with renal insufficiency. J Vasc Interv Radiol 2000; 11(1):35–43.
57. Nyman U, Elmstahl B, Leander P, et al. Are gadolinium-based contrast media really safer than iodinated media for digital subtraction angiography in patients with azotemia?Radiology 2002; 223(2):311–318.
58. Le Blanche AF, Tassart M, Deux JF, et al. Gadolinium-enhanced digital subtraction angiography of hemodialysis fistulas: a diagnostic and therapeutic approach. AJR Am J Roentgenol 2002; 179(4):1023–1028.
59. Prince MR, Arnoldus C, Frisoli JK. Nephrotoxicity of high-dose gadolinium compared with iodinated contrast. J Magn Reson Imaging 1996; 6(1):162–166.
60. Puls R, Knollmann F, Werk M, et al. [Multi-slice spiral CT: 3D CT angiography for evaluating therapeutically relevant stenosis in peripheral arterial occlusive disease.] Rontgenpraxis 2001; 54(4):141–147.
61. Ofer A, Nitecki SS, Linn S, et al. Multidetector CT angiography of peripheral vascular disease: a prospective comparison with intraarterial digital subtraction angiography. AJR Am J Roentgenol 2003; 180(3):719–724.
62. Heuschmid M, Krieger A, Beierlein W, et al. Assessment of peripheral arterial occlusive disease: comparison of multislice-CT angiography (MS-CTA) and intra-arterial digital subtraction angiography (IA-DSA). Eur J Med Res 2003; 8(9):389–396.
63. Mesurolle B, Qanadli SD, El Hajjam M, et al. Occlusive arterial disease of abdominal aorta and lower extremities: comparison of helical CT angiography with trans-catheter angiography. Clin Imaging 2004; 28(4):252–260.
64. Ota H, Takase K, Igarashi K, et al. MDCT compared with digital subtraction angiography for assessment of lower extremity arterial occlusive disease: importance of reviewing cross-sectional images. AJR Am J Roentgenol 2004; 182(1):201–209.
65. Portugaller HR, Schoellnast H, Hausegger KA, et al. Multislice spiral CT angiography in peripheral arterial occlusive disease: a valuable tool in detecting significant arterial lumen narrowing?Eur Radiol 2004; 14(9):1681–1687.
66. Bui TD, Gelfand D, Whipple S, et al. Comparison of CT and catheter arteriography for evaluation of peripheral arterial disease. Vasc Endovascular Surg 2005; 39(6):481–490.
67. Edwards AJ, Wells IP, Roobottom CA. Multidetector row CT angiography of the lower limb arteries: a prospective comparison of volume-rendered techniques and intra-arterial digital subtraction angiography. Clin Radiol 2005; 60(1):85–95.
68. Willmann JK, Wildermuth S. Multidetector-row CT angiography of upper- and lower-extremity peripheral arteries. Eur Radiol 2005; 15(suppl 4):D3–D9.
69. Schertler T, Wildermuth S, Alkadhi H, et al. Sixteen-detector row CT angiography for lower-leg arterial occlusive disease: analysis of section width. Radiology 2005; 237(2):649–656.
70. Fraioli F, Catalano C, Napoli A, et al. Low-dose multidetector-row CT angiography of the infra-renal aorta and lower extremity vessels: image quality and diagnostic accuracy in comparison with standard DSA. Eur Radiol 2006; 16(1):137–146.
71. Sun Z. Diagnostic accuracy of multislice CT angiography in peripheral arterial disease. J Vasc Interv Radiol 2006; 17(12):1915–1921.
72. Tepel M, van der GM, Schwarzfeld C, et al. Prevention of radiographic-contrast-agent-induced reductions in renal function by acetylcysteine. N Engl J Med 2000; 343(3):180–184.

6 Risk Factor Modification in the Management of Critical Limb Ischemia

Roger Walcott
Georgetown University Hospital, Washington Hospital Center, and Washington DC VA Medical Center, Washington, D.C., U.S.A.

Robyn A. Macsata
Washington DC VA Medical Center, Washington, D.C., U.S.A.

Anton N. Sidawy
Washington DC VA Medical Center, and Georgetown and George Washington Universities, Washington, D.C., U.S.A.

INTRODUCTION

Peripheral arterial disease (PAD) is the peripheral manifestation of atherosclerosis and affects over eight million Americans. The most common symptoms of PAD are intermittent claudication and critical leg ischemia (CLI). CLI is limb threatening; symptoms manifest as rest pain and tissue loss, including nonhealing ulcers and gangrene. Of paramount importance, patients with PAD are not only at risk of limb loss but also at increased risk of cardiac and cerebral morbidity and mortality. Patients with PAD have a mortality of 4.8% per year, a 2.5-fold rise in risk from age-matched controls. In patients with known coronary artery disease (CAD), the presence of PAD is an independent risk factor for death, raising the risk 25% even when other known risk factors are controlled (1).

Aggressive treatment of atherosclerosis can slow or halt progression of PAD, even in patients with advanced disease, including CLI. Treatment goals must focus on the effects of atherosclerosis in the peripheral circulation and the systemic nature of the disease, including coronary and carotid arterial occlusive diseases. Therefore, all patients presenting for treatment of lower extremity atherosclerosis must undergo rigorous assessment of cardiovascular risk factors and appropriate therapies must be instituted to reduce the risks of progression of PAD to CLI.

PATHOPHYSIOLOGY OF ATHEROSCLEROSIS

The pathophysiology of atherosclerosis is similar in the peripheral circulation to that in the coronary and cerebral arterial beds; the same risk factors, including diabetes, hypercholesterolemia, tobacco use, and hypertension (HTN) are involved.

Under ideal circumstances, the arterial endothelium serves as a barrier to atherosclerosis by serving as a "Teflon" coat that prevents circulating atherogenic lipoproteins from entering the arterial wall and maintains normal arterial hemodynamics. Endothelial damage results from the above-mentioned modifiable risk factors. Once injured, the endothelium secretes a number of deleterious cytokines that promote the entry of circulating macrophages into the arterial wall, stimulates macrophage proliferation and conversion to tissue macrophages. The endothelium becomes permeable to the circulating atherogenic lipoproteins, low-density lipoprotein (LDL), very low density lipoprotein (VLDL) remnants, intermediate density lipoprotein (IDL), and chylomicron remnants, which then penetrate the intima of the arterial wall. Once internalized, these lipids are absorbed through specific scavenger receptors into the fixed tissue macrophages, transforming the macrophages into lipid-filled foam cells (2). Groups of foam cells accumulate underneath the endothelium becoming the initial lesion of atherosclerosis, the fatty streak.

As this process continues, the foam cells undergo the process of apoptosis, or cell death, which allows the contained lipid to spill out to form the lipid core of an atherosclerotic plaque. Some plaques continue to grow, become fibrotic, and intrude onto the arterial lumen. Clinically, in the lower extremities, this manifests initially as claudication; as the lumen becomes further narrowed, rest pain and tissue loss may develop. These fibrotic plaques are thought to be stable, and are not the cause of the majority of acute clinical events such as myocardial infarction (MI) or stroke, but play a significant role in the PAD process.

Other plaques accumulate a large lipid core, which induces an intense local inflammatory reaction as this lipid is oxidized and results in the infiltration of additional macrophages and inflammatory cells. These unstable plaques, which often remain small and do not cause a critical level of lumen compromise, are also known as vulnerable plaques. The vulnerable plaque is covered by a thin fibrous cap, which is prone to ulcerate or rupture. When this occurs, a platelet-rich clot rapidly forms on top of the plaque, producing the complete obstruction of the involved artery, resulting in acute ischemia in the lower extremity, a myocardial infarct in the coronary circulation, or stroke in the cerebral circulation.

NON-PHARMOCOLOGIC THREATMENT OF ATHEROSCLEROTIC RISK FACTORS
Therapeutic Lifestyle Change

The Adult Treatment Panel III (ATP III) issued by the National Cholesterol Education Program (NCEP) on cholesterol management recommends therapeutic lifestyle change (TLC) as an essential modality in the clinical management of hypercholesterolemia (3). The guidelines state that any person at high risk or moderately high risk who has lifestyle-related risk factors is a candidate for TLC. Severe risk factors include the presence of PAD, heavy cigarette smoking, poorly controlled HTN, diabetes mellitus, strong family history of premature coronary heart disease (CHD), or very low high-density lipoprotein (HDL) cholesterol. TLCs include the following components: reduced intake of saturated fats and cholesterol, therapeutic dietary options for enhancing LDL lowering, losing as little as 7% of body weight, and exercising regularly (brisk walking for 150 min/wk) (3).

Dietary modifications include high amounts of fruits and vegetables, legumes, and whole grains as part of a low-fat diet. These modifications have been shown to reduce LDL and total cholesterol (4). For example, one study examined the effects of reducing dietary saturated fatty acids from 15% of total calories to 6.1% of total calories. On the diet low in saturated fatty acids, LDL cholesterol was reduced by 11% (5). NCEP recommends the reduction of saturated fats to less than 7% of total calories and cholesterol to less than 200 mg/day. The addition of spreads and other dietary products containing plant sterols or stanols, which are available on the shelves of most grocery stores, has been shown to reduce total and LDL-C by 10% to 15%. Soluble fiber supplements are also suggested as adjuncts to dietary therapy. ATP III outlines maximal dietary therapy including balancing energy intake and expenditure to maintain desirable body weight/prevent weight gain, which all together can reduce LDL-C by 25% to 30%. Lipid panels should be rechecked at six-week intervals, and if lipid goals are not achieved by three to six months, drug therapy should be considered for those patients not already being treated.

Physical activity favorably modifies several risk factors; it has been reported to lower LDL and triglyceride levels, raise HDL cholesterol, improve insulin sensitivity, and lower blood pressure (6). Therefore, as part of a comprehensive lifestyle approach to atherosclerosis, daily energy expenditure should include at least moderate physical activity, contributing about 200 kcal/day to the balance of energy intake and expenditure. Exercise specialists in addition to nutrition professionals can be utilized to assist patients in achieving their TLCs.

PHARMOCOLOGIC TREATMENT OF ATHEROSCLEROTIC RISK FACTORS
Diabetes Mellitus
The greatest risk factor for PAD and the subsequent development of CLI is diabetes. A 1% increase in hemoglobin A1c (HbA1c) correlates with a 8% increase in PAD and a 28% increase in risk of death (7). Fifty percent of diabetics will be affected by a manifestation of diabetic foot (neuropathy, ischemia, or infection); 15% of diabetics will experience a foot ulcer in their lifetime; 20% of those affected with a foot ulcer will progress to an amputation. This confers an amputation relative risk 40 times greater for diabetics than nondiabetics, and a reamputation rate of over 60% at five years. Also, patients with nondiabetic range dysglycemia (i.e., abnormal glucose levels in response to a glucose challenge but normal fasting glucose levels) are at an increased risk of neuropathy and PAD (8). Therefore, proper management of diabetics and prediabetics with lifestyle changes including dietary modification, exercise, and smoking cessation as well as medical management is of the utmost importance (3,9).

Pathophysiology
The principle mechanisms involved in the peripheral manifestations of diabetes include neuropathy, ischemia, and infection.

Neuropathy
The most common neuropathy associated with diabetes is termed distal symmetric neuropathy (DSN) or so-called "diabetic neuropathy." The pathophysiology is felt to arise from both vascular and metabolic factors (10). Factors likely to play a role include formation of oxygen radicals, the polyol pathway, nonenzymatic glycation, and protein kinase C activation. Formation of oxygen radicals through hyperglycemia occurs though the polyol cascade or through nonenzymatic glycation. Also, nicotinamide adenine dinucleotide phosphate (NADPH), a free radical scavenger, is depleted in states of polyol cascade over activity. Oxygen radical species are directly toxic to the nerve cell and may

reduce the epineuronal blood flow through depletion of nitric oxide (NO), with effects on both the autonomic as well as the sensorimotor nerves. The polyol pathway not only produces free radicals, it is implicated in the deposition of sorbitol that is felt to contribute to neuropathy.

High glucose levels also lead to the accumulation of advanced glycation end products, including Amadori products among other molecules. In high levels, these cause a disruption in normal metabolism at the cellular level. One way in which this occurs is by Amadori product's ability to absorb NO, potentially impairing NO-dependent vasodilation in the epineurium, leading to ischemia and neuropathy (11). Demyelination of peripheral nerves has also been associated with nonenzymatic glycation, with increased end products of glycation, as well as increased tubulin in peripheral nerves.

Sensorimotor neuropathy initially involves the lower extremities and progresses centrally; two theories of Charcot foot development exist, including the neurotraumatic and neurovascular reflex theory. The neurotraumatic theory of Charcot foot postulates that neuropathy leads to the loss of protective mechanisms of painful sensation as well as muscle loss, which leads to prominent metatarsal heads and clawing of the toes. It also worsens the process of joint and bone destruction by repeated trauma, leading to further ligamentous laxity and joint instability. The resultant abnormal pressure points and foot deformities predispose patients to ulceration. As the deformity worsens, the patient develops midfoot collapse with loss of the plantar arch, leading to a rocker-bottom contour to the foot. Coupled with a decreased ability both to detect and to mount an immune response to infection, this creates a treacherous clinical situation.

The neurovascular reflex theory of the development of Charcot foot proposes a vascular etiology, though likely both mechanisms contribute to Charcot foot. Autonomic denervation leads to loss of sympathetic tone and capillary arteriovenous shunting. As a result, there is increased flow to the bone. As a result of this increased blood flow, the bone becomes demineralized and weak, leading to osteoarthropathy. Autonomic neuropathy results in inappropriate vasodilatation and vasoconstriction, improper sweating, and drying of the skin. The dry skin is more likely to crack and open, creating a potential site of entry for bacteria into the foot.

Ischemia

Microvascular ischemia. Microvascular ischemia is a nonocclusive microcirculatory impairment that typically involves the capillaries and arterioles of the kidneys (nephropathy), eye (retinopathy), and peripheral nerves (causing neuropathy). This should not be confused with the term "small vessel disease," which refers to the common misconception of an untreatable occlusive lesion in the microcirculation. Dispelling the notion of small vessel disease has been fundamental to diabetic limb salvage, because arterial reconstruction is almost always possible and successful in these patients. Multiple structural and physiologic abnormalities result in microvascular impairment. Endothelial dysfunction and the response to NO are diminished in diabetics, and hyperglycemia may be responsible for some of these abnormalities. Thickening of the capillary basement membrane is the dominant structural change in neuropathy as well as retinopathy. It is postulated that this thickening may impair migration of leukocytes and the hyperemic response to injury, whereby increasing the risk of infection in the diabetic foot. It is important to note that this does not lead to narrowing of the capillary lumen. However, capillary blood flow and the maximal hyperemic response to stimuli are reduced in the diabetic foot, suggesting a functional impairment. In the nondiabetic, injury-mediated nociceptive C fiber stimulation results in adjacent neurogenic release of vasoactive peptides, leading to vasodilation and increased blood flow to the area of injury. Loss of this axonal reflex may lead to a blunted response to injury.

Macrovascular ischemia. Macrovascular disease in the diabetic is morphologically similar to that in the nondiabetic patient. PAD is more aggressive in diabetics, and the severity of PAD appears to be related to both the duration of hyperglycemia and glycemic control. The atherosclerotic process is accelerated in diabetics, with earlier and more numerous fatty streaks, which evolve into fibrofatty plaques. These lead to fibrin and calcium deposition, which predispose to plaques to fissure and hemorrhage. It is also evident that fatty acids and triglycerides accumulate inappropriately in cardiac and other tissues.

In diabetics, atherosclerotic lesions have a typical distribution and pattern of occlusion. Typically, these patients have occlusive disease of the infrageniculate or tibioperoneal arteries with sparing of the pedal vessels; the arteries above the knee are more likely to be uninvolved (Fig. 1). As stated earlier, arterial reconstruction is almost always possible with the use of venous bypasses

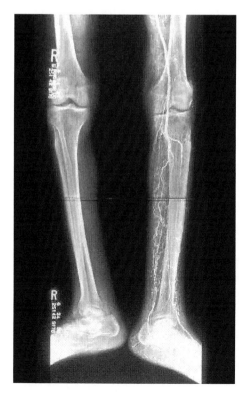

FIGURE 1 Diabetic tibioperoneal occlusive disease with sparing of pedal arteries.

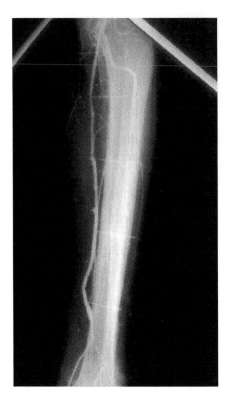

FIGURE 2 Below-knee popliteal artery to posterior tibial artery bypass using in situ saphenous vein.

to the pedal vessels (Fig. 2). Five-year patency rates for tibial bypasses performed with vein range from 50% to 70%, with secondary patency rates as high as 80%. Patency of bypasses to the pedal vessels ranges from 35% to 65%, with secondary patency rates over 60% (12).

Infection

Diabetes mellitus is associated with defective humoral and cellular immunity, leading to decreased neutrophil chemotaxis, decreased phagocytosis, impaired bacterial killing, and abnormal lymphocyte function. These factors all lead to increased susceptibility of the diabetic patient to infection. Of equal importance, when infection occurs, diabetic patients may not have pronounced symptoms and physical examination findings such as redness and erythema. Quite often, diabetic patients have extensive infection before recognition by the patient or treating physician, which ultimately leads to their increased risk of limb loss.

The microbiology of diabetic foot infections can be complex with multiple aerobic and anaerobic species involved. Staphylococci and streptococci are the most common bacteria isolated, but even in uncomplicated infections, these are the sole pathogen in less than 50% of cases. As the severity of infection worsens, anaerobes and gram-negative bacteria increase, including Klebsiella, Proteus, and Pseudomonas species.

THERAPEUTIC GOALS

Patients with vascular disease should be screened carefully for diabetes. Since a fasting glucose of 126 mg/dL will miss 20% to 30% of diabetic patients, HbA1c should be checked. Strict glycemic control with a target HbA1c level of less than 6.5% in all patients with PAD is recommended on the basis of data showing a nearly 60% reduction in microvascular complications (13). The U.K. Prospective Diabetes Study (UKPDS) showed a 35% reduction in the complication rate with every 1% decrease in HbA1c (7).

Pharmacotherapy

Sulfonylureas

Sulfonylureas act by increasing pancreatic output of insulin and enhancing receptor sensitivity. Second-generation, shorter-acting agents include glipizide, glyburide, and glimepiride. The dose of a sulfonylurea is gradually increased from a low baseline at weekly intervals until the highest recommended dose is attained. At that dose, if normoglycemia is not obtained, consideration is given to combining the sulfonylurea with one of the other oral hypoglycemics or insulin.

Biguanide

Metformin, the prototype biguanide, exerts its effect by increasing peripheral glucose uptake and utilization and decreasing hepatic glucose production. It lowers blood glucose but carries the risk of fatal lactic acidosis in patients with renal, hepatic, or cardiac dysfunction. Therefore, metformin should be temporarily discontinued when intravenous radiologic contrast agents are used or when major surgery or septic conditions may result in hypoperfusion. Thirty percent of patients taking biguanides experience severe gastrointestinal (GI) side effects, such as diarrhea, nausea, and anorexia. As with the sulfonylureas, dosing begins low and is gradually increased until the target control is reached; the addition of other agents and insulin is reserved for those in whom the maximum dose of biguanide does not achieve the target glucose level.

α-Glucosidase Inhibitors

The class of oral hypoglycemics known as α-glucosidase inhibitors, including acarbose and miglitol, may be used in conjunction with diet control to lower blood glucose. These agents decrease postprandial plasma glucose by slowing the digestion of carbohydrates and delaying the absorption of glucose into the bloodstream. Diarrhea, flatulence, and abdominal pain are common side effects and often lead to the discontinuance of these drugs. However, with continued use of these agents, many of the side effects may diminish, leading to the recommendation that α-glucosidase inhibitors be initiated at low doses to help encourage patient compliance with therapy.

Thiazolidinediones

Thiazolidinediones are also often referred to as the "glitazones." Troglitazone, the first of the thiazolidinediones, is thought to act by enhancing the action of both endogenous insulin and exogenous insulin by improving sensitivity to insulin in muscle and adipose tissue and by inhibiting hepatic glucose production. Initially, troglitazone was approved only for use in patients with type 2 diabetes who require insulin therapy and was not approved for monotherapy use. Severe side effects, including significant liver dysfunction and failure and neutropenia, led to the withdrawal of troglitazone from the market. Rosiglitazone and pioglitazone, approved for use by the U.S. Food and Drug Administration (FDA) in 1997, have become important elements in the treatment of type 2 diabetes.

Meglitinides

Two drugs in the class known as meglitinides are now available: repaglinide, derived from benzoic acid and approved by the FDA in 1997; and nateglinide, derived from D-phenylalanine and approved in 2000. These agents raise insulin levels rapidly by stimulating the β-cells via mechanisms different from those seen with sulfonylureas. Meglitinides enhance insulin release from the pancreas over a short time only when the glucose level is high. Therefore, the risk of hypoglycemia is lower than with sulfonylureas. Their activity more closely mimics normal first-phase insulin release when food is eaten by a person without diabetes. Peak drug activity is seen in one hour, and their short action time (3 hours) makes these agents ideal for matching the glucose load imposed after a carbohydrate-rich meal.

Insulin

Exogenous subcutaneous insulin remains a mainstay for the patient with refractory type 2 diabetes. Hypoglycemia, the most common adverse effect reported by those who take insulin, has been reported to occur in up to 26% of patients, with a mean of approximately two episodes per year. Additionally, one can expect considerable weight gain with the commencement of insulin therapy. Further, rapid glucose control with aggressive insulin administration can exacerbate proliferative retinopathy in 5% of patients. Current recommendations for patients with diabetic retinopathy call for reductions in HbA1c by 2% per year, with retinal examinations every six months to avoid this complication.

Insulin therapy commences in patients with type 2 diabetes when oral therapy has failed, which is signified by HbA1c levels approaching 8% despite optimal oral therapy. Optimal management continues the oral agent in conjunction with insulin therapy. The majority of patients benefit from the addition of a sulfonylurea or metformin in combination with insulin, and this regimen generally reduces insulin dose by approximately 25% and by as much as 50% in some individuals. Emphasis is placed on target HbA1c level, reduced hypoglycemia, and reduced weight gain, not lower insulin dose.

Treatment of Combined Risk Factors

Glucose control alone does not confer maximal improvements in macrovascular outcomes. When blood pressure, lipid profile, hyperglycemia, and microalbuminuria were all treated intensively, significant improvements were seen in cardiovascular event rates, including amputation and vascular surgery for peripheral arterial atherosclerosis (14).

Lipid management in diabetics poses unique challenges and takes on increased importance. Diabetics typically have higher triglyceride levels and lower HDL. Target LDL levels should optimally be less than 80 mg/dL (15). A fibrate or niacin may be needed to raise HDL levels. The routine use of a statin should be considered for all patients with diabetes irrespective of preexisting CAD or cholesterol levels, considering there was an approximate 25% reduction of a major vascular event associated with statin use in one recent trial (16).

THE METABOLIC SYNDROME (SYNDROME X)

Hyperinsulinemia and glucose intolerance combine to cause metabolic, hemodynamic, and vascular sequelae. This phenomenon and related diagnostic features are referred to as the metabolic syndrome. It was defined by the NCEP as the presence of three or more of the following: (*i*) waist circumference greater than 102 cm in men and 88 cm in women, (*ii*) serum triglyceride level at least 150 mg/dL, (*iii*) HDL cholesterol level less than 40 mg/dL in men and less than 50 mg/dL in women, (*iv*) blood pressure of at least 130/85 mmHg, and (*v*) fasting serum glucose value of at least 110 mg/dL (17). Treatment of the metabolic syndrome is evolving and includes early diagnosis, emphasis on the avoidance of obesity, especially abdominal obesity, and regular exercise. Dietary recommendations should include avoiding saturated fat and carbohydrates, which cause insulin secretion and increasing intake of plant stanol or sterol esters, as discussed earlier.

Insulin sensitizers including the thiazolidinediones may help in combating insulin resistance, and the α-glucosidase inhibitors may improve insulin action. Statins have also been shown to improve insulin sensitivity, including simvastatin in the Scandinavian Simvastatin Survival Study (4S) (18). Just as in diabetes, fibrates can be used to raise HDL levels and lower triglyceride levels, abnormalities that are common in the metabolic syndrome. Angiotensin-converting enzyme (ACE) inhibitors are a good option as they have been shown to slow the development of micro- and macrovascular disease and are insulin sensitizing. Aspirin has been recommended to treat the prothrombotic state (19) as well as cessation of smoking in patients with the metabolic syndrome.

DYSLIPIDEMIA

Statin therapy has proven to be effective in improving pain-free walking time in patients with intermittent claudication (20,21). Patients treated with 80 mg of atorvastatin for one year had a 63% improvement in pain-free walking time compared with placebo. No significant improvement in ankle-brachial index was seen. The mechanism by which pain-free walking time improves is not clear, but statin-induced improvement of endothelium-dependent vasodilation in the microcirculation may be one potential mechanism (22). The 4S cited above also demonstrated a reduction in new or worsening intermittent claudication symptoms by 38% in patients on statin therapy compared with patients on placebo (23). The Heart Protection Study (HPS) included 6000 patients with PAD in which patients were randomized to either 40 mg of simvastatin daily or placebo. The average LDL-C difference between the placebo and treatment groups was 39 mg/dL during a mean follow-up of five years. The participants receiving simvastatin had a reduction in the number of carotid and peripheral revascularizations (24).

PATHOPHYSIOLOGY

Although dietary cholesterol and triglycerides are absorbed by different mechanisms within the GI tract, they are combined in single chylomicron particles for transport from the GI tract to the rest of the body with triglycerides comprising approximately 90% of the chylomicrons lipid content. These large lipoproteins are transported from the gut through the thoracic duct and into the bloodstream. Because of their very large size, when in significant concentration, chylomicrons account for the turbidity or "milkiness" of the plasma, known as postprandial lipemia. Chylomicrons are distinguished by the presence of one apo B-48 molecule in each chylomicron particle. In the bloodstream, the enzyme lipoprotein lipase (LPL) hydrolyzes the triglyceride contained within the chylomicron into free fatty acids, which are then stored in the adipocyte and muscle cells to be metabolized for future energy production. The remaining triglyceride poor chylomicron remnant contains only the absorbed dietary cholesterol, which is then transported to the liver for storage. Recent studies of atherosclerotic lesions have found apo B-48 within the plaque, implicating these chylomicron remnants as atherogenic particles.

The endogenous phase of lipoprotein metabolism involves the formation of VLDLs containing both cholesterol and triglycerides derived from stores of these two lipids within the liver and adipocytes. Each VLDL particle contains apolipoproteins from the C and E families and one molecule of apo B-100 per particle. Although not as large as chylomicrons, VLDL is large enough to cause lipemia when present in very high concentration. VLDL is released from the liver into the bloodstream where LPL again facilitates the removal of the triglyceride component of VLDL and presents it to the muscle cell as fuel for energy production. As the triglyceride is removed, two additional atherogenic lipoprotein particles are formed, VLDL remnants and IDL. These triglyceride-rich lipoprotein particles are atherogenic and play an important role in the accelerated atherosclerosis observed in the metabolic syndrome and type 2 diabetes mellitus. In addition to LPL, another lipase known as hepatic lipase participates in the conversion of VLDL to LDL, the most atherogenic of all lipoprotein particles. LDL binds to specific LDL receptors on the surface of each cell and facilitates the transfer of the remaining cholesterol to these cells where it can be stored for future use. The circulating LDL concentration within the plasma is determined by the number of LDL receptors on the various cells of the body, with the liver accounting for over 70% of this total receptor number. In turn, the number of LDL receptors is regulated by the intracellular concentration of cholesterol within each cell. When the intracellular cholesterol content of the cells is low, LDL receptor synthesis is upregulated, receptor numbers increase, and the LDL concentration of the circulating plasma diminishes. On the other hand, when intracellular cholesterol is increased, LDL receptor synthesis is downregulated, receptor numbers diminish, and LDL within the circulation rises. When plasma LDL is present in excess, atherosclerosis results in proportion to the degree of circulating LDL.

HDL is synthesized by the liver and intestine as apolipoprotein A-1, which is then released into the bloodstream as a lipid-poor discoid particle. As it circulates, stored cholesterol is released from the peripheral cells through the action of a specific transporter known as ATP binding cassesstte transporter A1 (ABCA-1) (25). As cholesterol is absorbed by the discoid A-1 and converted to cholesterol ester under the influence of lecithin cholesterol amino transferase (LCAT), HDL becomes a spherical particle. Additional cellular cholesterol is then added by another cassette transporter, ABCG-1 and through the action of the receptor scavenger-receptor class B (SRB)-1. The HDL particle can then return to the liver, where it binds to hepatic SRB-1 and releases its cholesterol, or it can exchange a portion of its cholesterol content for triglyceride from VLDL through the chemical action of the cholesterol ester transfer protein (CETP). The exchanged cholesterol can then be transported back to the liver by LDL. This process is known as "reverse cholesterol transport" and plays an important role in the antiatherogenic properties of the HDL particle.

THERAPEUTIC GOALS
Patients with CLI are in the high-risk category when determining goals of TLC and drug therapy. Their LDL-C goal is less than 100 mg/dL, with an optional goal of less than 70 mg/dL. They should initiate TLC and consider drug therapy at LDL levels over 100 mg/dL.

PHARMACOTHERAPY
Statins
The HMG-CoA (3-hydroxy-3-methylglutaryl coenzyme A) reductase inhibitors (statins) are the most effective class of drugs for treating elevated LDL-C levels. This class of medications has been shown to reduce LDL-C by 18% to 60%, raise HDL-C by 5% to 15%, and decrease triglycerides by 7% to 30%. As discussed previously, statins are proven to reduce risk of CHD, stroke, and PAD as well as decrease mortality. They are also proven to be safe with very low levels of major adverse events. Reduction in LDL-C is dose dependent and log linear. The starting dose of each statin produces 75% to 80% of the maximal LDL-C reduction, and with each subsequent doubling of the dose, an additional 6% reduction in LDL-C is achieved. Rarely patients can experience myopathy (0.1%), which if strongly suspected warrants measurement of a total creatinine phosphokinase (CPK) and, if significantly elevated (>5× ULN), discontinuation of the medication.

Recent studies have focused on possible plaque regression with use of lipid-lowering agent. This was seen in the Stop Atherosclerosis in Native Diabetics Study (SANDS) trial, which used combination therapy to achieve prespecified lipid goals for LDL-C and non-HDL-C for primary prevention in a small group of participants with type 2 diabetes mellitus (26). This trial used the end point of change in carotid intimal medial thickness (CIMT) as a surrogate for the control of atherosclerosis. In the most aggressive group with lipid goals of less than 70 mg/dL for LDL-C and less than 100 mg/dL for non-HDL-C, CIMT regression was achieved. However, larger prospective studies with clinical end points to include PAD are still needed to evaluate the outcome benefits of combination therapy.

Niacin
Niacin or nicotinic acid was the first pharmacologic agent demonstrated to reduce cholesterol. This class of drugs favorably affects all lipids and lipoproteins, with 15% to 35% increases in HDL-C and 5% to 25% decreases in LDL-C. Niacin alters lipid levels by inhibiting lipoprotein synthesis and improving the clearance of triglyceride-rich lipoproteins from the circulation.

Niacin is also the most effective agent at raising HDL-C levels. Because of the significant incidence of a "flushing" reaction at the initiation of therapy, niacin is usually started at a low dose and titrated over time. The use of an aspirin given one hour prior to niacin dosing helps to prevent flushing, and newer forms of extended-release (ER) niacin are available with a reduced propensity for flushing. Although available over the counter, these prescription forms of ER niacin are most commonly used. Initial dosage should be 500 mg ER by mouth nightly for four weeks, then increased by 500 mg/day every four weeks on the basis of effect and tolerance. The maximum dose is 2 g/day ER. It is contra-indicated in gout and chronic liver disease and should not be used cautiously at higher doses in diabetics as it may worsen insulin resistance. Major side effects include flushing, hyperuricemia/gout, hyperglycemia, and upper GI distress among others.

Fibrate
The fibrates, gemfibrozil and fenofibrate, are used in treating hyper-triglyceridemia and to increase HDL-C. The therapeutic effect of these drugs is a decrease in triglyceride levels of 25% to 50% and an increase in HDL-C of 5% to 15%. In addition, fenofibrate may also decrease LDL-C by 10% to 20%. An increase in LDL-C is often seen with gemfibrozil when used to treat very high levels of triglycerides, but this is not seen as frequently with fenofibrate. Although several prospective controlled trials have shown a reduction in the progression of atherosclerosis and a decreased incidence of cardiovascular morbidity and mortality, none of the fibrate trials have demonstrated a decrease in total mortality. Gemfibrozil is taken 30 minutes before morning and evening meals as a 600-mg tablet. Fenofibrate is started at 54 mg by mouth with food once daily, and the dosage can be increased to 160 mg/day.

Bile Acid Sequestrants
The bile acid sequestrants include colestipol, cholestyramine, and a more recently developed form, colesevelam. Historically, cholestyramine and coles-tipol were also among the first group of drugs used to treat total cholesterol (TC) and LDL-C. These drugs may be used as monotherapy, but are more often used in combination with statin therapy. They have extremely low rates of systemic toxicity as they are not absorbed, but remain in the GI tract. The initial agents in this class were associated with significant levels of dyspepsia, and constipation, which limited their tolerability. Colesevelam has significantly reduced these side effects and increased the compliance of individuals to use these drugs. It also has the advantage of being formulated as a tablet, whereas the earlier agents in this class had to be given as a granular powder mixed in liquid, which further limited their therapeutic utility. Doubling the dose of a statin may only achieve a 6% further reduction in LDL-C as noted above, but adding a sequestrant to a statin can further lower LDL-C by 12% to 16% (27).

Ezetimibe
Ezetimibe is the first in a new class of pharmacologic agents for reducing TC and LDL-C. It specifically interferes with the absorption of cholesterol from the GI tract resulting in a 15% to 20% reduction in LDL-C as monotherapy. In addition

to its use as monotherapy, ezetimibe is often used with a statin with a further LDL-C reduction of 20% to 25%, with added beneficial effects on triglycerides and HDL-C. Although its efficacy in reducing atherosclerotic events was recently questioned by the results of the ENHANCE trial, a small study of the effect of ezetimibe plus simvastatin versus simvastatin alone on CIMT, the National Lipid Association (NLA) has stated that the results of this trial do not warrant a change in the use of ezetimibe to reduce LDL-C. The NLA's recommendation was based on the fact that ezetimibe effectively lowered LDL-C and triglycerides without any significant adverse effects. Further studies of ezetimibe are now in progress, which will look at the clinical cardiovascular outcomes of this drug as lipid-lowering therapy. Ezetimibe is administered as a 10-mg once-daily tablet.

ω-3 Fatty Acids

Polyunsaturated fatty acids of the ω-3 type occur in fish and other marine animals, soybeans, other vegetables. Varying strengths of evidence exist to support ω-3 fatty acid consumption. ATP III supports the American Heart Association's (AHA) recommendation that fish, particularly those high in ω-3 fatty acids, should be included as part of a CHD risk-reduction diet (28). Fish also is low in saturated fat and may be cardioprotective. A number of observational studies have suggested that the regular consumption of fish reduces the risk of CHD. In addition, the ω-3 fatty acids, eicosapentaenoic acid (EPA) and DHA at a dose of 1 gm daily, were demonstrated in the GISSI trial to significantly reduce the risk for sudden death in individuals with underlying CHD. The Lyon Heart Trial included increased levels of α-linolenic as part of a "Mediterranean" diet and these subjects had fewer coronary events (29,30). Higher doses of EPA and DHA, 3 or more g daily, have a significant hypotriglyceridemic effect without significant adverse events. However, more definitive trials are necessary prior to strongly recommending high doses of ω-3 fatty acids.

Combination Drug Therapy

A combination of agents will be required for many patients, especially those with very elevated LDL-C levels or a mixed dyslipidemia such as the atherogenic dyslipidemia that is characteristic of type 2 diabetes and the metabolic syndrome. A combination of a statin plus an agent that blocks the intestinal absorption of cholesterol is particularly effective in decreasing LDL-C levels. Both ezetimibe and the bile acid sequestrants can be safely added to the maximal dose of a statin or can be used with lower doses to reach LDL-C therapeutic goals. Some patients will not tolerate the maximal dose of any statin, and one or both of these intestinally acting agents will allow the attainment of LDL-C goals when added to a submaximal dose of a statin. In addition, ER niacin can be combined with a statin, one of the intestinally acting drugs, or can be used in combination with both classes of drug to reach LDL-C targets in patients with very high LDL-C levels, such as those with heterozygous familial hypercholesterolemia. Statin therapy may also be combined with fenofibrate, niacin, or ω-3 fatty acids to achieve control in patients with combined hyperlipidemia, yielding superior results over monotherapy. Gemfibrozil should never be used with a statin because of its inhibition of statin metabolism increasing the toxicity of all statins. Niacin has also shown to be effective in combination with statin therapy.

Drugs Under Development
One of the most effective HDL-raising agents is niacin, but the tolerability of niacin has been severely limited by flushing and cutaneous side effects. An enteric-coated form of ER niacin is now available, which reduces the flushing frequency and intensity. In addition, recent studies have demonstrated that the flushing reaction is mediated by the production of prostaglandin D, which binds to a specific receptor in the skin and results in the flushing reaction. Laropiprant is a selective prostaglandin D receptor antagonist that substantially reduces the frequency and intensity of niacin-induced flushing. Daily oral doses of ER niacin plus laropiprant 2 g have been well tolerated in early studies (31). It is antici- pated that the use of these two newer forms of niacin therapy will improve patient compliance and allow a wider use of niacin to increase HDL-C.

TOBACCO USE
Smoking is an independent risk factor for the development of CLI (32,33). Patients who stop smoking reduce their risk for developing CLI or major amputation (34–36). Amputation rates can be decreased to 11% from 28%. Furthermore, smoking confers a threefold increased risk of graft failure in patients who continue to smoke after lower extremity revascularization via open surgical bypass (37). Similar to diabetes and hypercholesterolemia, smoking also increases cardiac and cerebral mortality. If fact, smoking as few as one to four cigarettes a day substantially increases the risk of cardiovascular and all-cause mortality (38). Nonsmokers with PAD have double the five-year survival rate over smokers.

PATHOPHYSIOLOGY
The mechanism of smoking-induced atherogenesis is not completely under- stood. Almost 5000 chemicals are found in cigarette smoke. Cigarette smoke has been shown to cause endothelial cell swelling and bleb formation, greater for- mation of luminal surface projections, subendothelial edema, widening of endothelial junctions, and thickening of the basement membrane. Studies with nicotine alone have demonstrated similar effects, along with a higher frequency of endothelial cell death and a lower rate of cell replication. This abnormal capability for endothelial cell regeneration results in an impaired ability to repair sites of endothelial cell damage. Thus, cigarette smoke is not only toxic to the endothelial cell, causing injury and death, but also inhibits the ability of the endothelium to repair the injury induced by the cigarette smoke.

In addition to direct injury to the endothelium, smoking can indirectly damage the endothelium, resulting in abnormalities of endothelial function. Smokers have been shown to have abnormal levels of plasma lipoproteins; as discussed previously, lipoprotein elevation initiates endothelial cell injury. Cigarette smoking is associated with abnormal prostaglandin production, resulting in an imbalance between prostacyclin and thromboxane A_2. The imbalance reduces the antithrombotic potential of the endothelial surface by inducing platelet aggregation and adherence. Also, smoking inhibits the

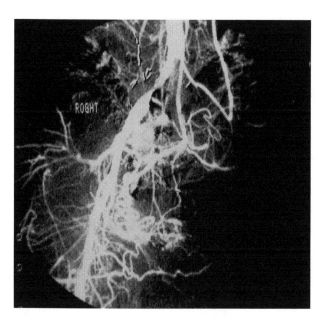

FIGURE 3 Aortoiliac occlusive disease in a 45-year-old smoker with complete occlusion of left iliac system and severe stenosis of the right common iliac artery.

production of NO, which has adverse effects on vasomotor regulation, smooth muscle cell (SMC) proliferation, and platelet and macrophage adhesion.

Unlike diabetics who often localize disease to their tibial vessels, smokers often manifest clinically with localized aortoiliac occlusive disease with a relative absence of disease in the lower extremity arteries (Fig. 3).

THERAPEUTIC GOAL
The goal for patients with CLI who smoke is complete cessation.

TREATMENT
A successful tobacco cessation strategy includes both behavioral therapy and pharmacotherapy (39).

Behavioral Therapy
Vascular surgeons are well positioned to provide motivation to the patient and to initiate cessation strategies when patients are faced with a life- or limb-threatening disorder. Telling patients that smoking is associated with accelerated disease, limb loss, and death may be particularly effective in helping patients find the motivation to remain abstinent. In addition to providing motivation to quit, the surgeon must be prepared to provide smoking cessation strategies such as a referral to behavioral therapist or a prescription for nicotine replacement therapy at each clinical encounter (40). An effective strategy can achieve cessation rates of 25% to 30% at one year (41).

The U.S. Department of Health and Human Services/Public Health Service Guideline, *Treating Tobacco Use and Dependence*, emphasizes that counseling is quite successful in helping patients quit smoking, whether administered in an individual, group, or telephone setting (42). The 2000 guideline documents that clinical interventions as brief as three minutes can substantially increase cessation success. There is a strong dose-response relationship between the intensity of tobacco dependence counseling and its effectiveness. Treatments involving person-to-person contact (i.e., via individual, group, or proactive telephone counseling) are consistently effective, and their effectiveness increases with treatment intensity (e.g., the number of minutes of contact). While even a brief intervention is effective in increasing quitting rates, there is a dose-response relationship between treatment duration and its effectiveness. Because clinicians frequently have limited time with patients, adjuvant staff may be utilized to maximize the impact of treatment. Guideline analysis suggests that a wide variety of health care professionals can effectively implement these brief strategies. Adjuvant staff (e.g., physician assistants, nurses, and medical assistants) reinforce the brief clinician cessation message and provide follow-up and support services to patients attempting to quit. Quit rates at one year are approximately 20% for patients who complete a program, but the best cessation rates are obtained when a multi-pronged approach is used.

Pharmacotherapy
Nicotine Replacement
Nicotine is a potent psychoactive drug and symptoms of withdrawal include dysphoria, depression, insomnia, anxiety, irritability, restlessness, and weight gain. Therefore, nicotine replacement therapy is important to bridge patients to cessation while they undergo concurrent behavioral therapy, and increases the odds of quitting 1.5- to 2-fold (43). Nicotine replacement therapy is safe for patients and does not cause coronary vasospasm, myocardial ischemia, or major changes in heart rate or blood pressure that are associated with smoking (44). Nicotine replacement is available in gum, lozenge, transdermal patch, nasal spray, and inhaler.

Bupropion SR
Bupropion is an atypical antidepressant and can be used as a sole agent or combined with nicotine replacement therapy. Treatment with bupropion SR doubles quit rates at one year versus that of placebo (45). Bupropion is contraindicated in patients with a seizure disorder because it lowers the seizure threshold, but has a good safety profile. Common side effects are insomnia, dry mouth, and nausea.

Varenicline
Varenicline (Chantix) is a partial agonist of the $\alpha4\beta2$ nicotinic acetylcholine receptor. It acts by stimulating dopamine release in the brain and blocks nicotine from binding to the nicotine receptor. This results in relief of nicotine withdrawal symptoms and cigarette cravings as well as decreases the reinforcement and reward associated with smoking. It gained FDA approval for smoking cessation in May 2006. Varenicline appears to have a slight advantage in continuous abstinence rates over bupropion SR at three and six months, but perhaps less so at later intervals (46,47). Serious neuropsychiatric symptoms have occurred in

patients taking Chantix. These symptoms include changes in behavior, agitation, depressed mood, suicidal ideation, and attempted and completed suicide.

HYPERTENSION

The relationship between HTN and PAD was definitively established with the PAD Awareness, Risk, and Treatment: New Resources for Survival (PARTNERS) program, a multicenter, cross-sectional study conducted at 27 sites (48,49). Observations from this program showed 92% of enrolled individuals had both HTN and PAD. The NCEP ATP III (NCEP ATP III) guidelines do not specify a class of medication to be used to control blood pressure, but evidence favors ACE inhibitors and β-blockers if there is concurrent coronary disease. Contrary to historical opinion, a meta-analysis of 11 randomized trials showed that β-blockers do not adversely effect walking capacity or the symptoms of intermittent claudication in patients with mild to moderate PAD.

While large trials on the efficacy of antihypertensive therapy in slowing progression of PAD to CLI are yet to be conducted, intensive blood pressure lowering strategies are effective in improving cardiovascular outcomes (50,51).

PATHOPHYSIOLOGY

HTN induces morphologic as well as functional changes in the endothelium. Endothelial cells from hypertensive patients are edematous and project farther into the lumen of the vessel than normal. Vessels from hypertensive patients demonstrate vascular SMC proliferation along with thickening of the basement membrane, subendothelial accumulation of fibrin, and increased fibronectin in the extracellular matrix. Levels of growth factors such as transforming growth factor (TGF)-β and platelet-derived growth factor (PDGF) are increased, contributing to vascular SMC proliferation. Endothelium-dependent relaxation is impaired in hypertensive patients via abnormalities of NO metabolism. The effect of an acetylcholine infusion on the release of NO is significantly reduced in hypertensive patients. It appears that the severity of the endothelial dysfunction associated with HTN is related to the degree of blood pressure elevation.

Atherosclerosis is seen only in vessels subjected to arterial pressure. Atherosclerosis does not develop in veins but commonly occurs in vein grafts placed into the arterial circulation.

Therapeutic Goals

The American College of Cardiology (ACC)/AHA 2005 guidelines identify a goal blood pressure of less than 140/90 mmHg (52). If patients also have chronic kidney disease, congestive heart failure, or diabetes, the goal should be less than 130/80 mmHg. Frequently multiple medications will be required. Initial treatment should include a β-blocker and/or ACE inhibitors.

Pharmocotherapy

Angiotensin-Converting Enzyme Inhibitors

ACE inhibitors have been proven to confer a 22% relative risk reduction in the composite end points of MI, stroke, or cardiovascular death in patients with PAD over a five-year period (53). In this trial, the Heart Outcomes Prevention Evaluation (HOPE) trial, of over 9000 high-risk patients, randomization was to a ramipril group or placebo. Nearly half of the enrolled patients had PAD, claudication, or an ankle-brachial index less than 0.9, and this group benefited just as much as the larger group, and this benefit was independent of the effect of ramipril on blood pressure. The trial was concluded after two years, given the dramatic benefit of ramipril. Another trial has also shown that an ACE inhibitor may lead to improvements in walking distance by increasing peripheral perfusion (54). ACE inhibitors also have vascular protective effects similar to statins. ACE inhibitors potentially stabilize atherosclerotic plaque, improve endothelial vasomotor dysfunction, and show improvement in vessel wall function (55,56). In addition, the Study to Evaluate Carotid Ultrasound Changes in Patients Treated with Ramipril and Vitamin E (SECURE), ramipril reduced the intima-to-media ratio of carotid arteries in high-risk patients (57).

The ACC/AHA guidelines recommend treating all persons with atherosclerotic vascular disease with ACE inhibitors to reduce cardiovascular mortality and morbidity, unless contraindicated (58). Ramipril is the only agent specifically indicated for cardiovascular event protection. In the HOPE trial, the cardioprotective dose was 10 mg/day. Side effects of ACE inhibitors include dry cough, and an angiotensin receptor blocker (ARB) can be used as an alternative choice.

β-Adrenergic Antagonists

β-Blocker therapy reduces the incidence of new coronary events in patients with CAD and concurrent symptomatic PAD by 53% (59). These results were from an observational study of 575 men and women with symptomatic PAD and prior MI. Twelve percent of patients had adverse side effects requiring cessation of the medication. While the specific β-blocker was not named, biaoprolol (Ziac) had been used effectively with a starting dose of 2.5 mg/day, which can be adjusted to as high as 40 mg/day. Contraindications include asthma, bradycardia, heart block, and congestive heart failure.

Diuretics

A diuretic may be used to treat HTN with the addition of potassium-sparing agents if hypokalemia is noted during the first six months of treatment. They are also commonly used as adjuncts to other antihypertensive drugs and are especially useful in patients with hypercalciuria, calcium stones, and osteoporosis because they decrease calcium excretion. The first group of diuretics includes the thiazides, of which the prototype is hydrochlorothiazide, and chlorthalidone. Lower-dose thiazides are quite effective but usually take three to four weeks to reduce blood pressure. The second group of drugs includes the loop diuretics, of which the prototype is furosemide. Although the latter has been used in the direct treatment of HTN, it usually is used in individuals who are azotemic where volume or cardiac failures are issues.

Calcium Channel Blockers

Calcium channel blockers have frequently been administered to control mild or modest HTN. These drugs interfere with angiotensin II and α2-adrenergic-mediated vasoconstriction, and they may also affect α1-adrenergic vasoconstriction by blocking cellular Ca^{2+} entry. These drugs work well in both black and white patients. There are two major types of calcium channel blockers: the dihydropyridines (e.g., nifedipine and amlodipine), which are potent vaso-dilators and the non-dihydropyridines (e.g., verapamil), which have cardiac-depressant activity, and diltiazem, which has both less vasodilator activity than nifedipine and less cardiac depression than verapamil. Although these differ-ences result in different kinds of side effects, the degree of blood pressure control tends to be roughly equivalent. The non-dihydropyridine agents reduce cardiac contractility as well as peripheral vasoconstriction. Their use has been most often as an effective alternative to β-blockers. The dihydropyridine class has selective vasodilators, do not have the significant cardiac-depressive effects, and may be more appropriate for use when cardiac depression is to be avoided or when mild cardiac stimulation might prove beneficial. Renal insufficiency does not have a major effect on the pharmacokinetics of these drugs. Calcium channel blockers are effective antihypertensive agents that do not produce hyperlipidemia or insulin resistance and do not interfere with sympathetic function. Important side effects of these agents include depression of cardiac contractility, rate, automaticity, and impulse conduction, all of which have made these drugs potentially hazardous in patients with second- or third-degree heart block (verapamil and diltiazem) and congestive heart failure with moderate to marked systolic dysfunction.

Angiotensin II Receptor Blockers
Although not as extensively studied as ACE inhibitors, ARBs appear to have similar efficacy both as antihypertensives and as medications that can decrease cardiovascular morbidity and mortality in high-risk patients. They have also been shown to have similar benefit in high-risk type 2 diabetic patients and may preserve renal function in this group. Two major trials—the Irbesartan Diabetic Nephropathy trial and the Reduction in End Point in Non-insulin-Dependent Diabetes Mellitus with the Angiotensin II Antagonist Losartan (RENAAL) trial—demonstrated a clear benefit in terms of renoprotection with ARBs in patients with nephropathy due to type 2 disease (60). These receptor blockers are a reasonable alternative to ACE inhibitors, with fewer or no typical ACE inhibitor side effects. Their action in blocking angiotensin II receptors results in the reduction of angiotensin II–mediated vasoconstriction and a secondary decrease in aldosterone release. The angiotensin I receptor is selectively blocked with these agents, and it is this receptor that mediates most all of the actions of angiotensin II. These ARBs lack the potential beneficial effects of enhancing bradykinin metabolism accompanying ACE inhibitors. These ARBs may be particularly useful in reducing proteinuria in nephrotic states. Like the ACE inhibitors, diuretics are logical drugs to be added to these receptor blockers to control HTN in many patients.

HYPERCOAGULABILITY
Hypercoagulability disorders can have devastating clinical sequelae, and vas-cular surgeons should be prepared to diagnose and treat these disorders. Arterial thromboses, the focus of this section, are primarily related to environ-mental and acquired risk factors. Alternatively, up to 30% of venous thromboses occur in patients with inherited molecular defects, which are beyond the scope of this chapter (Table 1).

TABLE 1 Thromboses Due to Hypercoagulable States

Inherited prothrombotic conditions	Acquired prothrombotic conditions
Activated protein C resistance (factor V Leiden)	Antiphospholipid antibody syndrome
Prothrombin G20210A mutation	Heparin-induced thrombocytopenia
Deficiencies of antithrombin, protein C, protein S	Hyperhomocysteinemia
Elevated procoagulant factors VIII, IX, XI	Hyperfibrinogenemia
	Defective fibrinolysis
	Lipoprotein(a)
	Abnormal platelet aggregation
	Elevated plasminogen activator inhibitor 1

Arterial thromboses are associated with atherosclerotic vessel changes in a setting of specific risk factors such as diabetes, hyperlipidemia, or tobacco use. Arterial thrombosis in the absence of these risk factors, in younger patients, or patients with multiple failed bypass grafts should initiate an investigation for acquired procoagulant states. These conditions include the antiphospholipid antibody syndrome, heparin-induced thrombocytopenia (HIT), hyperhomocysteinemia, hyperfibrinogenemia, and less commonly defective fibrinolysis, lipoprotein(a), abnormal platelet aggregation, and elevated plasminogen activator inhibitor 1(PAI-1).

Components of the laboratory investigation in patients with a suspected hypercoagulable state manifested in the arterial circulation should include fasting homocysteine levels, antiphospholipid and anticardiolipin antibody (ACA) titers, β2-glycoprotein I antibody levels, an activated partial thromboplastin time (aPTT) and dilute Russell viper venom time, testing for antiheparin antibodies, clottable fibrinogen and fibrinogen antigen, lipoprotein(a) levels, PAI-1, and a prothrombin time. Table 2 includes laboratory evaluation for both venous and arterial thromboses. These laboratory evaluations are ideally performed two to three weeks after discontinuation of anticoagulation. If this is not possible, a direct thrombin inhibitor may be used prior to laboratory investigation.

TABLE 2 Laboratory Evaluation for Hypercoagulable States

Antithrombin activity and antigen assay
Protein C activity and antigen assay
APC resistance assay and factor V Leiden py PCR
Prothrombin G20210A by PCR
β2-glycoprotein I antibodies[a]
Anitphospholipid and anticardiolipin antibody titer[a]
Measurement of fasting total plasma homocysteine levels[a]
Clottable fibrinogen and fibrinogen antigen[a]
Dilute Russell viper venom time[a]
Tissue thromboplastin inhibition time
Lipoprotein(a) level[a]
ELISA for antiheparin antibody[a]
aPTT[a]
PT[a]
D-dimer

[a]Most relevant in arterial thrombosis.

Antiphospholipid Antibody Syndrome

The antiphospholipid antibody syndrome consists of the presence of an elevated antiphospholipid antibody titer [either lupus anticoagulant (LA) or ACA] in association with episodes of thrombosis. Although the LA has been reported in 5% to 40% of patients with systemic lupus erythematosus, it can exist in patients without lupus and can be induced in patients by medications, cancer, and certain infectious diseases. Antiphospholipid antibody syndrome results in a 5- to 16-fold greater risk of arterial and venous thrombosis. Many possible thrombotic mechanisms have been suggested, including (*i*) inhibition of prostacyclin synthesis or its release from endothelial cells, (*ii*) inhibition of protein C activation by thrombin/thrombomodulin, (*iii*) increased PAI-1 levels, (*iv*) direct platelet activation, (*v*) coexistence of endothelial cell activation with antiphospholipid antibodies, and (*vi*) interference with the endothelial cell-associated anticoagulant activity of annexin V. Thrombosis can specifically involve the peripheral arterial circulation. Graft thrombosis has been observed in 27% to 50% of patients positive for antiphospholipid antibody.

The diagnosis is based on a prolonged aPTT with other coagulation tests within normal limits and the presence of an increased antiphospholipid or ACA titer and elevation of β2-glycoprotein. A prolonged dilute Russell viper venom time shortened by the addition of excess phospholipids confirms the presence of a LA. Heparin followed by anticoagulation with warfarin (international normalized ratio >3) is recommended to treat antiphospholipid antibody syndrome. In patients with LAs, heparin therapy is monitored by antifactor Xa levels.

Heparin-Induced Thrombocytopenia

HIT is an immune-mediated adverse response to heparin therapy. Heparin-dependent immunoglobulin G (IgG) antibodies are directed at platelet factor 4 (PF4) in complex with heparin, forming an immune complex. This immune complex binds to platelets. Platelet activation is triggered when the Fc portion of the IgG antibody bound to the heparin-PF4 complex reacts with the Fc receptor on adjacent platelets. In addition to platelet activation, aggregation and formation of procoagulant microparticles occurs. These events lead to thrombin generation and HIT-associated thrombosis. Activated platelets also induce an inflammatory state with macrophage and neutrophil activation and susbsequent endothelial adhesion.

HIT is defined as a platelet count less than $100 \times 10^9/L$ starting 4 to 14 days after heparin administration or a 30% to 50% drop in platelet count from preheparin baseline. The major significance of HIT is paradoxical thrombosis, occurring in 30% of patients with HIT and thrombocytopenia. Treatment should be instituted immediately in patients with HIT to prevent thrombosis with direct thrombin inhibitors, which inhibit the high level of thrombin generation. Long-term anticoagulation should include vitamin K antagonists, but these should only be started when the platelet count is greater than $100 \times 10^9/L$.

Hyperhomocysteinemia

The incidence of hyperhomocysteinemia in patients with PAD is as high as 60%, and as many as 30% of patients with premature PAD may have hyperhomocysteinemia. Elevated levels may be more strongly associated with PAD than with CAD, as found in a meta-analysis concluding that the odds ratio of having elevated homocysteine levels for CAD were 1.6 compared with 6.8 for PAD (61).

Homocysteine is an amino acid that can oxidize LDL cholesterol, which is subsequently found in foam cells and early atherosclerotic lesions. The formation of reactive oxygen species promotes endothelial dysfunction, as does homocysteines inhibition of NO production by endothelial cells (62). All these mechanisms may lead to accelerated atherosclerosis.

Patients with a strong family history of atherosclerotic disease that cannot be explained by their lipid profile should be tested for hyperhomocysteinemia (17). Elevated homocysteine levels can be treated with folic acid supplementation between 0.5 and 1.0 mg/day.

Hyperfibrinogenemia

Elevated fibrinogen levels are associated with increased blood viscosity, and multiple studies have illustrated elevated fibrinogen and blood viscosity to be independently associated with PAD (63). Increased fibrinogen is also associated with worsening symptomatic claudication, possibly secondary to the elevated blood viscosity and decreased oxygen delivery in the microcirculation (64). Potential causes include defective thrombin binding or resistance to plasmin-mediated breakdown. Laboratory evaluation should include a clottable fibrinogen activity-to-fibrinogen antigen ratio. Therapy includes exercise, as it is thought to potentially lower fibrinogen levels, which also may be one mechanism by which exercise alleviates claudication symptoms (65).

Lipoprotein(a)

Lipoprotein(a), associated with LDL, is atherogenic and prothrombotic. It inhibits plasminogen activation from initiating fibrinolysis and prevents plasminogen from binding to cells or fibrin.

MOLECULAR MARKERS ASSOCIATED WITH PROGRESSION OF ATHEROSCLEROSIS
C-Reactive Protein

C-reactive protein (CRP) is independently associated with PAD (66). Furthermore, an elevated level has been shown to be risk factor for the progression of PAD to CLI requiring revascularization (67). CRP can also be used to guide lipid therapy as the statins lower CRP levels. CRP is an independent predictor of future cardiovascular events in patients with established PAD.

Interleukin-6

The Edinburgh Artery Study measured CRP, interleukin-6 (IL-6), intercellular adhesion molecule 1 (ICAM-1), vascular adhesion molecule 1 (VCAM-1), and E-selectin at baseline (68). Valid ankle-brachial index (ABI) measurements were obtained at baseline and 5-year and 12-year follow-up examinations. At baseline, a significant trend was found between higher plasma levels of CRP (P0.05) and increasing severity of PAD. IL-6 at baseline was associated with progressive atherosclerosis at 5 years, and CRP, IL-6, and ICAM-1 were associated with changes at 12 years. Only IL-6 independently predicted ABI change at 5 years and 12 years in analyses of all inflammatory markers simultaneously. This suggests that while CRP, IL-6, and ICAM-1 are molecular markers associated with atherosclerosis and its progression, IL-6 showed more consistent results and stronger independent predictive value than the other markers. It is not currently part of the diagnostic evaluation of patients with CLI.

Prostaglandins

Vasodilator prostaglandins, including prostaglandin E (PGE)-1, iloprost, and ciprostene have been studied in placebo-controlled trials as potentially beneficial in patients with CLI with inconsistent results. Research is ongoing.

Angiogenic Growth Factors

Therapeutic angiogenesis evolved from work in the 1970s by Folkman, with his observations that the development and maintenance of an adequate microvascular supply was essential for the growth of neoplastic tissue. Since then it has been shown that stimulating angiogenesis can improve perfusion. Early-phase clinical studies support the safety of these approaches and provide indications of bioactivity in patients with CLI (69,70).

ANTIPLATELET THERAPY

An antiplatelet agent should be an integral part of any medication regimen for all patients with PAD barring contraindications. The Antithrombotic Trialists' Collaboration Groups determined that a daily aspirin resulted in a 23% risk reduction in nonfatal MI, stroke, and vascular death (71). Specifically, among 9214 patients with PAD in 42 trials there was a proportional reduction of 23% in serious vascular events ($p = 0.004$), with similar benefits among patients with intermittent claudication, those having peripheral grafting, and those having peripheral angioplasty. A Cochrane review also found aspirin to reduce the risk of peripheral arterial occlusion after revascularization procedures (72). A daily aspirin has resulted in an approximately 30% decrease in strokes in high-risk patients. Those older than 65 years show the most benefit. An 81-mg aspirin once a day is the recommended dose for patients with PAD. Higher doses have been associated with an increased risk of bleeding secondary to GI toxicity (73).

The second widely used antiplatelet agent is clopidogrel. Clopidogrel irreversibly inactivates the adenosine diphosphate P_2Y_{12} receptor on the surface of platelets, whereby preventing platelet aggregation. The Clopidogrel versus Aspirin in Patients at Risk of Ischemic Events (CAPRIE) trial prospectively compared aspirin 325 mg/day with clopidogrel 75 mg/day (74). At two-year follow-up, a small absolute improvement (3.71% vs. 4.86%) was seen in the clopidogrel group with respect to ischemic stroke, MI, and vascular death. Clopidogrel has also been shown to reduce cardiovascular events in diabetics (75). The Clopidogrel for High Atherothrombotic Risk and Ischemic Stabilization, Management and Avoidance (CHARISMA) trial compared dual antiplatelet therapy versus aspirin alone. In this trial, there was a suggestion of benefit (small but statistically significant) with clopidogrel and aspirin therapy combined in patients with symptomatic atherothrombosis and a suggestion of harm in patients with multiple risk factors (76,77).

All patients with peripheral vascular disease should be on 81 mg of aspirin daily. Dual antiplatelet regimens should be reserved for those patients at highest risk or who have already undergone revascularization for CLI.

PENTOXIFYLLINE AND CILOSTAZOL

While pentoxifylline and cilostazol have been advocated in claudicants, neither is used in the treatment of CLI. Pentoxifylline is a xanthine derivative possessing vasodilator and hemorheologic properties. Two placebo-controlled trials have evaluated pentoxifylline treatment in patients with CLI. In one trial, intravenous infusion of pentoxifylline was used and resulted in a slight decreased in pain, and in the other no benefit was shown (78,79). Therefore, Pentoxifylline is no longer used.

Cilostazol inhibits phosphodiesterase type 3, increasing cyclic adenosine monophosphate and causing vasodilatation, has antiplatelet effects, and acts to modify plasma lipoproteins. It has been shown to improve overall walking distance and quality of life. A 1999 meta-analysis of the effects of cilostazol reported increases of 50% in maximal walking distance compared with placebo and significant improvements in quality of life as measured by Rand Short Form 36 questionnaires (80). There seems to be a dose-response effect, with 100 mg twice daily being more efficacious than 50 mg twice daily. The main adverse effects include headache, palpitations, and diarrhea, leading approximately 15% of people to stop the medication. Congestive heart failure is a major contraindication to the use of cilostazol.

REFERENCES

1. Eagle KA, Rihal CS, Foster ED, et al. Long-term survival in patients with coronary artery disease: importance of peripheral vascular disease. The Coronary Artery Surgery Study (CASS) investigators. J Am Coll Cardiol 1994; 23:1091–1095.
2. Libby P, Hansson GK, Pober JS. Atherogenesis and inflammation. In: Chien K, ed. Molecular Basis of Cardiovascular Disease. Philadelphia: W.B. Saunders, 1999:349–366.
3. The Diabetes Prevention Program Research Group. Reduction in the incidence of type 2 diabetes with lifestyle intervention or metformin. N Engl J Med 2002; 346:393–403.
4. Gardner CD, Coulston AM, Chatterjee L, et al. The effect of a plant based diet on plasma lipids in hypercholesterolemic adults: a randomized trial. Ann Intern Med 2005; 142:725–733.
5. Ginsberg HN, Kris-Etherton P, Dennis B, et al. Effects of reducing dietary saturated fatty acids on plasma lipids and lipoproteins in healthy subjects: the DELTA study, protocol 1. Arterioscler Thromb Vasc Biol 1998; 18:441–449.
6. Helmrich SP, Ragland DR, Leung RW, et al. Physical activity and reduced occurrence of non-insulin-dependent diabetes mellitus. N Engl J Med 1991; 325:147–152.
7. Intensive blood-glucose control with sulphonylureas or insulin compared with conventional treatment and risk of complications in patients with type 2 diabetes (UKPDS 33) UK Prospective Diabetes Study (UKPDS) Group. Lancet 1998; 352:837–853.
8. Muntner P, Wildman RP, Reynolds K, et al. Relationship between HbA1c level and peripheral arterial disease. Diabetes Care 2005; 28:1981–1987.
9. Uusitupa M, Lindi V, Louherenta A, et al., for the Finnish Study Group. Long-term improvements in insulin sensitivity by changing lifestyles of people with impaired glucose tolerance. Diabetes 2003; 52:2532–2538.
10. Parkhouse N, LeQueen PM. Impaired neurogenic vascular response in patients with diabetes and neuropathic foot lesions. N Engl J Med 1988; 318:1306–1309.
11. Bucala R, Cerami A, Vlassara H. Advanced glycosylation end products in diabetic complications. Biochemical basis and prospects for therapeutic intervention. Diabetes Rev 1995; 3:258–268.

12. Sidawy AN. Diabetic Foot: Lower Extremity Arterial Disease and Limb Salvage. Philadelphia: Lippincott Williams & Wilkins, 2006.
13. The effect of intensive treatment of diabetes on the development and progression of long-term complications in insulin-dependent diabetes mellitus. The Diabetes Control and Complications Trial Research Group. N Engl J Med 1993; 329:977–986.
14. Gaede P, Vedel P, Larsen N, et al. Multifactorial intervention and cardiovascular disease in patients with type 2 diabetes. N Engl J Med 2003; 348:383–393.
15. Grundy SM, Cleeman JI, Merz CN, et al. Implications of recent clinical trials for the National Cholesterol Education Program Adult Treatment Panel III guidelines. Circulation 2004; 110:227–239.
16. Heart Protection Study Collaborative Group. MRC/BHF Heart Protection Study of cholesterol –lowering with Simvastatin in 5963 people with diabetes: a randomized placebo-controlled trial. Lancet 2003; 361:2005–2016.
17. Third Report of the National Cholesterol Education Program Expert Panel on Detection, Evaluation, and Treatment of High Blood Cholesterol in Adults (Adult Treatment Panel III) (NIH Publication 01-3670). Bethesda: National Institutes of Health, 2001.
18. Ballantyne CM, Olsson AG, Cook TJ, et al. Influence of low high-density lipoprotein cholesterol and elevated triglyceride on coronary heart disease events and response to simvastatin therapy in 4S. Circulation 2001; 104:3046–3051.
19. Hennekens CH, Dyken ML, Fuster V. Aspirin as a therapeutic agent in cardiovascular disease: a statement for healthcare professionals from the American Heart Association. Circulation 1997; 96:2751–2753.
20. Mohler ER, Hiatt WR, Crager MA, et al. Cholesterol reduction with atrovastatin improves walking distance in patients with peripheral arterial disease. Circulation 2003; 108:1481–1486.
21. Mondillo S, Ballo P, Barbati R, et al. Effects of simvastatin on walking performance and symptoms of intermittent claudication in hypercholesterolemic patients with peripheral vascular disease. Am J Med 2003; 114:359–364.
22. Kinlay S, Plutzky J. Effect if lipid-lowering therapy on vasomotion and endothelial function. Curr Cardiol Rep 1999; 1:238–243.
23. Pedersen TR, Kjekshus J, Pyorala K, et al. Effect of simvastatin on ischemic signs and symptoms in the Scandinavian Simvastatin Survival Study (4S). Am J Cardiol 1998; 81:333–335.
24. Heart Protection Study Collaborative Group. HPS Randomized trial of the effects of cholesterol-lowering with simvastatin on peripheral vascular disease and other major vascular outcomes in 20,536 people with peripheral arterial disease and other high-risk conditions. J Vasc Surg 2007; 45(4):645–654.
25. Brewer HB. Increasing HDL cholesterol levels. N Engl J Med 2004; 350:1491–1494.
26. Howard BV, Roman MJ, Devereux RB, et al. Effect of lower targets for blood pressure and LDL cholesterol on atherosclerosis in diabetes. The SANDS randomized trial. JAMA 2008; 299(14):1678–1689.
27. Knapp HH, Schrott H, Ma P, et al. Efficacy and safety of combination simvastatin and colesevelam in patients with primary hypercholesterolemia. Am J Med 2001; 110:352–360.
28. Kris-Etherton PM, Harris WS, Appel LJ. American Heart Association, Nutrition Committee. Fish consumption, fish oil, omega-3 fatty acids, and cardiovascular disease. Circulation 2002; 106:2742–2757.
29. de Lorgeril M, Salen P, Martin JL, et al. Mediterranean diet, traditional risk factors, and the rate of cardiovascular complications after myocardial infarction: final report of the Lyon Diet Heart Study. Circulation 1999; 99:779–785.
30. von Schacky C, Angerer P, Kothny W, et al. The effect of dietary Ω-3 fatty acids on coronary atherosclerosis: a randomized, double-blind, placebo-controlled trial. Ann Intern Med 1999; 130:554–562.
31. Paolini JF, Mitchel YB, Reyes R, et al. Effects of laropiprant on nicotinic acid-induced flushing in patients with dyslipidemia. Am J Cardiol 2008; 101(5):625–630.
32. Cronenwett JL, Warner KG, Zelenock GB, et al. Intermittent claudication: current results of nonoperative management. Arch Surg 1984; 119:430–436.

33. Hirsch AT, Treat-Jacobson D, Lando HA, et al. The role of tobacco cessation, anti-platelet and lipid-lowering therapies in the treatment of peripheral arterial disease. Vasc Med 1997; 2:243–251.
34. Jonason T, Bergstrom R. Cessation of smoking in patients with intermittent claudication. Effects on the risk of peripheral vascular complications, myocardial infarction and mortality. Acta Med Scand 1987; 221:253–260.
35. Leng GC, Papacosta O, Whincup P, et al. Femoral atherosclerosis in an older British population: prevalence and risk factors. Atherosclerosis 2000; 152:167–174.
36. Hobbs SD, Bradbury AW. Smoking cessation strategies in patients with peripheral arterial disease: an evidence-based approach. Eur J Vasc Endovasc Surg 2003; 26: 341–347.
37. Willigendael EM, Teijink JA, Bartelink ML, et al. Smoking and the patency of lower extremity bypass grafts: a meta-analysis. J Vasc Surg 2005; 42:67–74.
38. Bjartveit K, Tverdal A. Health consequences of smoking 1-4 cigarettes per day. Tob Control 2005; 14:315–320.
39. Rehring T, Stolepart R, Whitton Hollis H Jr. Pharmacologic risk factor management in peripheral arterial disease: a vade mecum for vascular surgeons. J Vasc Surg 2008; 47:1108–1115.
40. Anderson JE, Jorenby DE, Scott WJ, et al. Treating tobacco use and dependence: an evidence-based clinical practice guideline for tobacco cessation. Chest 2002; 121:932–941.
41. Fiore MC. US public health service clinical practice guideline: treating tobacco use and dependence. Respir Care 2000; 45:1200–1262.
42. Fiore MC, Bailey WC, Cohen SJ, et al. Treating Tobacco Use and Dependence: Clinical Practice Guideline. Rockville: U.S. Department of Health and Human Services, Public Health Service, 2000.
43. Silagy C, Lancaster T, Stead L, et al. Nicotine replacement therapy for smoking cessation. Cochrane Database Syst Rev 2004:CD000146.
44. Ford Cand Zlabek J. Nicotine replacement therapy and cardiovascular disease. Mayo Clin Proc 2005; 80:652–656.
45. Hughes JR, Stead LF, Lancaster T. Antidepressants for smoking cessation. Cochrane Database Syst Rev 2007:CD000031.
46. Gonzales D, Rennard S, Nides M, et al. Varenicline, an alpha4beta2 nicotinic ace-tylcholine receptor partial agonist, vs sustained-release bupropion and placebo for smoking cessation: a randomized controlled trial. JAMA 2006; 296:47–55.
47. Jorenby D, Hays J, Rigotti N, et al. Efficacy of varenicline, an alpha4beta2 nicotinic acetylcholine receptor partial agonist, vs placebo or sustained-release bupropion for smoking cessation: a randomized controlled trial. JAMA 2006; 296:56–63.
48. Hirsch AT, Criqui MH, Treat-Jacobson D, et al. Peripheral arterial disease detection, awareness, and treatment in primary care. JAMA 2001; 286:1317–1324.
49. Olin JW. Hypertension and peripheral arterial disease. Vasc Med 2005; 10:241–246.
50. Chobanian AV, Bakris GL, Black HR, et al. The seventh report of the Joint National Committee on Prevention, Detection, Evaluation, and Treatment of High Blood Pressure: the JNC 7 report. JAMA 2003; 289:2560–2572.
51. Mehler PS, Coll JR, Estacio R, et al. Intensive blood pressure control reduces the risk of cardiovascular events in patients with peripheral arterial disease and type 2 diabetes. Circulation 2003; 107:753–756.
52. Hirsch AT, Haskal ZJ, Hertzer NR, et al. ACC/AHA 2005 guidelines for the man-agement of patients with peripheral arterial disease (lower extremity, renal, mes-enteric, and abdominal aortic): executive summary a collaborative report from the American Association for Vascular Surgery/Society for Vascular Surgery, Society for Cardiovascular Angiography and Interventions, Society for Vascular Medicine and Biology, Society of Interventional Radiology, and the ACC/AHA. J Am Coll Cardiol 2006; 47:e1–192.
53. Yusuf S, Sleight P, Pogue J, et al. Effects of an angiotensin-converting-enzyme inhibitor, ramipril, on cardiovascular events in high-risk patients. The Heart Out-comes Prevention Evaluation Study investigators. N Engl J Med 2000; 342:145–153.

54. Catalano M, Libretti A. Captopril for the treatment of patients with hypertension and peripheral vascular disease. Angiology 1985; 36:293–296.
55. Brown NJ, Vaughan DE. Angiotensin-converting enzyme inhibitors. Circulation 1998; 97:1411–1420.
56. Mancini GB, Henry GC, Macaya C, et al. Angiotensin-converting enzyme inhibition with quinapril improves endothelial vasomotor dysfunction in patients with coronary artery disease. The Trend (Trial on Reversing Endothelial Dysfunction) study. Circulation 1996; 94:258–265.
57. Lonn E, Yusuf S, Dzavik V, et al. Effects of ramipril and vitamin E on atherosclerosis: the study to evaluate carotid ultrasound changes in patients treated with ramipril and vitamin E (SECURE). Circulation 2001; 103(7):919–925.
58. Smith SC Jr., Blair SN, Bonow RO, et al. AHA/ACC Guidelines for preventing heart attack and death in patients with atherosclerotic cardiovascular disease: 2001 update. Circulation 2001; 104:1577–1579.
59. Aronow WS, Ahn C. Effect of beta blocker on incidence of new coronary events in older persons with prior myocardial infarction and symptomatic peripheral arterial disease. Am J Cardiol 2001; 87:1284–1286.
60. Lewis EJ, Hunsicker LJ, Clarke WR, et al. Renoprotective effect of the angiotensin receptor antagonist irbesartan in patients with nephropathy due to type 2 diabetes. N Engl J Med 2001; 345:851–860.
61. Taylor LM, Moneta GL, Sexton GJ, et al. Prospective blinded study of the relationship between plasma homocysteine and progression of symptomatic peripheral arterial disease. J Vasc Surg 1999; 29(1):8–19.
62. Stuhlinger MC, Oka RK, Graf EE, et al. Endothelial dysfunction induced by hyperhomocyst(e)inemia: role of asymmetric dimethyl-arginine. Circulation 2003; 108: 933–938.
63. Lee AJ, Lowe GDO, Woodward M, et al. Fibrinogen in relation to personal history of prevalent hypertension, diabetes, stroke, intermittent claudication, coronary heart disease, and family history: the Scottish Heart Health Study. Br Heart J 1993; 69:338–342.
64. Lowe GDO, Fowkes FGR, Dawes J, et al. Blood viscosity, fibrinogen, and activation of coagulation and leukocytes in peripheral arterial disease and the normal population in the Edinburgh Artery Study. Circulation 1993; 87:1915–1920.
65. Gardner AW, Killewich LA. Association between physical activity and endogenous fibrinolysis in peripheral arterial disease: a cross-sectional study guidelines. Circulation 2004; 110:227–239.
66. Collaborative meta-analysis of randomised trials of antiplatelet therapy for prevention of death, myocardial infarction, and stroke in high risk patients. BMJ 2002; 324:71–86.
67. Dorffler-Melly J, Koopman MM, Adam DJ, et al. Antiplatelet agents for preventing thrombosis after peripheral arterial bypass surgery. Cochrane Database Syst Rev 2003; 3:CD000535.
68. Campbell CL, Smyth S, Montalescot G, et al. Aspirin dose for the prevention of cardiovascular disease: a systematic review. JAMA 2007; 297:2018–2024.
69. A randomised, blinded, trial of clopidogrel versus aspirin in patients at risk of ischaemic events (CAPRIE) CAPRIE steering committee. Lancet 1996; 348:1329–1339.
70. Bhatt DL, Marso SP, Mirsch AT, et al. Amplified benefit of clopidogrel versus aspirin in patients with diabetes mellitus. Am J Cardiol 2002; 90:625–628.
71. Bhatt DL, Fox KA, Hacke W, et al. Clopidogrel and aspirin versus aspirin alone for the prevention of atherothrombotic events. N Engl J Med 2006; 354:1706–1717.
72. Bhatt DL, Flather MD, Hacke W, et al. Patients with prior myocardial infarction, stroke, or symptomatic peripheral arterial disease in the CHARISMA trial. J Am Coll Cardiol 2007; 49:1982–1988.
73. The European Study Group. Intravenous pentoxifylline for the treatment of chronic critical limb ischaemia. Eur J Vasc Endovasc Surg 1995; 9:426–436.
74. Efficacy and clinical tolerance of parenteral pentoxifylline in the treatment of critical lower limb ischemia. A placebo controlled multicenter study. Norwegian Pentoxifylline Multicenter Trial Group. Int Angiol 1996; 15:75–80.

75. Thompson PD, Zimet R, Forbes WP, et al. Meta-analysis of results from eight randomized, placebo-controlled trials on the effect of cilostazol on patients with intermittent claudication. Am J Cardiol 2002; 90:1314–1319.
76. Ridker PM, Stampfer MJ, Rifai N. Novel risk factors for systemic atherosclerosis: a comparison of C-reactive protein, fibrinogen, homocysteine, lipoprotein(a), and standard cholesterol screening as predictors of peripheral arterial disease. JAMA 2001; 285:2481–2485.
77. Ridker PM, Cushman M, Stampfer MJ, et al. Plasma concentration of C-reactive protein and risk of developing peripheral vascular disease. Circulation 1998; 97:425–428.
78. Tzoulaki I, Murray GD, Lee AJ. C-reactive protein, interleukin-6, and soluble adhesion molecules as predictors of progressive peripheral atherosclerosis in the general population: Edinburgh Artery Study. Circulation 2005; 112(7):976–983.
79. Rajagopalan S, Olin J, Deitcher S, et al. Use of a constitutively active hypoxia-inducible factor-1 transgene as a therapeutic strategy in no-option critical limb ischemia patients: phase I dose-escalation experience. Circulation 2007; 115:1234–1243.
80. Rajagopalan S, Mohler ER III, Lederman RJ, et al. Regional angiogenesis with vascular endothelial growth factor in peripheral arterial disease: a phase II randomized, double-blind, controlled study of adenoviral delivery of vascular endothelial growth factor 121 in patients with disabling intermittent claudication. Circulation 2003; 108:1933–1938; Angiology 2002; 53:367–374.

7 Endovascular Therapy of Superficial Femoral Artery and Popliteal Lesions in Critical Limb Ischemia

Patrick Peeters, Willem Willaert, and Jürgen Verbist
Department of Cardiovascular and Thoracic Surgery, Imelda Hospital, Bonheiden, Belgium

Koen Deloose and Marc Bosiers
Department of Vascular Surgery, AZ St-Blasius, Dendermonde, Belgium

INTRODUCTION

In most developed countries, the incidence of severe limb ischemia is estimated to be approximately 50 to 100 patients per 100,000 every year. Despite advances in medical therapy, the prospects are that this number will most likely even increase in the near future, due to an ageing population, the increasing prevalence of diabetes, and the sustained tobacco consumption (1,2).

Whereas, intermittent claudication generally involves a benign natural evolution with a low risk of amputation, the presence of critical limb ischemia (CLI) implies a much more extensive underlying arterial disease with much more serious short- and long-term consequences (3). Because CLI is usually the result of multivessel disease, its presentation always mandates an aggressive treatment strategy to prevent tissue and, eventually, limb loss (4).

In patients with CLI, surgical femoropopliteal bypass has been established as an accepted therapy with reported limb salvage rates approaching 90% (5,6). As presented in Table 1, it offers better patency rates in claudicants compared to patients with CLI caused by long femoropopliteal occlusions (7,8).

Despite the good results often reported in surgical series, the success of surgery has not been universal, and surgical intervention is not always feasible in this patient population threatened by other comorbidities related to the generalized atherosclerotic process (9–11). It should always be questioned whether the benefit of a surgical intervention surpasses the anesthetic and other procedural risks. It is generally accepted that surgical mortality should be less than 5%, but in the group of CLI, 6% is reported (7,12). In addition, a distal anastomosis cannot always be achieved due to lack of a target vessel or infected distal anastomosis area. Furthermore, traditional reporting standards, such as graft patency, limb salvage, and mortality do not reflect the true outcome of infrainguinal bypass surgery. In a recent study, 48.9% of the 318 patients who underwent infrainguinal bypass surgery for CLI had to be reoperated on within the initial three months. In 54%, wound healing exceeded three months (13). Endovascular treatments have surfaced as an acceptable alternative to surgical reconstruction.

The BASIL (Bypass Versus Angioplasty in Severe Ischaemia of the Leg) trial in 2005 compared the use of bypass surgery versus angioplasty as a first-line intervention in patients with CLI (14). In the angioplasty group, the superficial femoral artery (SFA) was treated in 162 patients (80%). In 126 of these

TABLE 1   Five-Year Primary Patency Data From Meta-Analysis for Infrainguinal Bypass Grafts

	Intermittent claudication	Critical limb ischemia
Vein bypass (any level)	80%	66%
PTFE (above knee)	75%	47%
PTFE (below knee)	65%	33%

Abbreviation: PTFE, polytetrafluoroethylene.
Source: From Ref. 7.

patients (62%), more distally located vessels also underwent angioplasty. The authors saw no difference in amputation ratio, mortality, or health-related quality of life between the two treatment groups. However, in this particular trial, half of the patients presenting with CLI were deemed unsuitable for any surgical or endovascular revascularization. Only 10% of the patients were actually randomized and the authors concluded that a large percentage of patients had probably undergone primary amputation. As reflected by the inclusion characteristics of this trial, it is very difficult to conduct a study of which the results can be generalized to an entire, heterogenic population of patients with CLI. Nevertheless, the authors of the BASIL trial concluded that patients with a life expectancy of less than two years with significant comorbidity should be offered angioplasty first if the local technical expertise is available. If the patient is expected to live more than two years and is free from severe concomitant disease, the apparent improved durability and reduced reintervention rate of surgery could outweigh the short-term considerations of increased morbidity and cost (BASIL).

The aim of this chapter is to give an overview of the established and evolving endovascular techniques available for treating the disease of the femoropopliteal region and the results that can be anticipated in patients with CLI.

THE DIFFERENT ENDOVASCULAR TECHIQUES AND THEIR RESULTS

Endovascular treatment has undergone a significant evolution over the past 20 years. Whereas in the beginning only stand-alone percutaneous transluminal angioplasty (PTA) was applied for endovascular SFA treatment, the armamentarium of the interventionalist has been clearly expanded today. Thanks to advances in interventional tools such as nitinol stents, covered stents, and excimer laser, and with the adoption of coronary interventional techniques in the peripheral arteries, subintimal angioplasty, and debulking with remote endarterectomy with or without lining up, possibilities are created to effectively treat even long total occlusions. Importantly, the morbidity and mortality rates associated with endovascular therapy are minimal and even reported to be zero (15), and most endovascular procedures do not prohibit future surgical bypass or additional endovascular intervention. Consequently, the application of endovascular materials and techniques has become common practice worldwide.

Despite this vast array and application of endovascular possibilities for femoropopliteal treatment of patients with CLI, literature about this subject is limited and review shows different patient populations for different treatment modalities. For example, PTA is generally used to treat short lesions, while endografts and subintimal angioplasty are generally used for longer occlusions.

For this reason, patency rates for the different treatment modalities cannot be directly compared (16).

In January 2000, the TransAtlantic Inter-Society Consensus (TASC) document was published to create a standard of classification and care for managing peripheral arterial disease (PAD), including CLI. The original TASC 2000 document (12) discouraged the primary use of stents in the SFA and stated that when PTA alone resulted in significant recoil or dissection, additional stenting could be valuable as a bailout procedure after technical failure. However, the Inter-Society Consensus for the management of peripheral arterial disease, TASC II document, published in January 2007, not only states that there is general agreement that for acute failure of PTA of an SFA lesion, stent placement is indicated, but also that stenting results after one year are superior to PTA results for femoropopliteal lesions indicated for endovascular therapy (17).

Angioplasty

Angioplasty balloons have undergone various improvements since their first use in the peripheral arterial system. They have become notably longer and have lower crossing profiles. Although PTA has a technical success rate approaching 100% and is associated with a low risk of complications, the late clinical failure after one year remained problematic. Restenosis occurs in up to 50% of the cases and exceeds 70% in longer lesions (>100 mm) (18). This led to the development of novel techniques such as stents and alternative PTA catheters such as cryoplasty balloons, coated balloons, cutting balloons, and scoring balloons.

CLI often originates in the presence of chronic total occlusions. The goal of endovascular treatment of such lesions is to transverse the occlusion, which is typically done transluminally but sometimes requires a subintimal approach. Subintimal angioplasty was first reported more than 20 years ago. Its use was initially limited in the femoropopliteal segment; however, nowadays it is also applied infrapopliteally.

A recent systematic review by Met et al. (19) showed that subintimal angioplasty is a safe procedure and more effective in patients with CLI compared with claudicants. Although primary patency rates as low as 50% were noted, limb salvage rates were between 85% and 90% at one year. This was confirmed by Bolia (20), who reported primary success rates between 80% and 90% in the infrainguinal and the infrapopliteal segment with high limb salvage rates between 85% and 90% at one year. Subintimal angioplasty has proven to be very valuable for CLI patients, and moreover it is a very cost-effective technique.

Stent Placement

The femoropopliteal arterial region is subject to many biomechanical forces, which can potentially compromise the results with endovascular techniques in this region compared with other arterial segments. The femoral tract is unique as it undergoes flexion, torsion, compression, and elongation with movement. Any endovascular stent or graft, which is implanted permanently, has to be resistant to these forces (17).

Although initial stenting results in the SFA were disappointing (21), the outcome of stent placement improved considerably with the introduction of nitinol stents. The superelasticity and thermal memory make them ideal for application in the SFA and the popliteal artery. In 2004, Mewissen (22) reported on 122 patients with CLI due to femoropopliteal lesions of a variable length between 4 and 28 cm who were treated with SMART stent (Cordis, Miami, Florida, U.S.) implantation. Favorable primary patency rates of 76% after one year and 60% after two years were found.

However, patency results could still be improved by limiting neointimal growth. In this context, drug-eluting stents were introduced to try to improve patency rates in peripheral arteries, as has been widely documented in the coronary circulation. Both sirolimus and paclitaxel have been used as eluting drugs.

Another issue was raised by FESTO trial, in which Scheinert et al. (23) reviewed 121 stents by plain radiographic screening, on average 10 months after they were placed. A variety of stents, SMART (Cordis), SelfX (Abbott/Jomed, Chicago, Illinois, U.S.), and Luminexx (C.R. Bard Inc., Murray Hill, New Jersey, U.S.) were utilized to treat lesions that were on average 15.7 cm in length. They found 25% stent fractures on average, but if the stented length exceeded 16 cm, more than 50% fractures were seen. According to Kaplan-Meier estimates, the primary patency rate at 12 months was significantly lower for patients with stent fractures (41.1% vs. 84.3%; $p = 0.0001$), demonstrating that fractures are associated with a higher rate of restenosis and occlusion (Fig. 1). Fractures were reported to be instigated by stiffer stent designs, and a higher number of stents were placed. To improve patency rates, more flexible nitinol stent designs have been developed.

Bare Stents
The FAST trial was a controlled, randomized trial that compared stand-alone PTA versus the use of a single Bard Luminexx 3 Vascular nitinol stent (C.R. Bard Inc.) in 244 patients with SFA lesions up to 10 cm. Only seven patients presented with CLI. However, the trial noted a trend in favor of stenting in diabetics, smokers, and patients with impaired distal runoff and heavily calcified lesions. Both last characteristics are evident in patients with CLI.

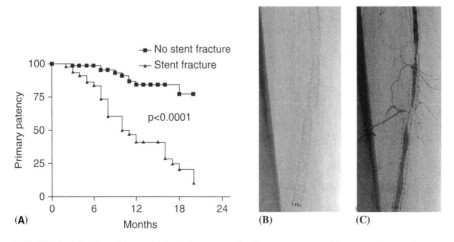

FIGURE 1 **(A)** Life table analysis of femoropopliteal stent patency. Absence of stent fracture correlates with significantly improved primary patency. **(B, C)** Angiographic demonstration of restenosis at two levels within a fractured SFA stent. *Source*: From Ref. 23.

Schillinger et al. (24) reported their results of nitinol stenting with the Absolute and Dynalink (Guidant, Indianapolis, Indiana, U.S.) stent versus PTA alone in long lesions (average 132 mm) of the SFA. Although only 3% of the patients presented with CLI, subgroup analysis showed no significant interaction between restenosis rate and stage of peripheral artery disease, implying that patients with CLI could benefit as much as claudicants from a PTA with stenting.

Drug-Eluting Stents

The Sirolimus-coated Cordis SMART nitinol self-expandable stent for the treatment of SFA disease (SIROCCO) trials (25,26) were randomized controlled studies, comparing the use of drug-coated stent versus bare nitinol stents in patients with chronic limb ischemia. Neither of the trials made any sub-analysis on the CLI population. The SIROCCO I trial randomized 36 patients but failed to reach the primary endpoint of improved in-stent mean percent diameter stenosis by quantitative angiography (22.6% in the sirolimus group vs. 30.9% in the control group; $p = $ NS). In a subgroup of five patients who received the slower-eluting sirolimus stent did appear to have a favorable outcome. The SIROCCO II trial randomized 57 patients to the slower-eluting sirolimus stents or control stents but also failed to reach significance with the same endpoints determined by quantitative angiography. Long-term follow-up of the slower-eluting formulation from SIROCCO I and II showed an early, statistically significant difference in the primary endpoint (mean stent diameter) but a loss of this difference at 18 months as determined by duplex sonography.

Currently, results from two breaking trials with drug-coated stents in the SFA are awaited to supply more evidence. First, the Cook Zilver PTX drug-eluting stent trial is a worldwide prospective study in SFA lesions up to 28 cm that combines results from a randomized arm comparing 240 PTA cases with 240 DES cases using the paclitaxel-coated Cook Zilver PTX stent (Cook Medical, Bloomington, Indiana, U.S.) and a nonrandomized arm including 550 patients treated with the same stent. At the 2008 CIRSE meeting in Copenhagen, Dr. Michael Dake presented a stent fracture rate of 1.5% and freedom of target lesion revascularization of 88% after one year. Second, the Strides study, a prospective nonrandomized European trial, enrolled 100 patients with femoropopliteal lesions up to 17 cm with the everolimus-eluting Dynalink-E (Abbott Vascular, Illinois, U.S.). Both trials are currently ongoing, and it is expected that their results will shed more light on the possible application of drug-eluting stents. A specific territory where drug-eluting stents may be most valuable is the small caliber crural vessels, where long lesions are frequently present. Further research is warranted.

Flexible Stent Designs

At the EuroPCR 2008 in Barcelona, Schillinger reported on the results of a trial with the Astron stent (Biotronik GmbH, Berlin, Germany), which is also characterized by a helically structured design, compared with PTA plus optional stenting. In a mixed population of 73 claudicants and CLI patients with SFA lesions up to 25 cm, primary patency rates were 48.9% in the cohort that received PTA plus optional stenting and 65.6% in the primary stenting group.

The DURABILITY trial is a prospective, nonrandomized, controlled trial to test the performance of the long stents (10–15 cm) in long SFA lesions (<14 cm). Only a minority of the patients (12.5%) in the trial had CLI, and no data on this specific subset are available yet. At the TCT 2008 conference in Washington, D.C., Dr. Dierk Scheinert presented a high 12-month primary patency rate of 91% and a fracture rate as low as 6%. This trial showed that stent elongation at the time of deployment compromises the durability and leads to lower patency in the long term as seven out of eight fractures occurred in stents that were elongated during deployment.

Nitinol Stent Grafts and Covered Stents

Stent grafts have been developed to imitate the surgical gold standard of a bypass by means of an endovascular approach. Initially, they were used for endovascular exclusion of arterial aneurysms, most frequently in the popliteal region. However, as restenosis rates have been high in long stenotic lesions of the SFA and popliteal region after PTA, interest in covered stents has grown to see if patency rates can be improved. As in open surgical bypass, the use of poly-tetrafluoroethylene (PTFE) material to cover the bare nitinol stents seemed to improve patency rates. The advantage of the system is that the PTFE cover acts as a barrier to intimal hyperplasia, something that is frequently seen after PTA.

In the only randomized trial of claudicants versus CLI treated with the Hemobahn, Hartung et al. (27) reported similar one-year primary patencies of 81.3% and 88.9%, respectively, if concomitant outflow-improving procedures were performed in the CLI group. The average lesion lengths were approximately 10 cm for both groups. However, as expected, the preoperative tibial outflow was significantly lower in the CLI group (with 0 to 1 tibial vessels in 18.7% of the claudicants and 88.9% of the CLI group). Outflow procedures, which primarily involved balloon angioplasty, were performed in 6.3% of the claudicants and 66.7% of the CLI group.

No large multicenter randomized trial results have been published evaluating the current Viabahn stent graft. The VIBRANT trial compares the results of the Viabahn prosthesis with bare nitinol stents. Results are still awaited.

Several small series have been published on the use of the Viabahn endoprosthesis for SFA treatment in patients with CLI. Railo and coworkers (28) reported on the use of the Viabahn PTFE-covered stent in a small series of 15 patients (73% CLI) and relatively short lesions (4–10 cm). They reported a primary patency of 93% at one year and 84% at two years. Bauermeister (29) evaluated the use of the Viabahn in 35 patients with more diffuse disease and a mean lesion length of 22 cm (74% with CLI). Approximately half of the patients had concomitant surgery in the form of common femoral surgical patching or ring-stripper procedure. A one-year primary patency of 73% by duplex scanning was reported. Kedora et al. (30) reported similar outcomes after Viabahn placement as compared with above the knee synthetic bypass for long lesions of the SFA (claudication and CLI). Primary and secondary patency rates at one year were approximately 75% and 85%, respectively.

Another stent graft recently investigated in a multicenter registry by Lenti et al. (31) is the aSpire stent (Vascular Architects Inc, San Jose, California, U.S.). Fifty percent of the treated limbs were in patients with CLI. In this multicenter experience, the one-year primary patency and secondary patency rates were

59% and 67%, respectively. Limb salvage rates in patients with CLI were also good (89.6%). The presence of CLI was associated with lower patency compared with claudicants (58% vs. 74%, respectively). CLI was the only significant factor affecting secondary patency but overall these patients also showed a favorable outcome with low morbidity. Intimal hyperplasia remained the primary cause for graft failure.

Cryoplasty

Cryoplasty, commercially available as the PolarCath (Boston Scientific, Natick, Massachusetts, U.S.), uses liquid nitrous oxide to inflate and cool the balloon to −10°C. The cooling of the vessel wall is hypothesized to induce apoptosis in the smooth muscle cells of the vessel wall, reduce elastic recoil, and decrease intimal hyperplasia, thus potentially reducing restenosis in the long term (32). The PolarCath system is available in balloon diameters of 2.5 to 8 mm and lengths from 2 to 10 cm. The smaller balloons are guided by 0.014″ wires and the larger through a 0.035″ wire.

No data are available on the efficacy of cryoplasty in patients with CLI. Although short and midterm patency rates in lesions shorter than 10 cm are comparable with PTA outcomes, it has not been established if the technique of cryoplasty offers any real advantage over PTA, with or without stenting.

Cutting and Scoring Balloons

The advantage of cutting balloons over regular PTA balloons is that they focus the dilation force at the tips of the atherotomes (4 microsurgical blades attached on the surface of the balloon). This allows for a more gentle dilatation of the vessel and less vessel wall disruption with less risk of major dissection, reduced elastic recoil, and more effective dilatation. It is thought to be more applicable in short calcified lesions or anastamotic or intragraft lesions. The cutting balloon (Boston Scientific, Natick, Massachusetts, U.S.) is now available in larger diameters (up to 8 mm) but its overall length of 1 or 2 cm still limits its use in long or diffuse SFA lesions.

Similarly, the exact role or advantage of the AngioSculpt scoring balloon (AngioScore, Inc, Fremont, California, U.S.) over traditional methods is also yet to be ascertained in the SFA region. The AngioSculpt is a semi-compliant balloon encircled by three spiral struts with a nitinol scoring element, which theoretically provides targeted scoring of lesions by concentrating the dilation force, thus minimizing barotrauma, elastic recoil, and uncontrolled dissection. This may improve the outcome of the intervention and reduce the number of stents required. The nitinol material is thought to increase device flexibility and therefore deliverability. The use of the AngioScore balloon is currently being investigated in a prospective, multicenter, nonrandomized clinical trial for the treatment of femoropopliteal stenotic disease (MASCOT).

Excimer Laser

The 308-nm excimer laser uses flexible fiberoptic catheters to deliver bursts of ultraviolet energy in short pulses. Tissue is ablated with direct contact, without a rise in temperature to surrounding tissue. An additional benefit of ultraviolet light is its ability to ablate thrombus material and to inhibit platelet aggregation (33).

Laser ablation can be used to treat occlusions and diffuse atherosclerotic disease, with less distal embolization and less need for bailout PTA and stenting. It can also be used in a step-by-step fashion to traverse chronic total occlusions in which the guidewire is advanced as far as possible, after which the laser can penetrate the occlusion further until a new channel is found by the wire.

In the Laser Angioplasty for Critical limb Ischemia (LACI) phase II clinical trial, 145 patients (155 critically ischemic limbs of which 92% were occluded) were treated with excimer laser (Spectranetics, Colorado Springs, Colorado, U.S.), with or without additional intervention. All patients included in this pivotal trial were poor candidates for surgical revascularization. As expected, the majority of patients had multilevel disease, and the mean treatment length was >16 cm. The SFA and popliteal segment were treated in 66% of the affected limbs. After six months, an excellent limb salvage rate of 93% was achieved (34).

These results were confirmed by the LACI Belgium trial, which used the same inclusion and exclusion criteria as the original LACI trial. This prospective, five-center Belgian study enrolled 48 patients who presented with 51 critically ischemic limbs and who were poor surgical bypass candidates. Initial treatment success was achieved in all 51 limbs. After 6 months, a limb salvage rate of 90.5% was reported, with a freedom of recurring CLI in 86% of the patients (35).

The results of the CLiRPath Excimer Laser to enlarge Lumen Openings (CELLO) clinical trial, evaluating the efficacy of the CLiRpath Excimer Laser system (Spectranetics) are awaited. Preliminary data presented at the TCT 2007 conference in Washington, D.C. by Dr. Rajesh Dave suggest a durability of the procedure through freedom from target lesion revascularization in 86% of the patients through six months following the initial procedure.

CONCLUSION AND FUTURE PERSPECTIVES

Not only because of the rapid development of endovascular techniques as outlined above but also because of changing practice patterns and changing patient and doctor preferences, it is difficult to evaluate the efficacy of the different treatment strategies in a randomized and controlled manner. Because there is a lack of hard level 1 data, it is not possible to give definitive guidelines and an evidence-based treatment approach for CLI. Despite this, in recent years there has been a notable shift in treating patients with CLI preferentially by endovascular means in most vascular practices. This has been done so with encouraging results.

For patients with CLI in relatively good health, with a reasonable life expectancy one can argue that surgical bypass with a venous conduit still remains the gold standard. It should be noted, however, that even a failed endovascular procedure does not prevent a subsequent open bypass. In this setting, the endovascular procedure can even sometimes be regarded as a bridge to bypass, alleviating rest pain and enabling minimal tissue loss to heal.

Adequate proximal inflow and the status of distal runoff vessels have been shown to affect the durability of both surgical bypass and endovascular procedures (36,37). Tibial patency may explain why both surgical and endovascular procedures appear to be more durable in claudicants than patients with CLI. With regard to stent grafts in general, adequate predilatation and postdilatation are of great importance to allow full stent placement and deployment. One must also not forget that where bare stents can preserve collaterals, covered stents cannot. However, complete coverage of atherosclerotic segments should always be favored against the preservation of collaterals. It appears appropriate to check the stent graft at regular intervals for follow-up evaluation, with ankle-brachial index and color-flow duplex scanning to evaluate vessel and graft narrowing to prevent late thrombosis of the graft.

Special interest to aggressive antiplatelet therapy must be maintained. Possibly there is a benefit to dual antiplatelet therapy to preserve longer-term patency after placement of covered stents and to prevent short-term thrombosis.

Over the past years, several reports on the efficacy of angioplasty in patients with CLI have been published, and they outline the trend to treat lesions by endovascular therapy in favor of surgery when technically feasible (38–40). Angioplasty with or without stenting has become more and more popular as primary and secondary revascularization method for CLI. In this setting, open surgery is reserved for failed endovascular revascularization or continuing signs of CLI. They show that the trend toward treating lesions resulting in CLI by endovascular means have not led to deterioration in treatment outcomes (38–42). Primary cumulative patency, limb salvage, and midterm survival rates for angioplasty were comparable to bypass surgery in spite of a high restenosis rate in the midterm after an endovascular approach. In general, it can be noted that when evaluating the results of different techniques in CLI patients, the short-term clinical improvement in CLI patients may be a more important outcome than long-term patency rates, as 50% of the patients die within five years because of their comorbidity.

Furthermore, studies show that preferential stenting in long lesions or occlusions in the SFA and popliteal region does seem better than angioplasty alone. It has become clear that the presence of stent fractures in longer lesions is associated with decreased patency rates. Further technical evolution of the design of stents and delivery devices may be able to improve results in the near future.

Neointimal hyperplasia is the most important factor in the outcome after PTA and stenting of the SFA and all other vascular beds. Stents themselves and stent fractures lead to an acceleration of the intimal hyperplasia. The introduction and further development of drug-eluting stents, absorbable metal stent, and helically structured stents (flexibility) will probably lead to ever better results for the endovascular therapy of patients with CLI. However, further research is needed, and at this moment in time definitive proof is not yet available. Future randomized trials should emphasize on studying the efficacy and results of this change in CLI management, although constant evolution of endovascular techniques will always make this difficult.

REFERENCES

1. Cavanagh PR, Lipsky BA, Bradbury AW, et al. Treatment for diabetic foot ulcers. Lancet 2005; 366:1725–1735.
2. Burns P, Gough S, Bradbury AW. Management of peripheral arterial disease in primary care. BMJ 2003; 326:584–588.
3. Lepantalo M, Matzke S. Outcome of unreconstructed chronic critical leg ischaemia. Eur J Vasc Endovasc Surg 1996; 11:153–157.
4. Dawson DL, Mills JL. Critical limb ischemia. Curr Treat Options Cardiovasc Med 2007; 9(2):159–170.
5. Taylor LM, Edwards JM, Porter JM. Present status of the reversed vein bypass grafting: five-year results of a modern series. J Vasc Surg 1990; 11:193–206.

6. Belkin M, Knox J, Donaldson MC, et al. Infrainguinal arterial reconstruction with nonreversed greater saphenous vein. J Vasc Surg 1996; 24:957–962.

7. Hunink MG, Wong JB, Donaldson MC, et al. Patency results of percutaneous and surgical revascularisation for femoropopliteal arterial disease. Med Decis Making 1994; 14:71–81.

8. Allen BT, Reilly JM, Rubin BG, et al. Femoropopliteal bypass for claudication: vein vs. PTFE. Ann Vasc Surg 1996; 10:178–185.

9. Muluk SC, Muluk VS, Kelley ME, et al. Outcome events in patients with claudication: a 15-year study in 2777 patients. J Vasc Surg 2001; 33:251–258.

10. Källerö KS, Berqqvist D, Cederholm C, et al. Late mortality and morbidity after arterial reconstruction: the influence of arteriosclerosis in popliteal artery trifurcation. J Vasc Surg 1985; 2:541–546.

11. Second European Consensus Document on Chronic Critical Limb Ischemia. Eur J Vasc Surg 1992; 6(suppl A):1–32.

12. Dormandy JA, Rutherford RB. Management of peripheral arterial disease (PAD). TASC Working Group. TransAtlantic Inter-Society Consensus (TASC). J Vasc Surg 2000; 31(1 pt 2):S1–S296.

13. Goshima KR, Mills JL, Hughes JD. A new look at outcomes after infrainguinal bypass surgery: traditional reporting standards systematically underestimate the expenditure of effort required to attain limb salvage. J Vasc Surg 2004; 39:330–335.

14. Adam DJ, Beard JD, Cleveland T, et al. Bypass versus angioplasty in severe ischaemia of the leg (BASIL): multicentre, randomised controlled trial. Lancet 2005; 366(9501):1925–1934.

15. Hynes N, Akhtar Y, Manning B, et al. Subintimal angioplasty as a primary modality in the management of critical limb ischemia: comparison to bypass grafting for aortoiliac and femoropopliteal occlusive disease. J Endovasc Ther 2004; 11:460–471.

16. Dorruci V. Treatment of superficial femoral artery occlusive disease. J Cardiovasc Surg 2004; 45:193–201.

17. Norgren L, Hiatt WR, Dormandy JA, et al.; TASC II Working Group. Inter-Society Consensus for the Management of Peripheral Arterial Disease (TASCII). Eur J Vasc Endovasc Surg 2007; 33(suppl 1):S1–S75.

18. Capek P, McLean GK, Berkowitz HD. Femoropopliteal angioplasty. Factors influencing long-term success. Circulation 1991; 83(suppl 2):I70–I80.

19. Met R, Van Lienden KP, Koelemay MJ, et al. Subintimal angioplasty for peripheral arterial occlusive disease: a systematic review. Cardiovasc Intervent Radioll 2008; 31(4):687–697.

20. Bolia A. Subintimal angioplasty in lower limb ischaemia. J Cardiovasc Surg (Torino) 2005; 46(4):385–394 (review).

21. Becquemin JP, Favre JP, Marzelle J, et al. Systematic versus selective stent placement after superficial femoral artery balloon angioplasty: a multicenter prospective randomized study. J Vasc Surg 2003; 37(3):487–494.

22. Mewissen MW. Self-expanding nitinol stents in the femoropopliteal segment: technique and mid-term results. Tech Vasc Interv Radiol 2004; 7(1):2–5.

23. Scheinert D, Scheinert S, Sax J, et al. Prevalence and clinical impact of stent fractures after femoropopliteal stenting. J Am Coll Cardiol 2005; 45:312–315.

24. Schillinger M, Sabeti S, Loewe C, et al. Balloon angioplasty versus implantation of nitinol stents in the superficial femoral artery. N Engl J Med 2006; 354(18):1879–1888.

25. Duda SH, Bosiers M, Lammer J, et al. Sirolimus-eluting versus bare nitinol stent for obstructive superficial femoral artery disease: the SIROCCO II trial. J Vasc Interv Radiol 2005; 16:331–338.

26. Duda SH, Bosiers M, Lammer J, et al. Drug-eluting and bare nitinol stents for the treatment of atherosclerotic lesions in the superficial femoral artery: long-term results from the SIROCCO trial. J Endovasc Ther 2006; 13:701–710.

27. Hartung O, Otero A, Dubuc M, et al. Efficacy of Hemobahn in the treatment of superficial femoral artery lesions in patients with acute or critical ischemia: a comparative study with claudicants. Eur J Vasc Endovasc Surg 2005; 30(3):300–306.

28. Railo M, Roth WD, Edgren J, et al. Preliminary results with endoluminal femoropopliteal thrupass. Ann Chir Gynaecol 2001; 90(1):15–18.
29. Bauermeister G. Endovascular stent-grafting in the treatment of superficial femoral artery occlusive disease. J Endovasc Ther 2001; 8(3):315–320.
30. Kedora J, Hohmann S, Garrett W, et al. Randomized comparison of percutaneous Viabahn stent grafts vs prosthetic femoral-popliteal bypass in the treatment of superficial femoral arterial occlusive disease. J Vasc Surg 2007; 45:10–16.
31. Lenti M, Cieri E, De Rango P, et al. Endovascular treatment of long lesions of the superficial femoral artery: results from a multicenter registry of a spiral, covered polytetrafluoroethylene stent. J Vasc Surg 2007; 45(1):32–39.
32. Yiu WK, Cheng SW, Sumpio BE. Vascular smooth muscle cell apoptosis induced by "supercooling" and rewarming. J Vasc Interv Radiol 2006; 17:1971–1977.
33. Lawrence JB, Prevosti LG, Kramer WS, et al. Pulsed laser and thermal ablation of atherosclerotic plaque: morphometrically defined surface thrombogenicity in studies using an annular perfusion chamber. J Am Coll Cardiol 1992; 19:1091–1100.
34. Laird JR, Zeller T, Gray BH, et al. Limb salvage following laser-assisted angioplasty for critical limb ischemia: results of the LACI multicenter trial. J Endovasc Ther 2006; 13:1–11.
35. Bosiers M, Peeters P, Van Elst F, et al. Excimer laser assisted angioplasty for critical limb ischemia: results of the LACI Belgium study. Eur J Vasc Endovasc Surg 2005; 29 (6):613–619.
36. Gallino A, Mahler F, Probst P, et al. Percutaneous transluminal angioplasty of the arteries of the lower limbs: a 5 year follow-up. Circulation 1984; 70:619–623.
37. Jeans WD, Armstrong S, Cole SE, et al. Fate of patients undergoing transluminal angioplasty for lower-limb ischemia. Radiology 1990; 177:559–564.
38. Dosluoglu HH, O'Brien-Irr MS, Lukan J, et al. Does preferential use of endovascular interventions by vascular surgeons improve limb salvage, control of symptoms, and survival of patients with critical limb ischemia? Am J Surg 2006; 192(5):572–576.
39. Kudo T, Chandra FA, Kwun WH, et al. Changing pattern of surgical revascularization for critical limb ischemia over 12 years: endovascular vs. open bypass surgery. J Vasc Surg 2006; 44(2):304–313.
40. Haider SN, Kavanagh EG, Forlee M, et al. Two-year outcome with preferential use of infrainguinal angioplasty for critical ischemia. J Vasc Surg 2006; 43(3):504–512.
41. Hynes N, Mahendran B, Manning B, et al. The influence of subintimal angioplasty on level of amputation and limb salvage rates in lower limb critical ischaemia: a 15-year experience. Eur J Vasc Endovasc Surg 2005; 30:290–299.
42. Nasr MK, McCarthy RJ, Hardman J, et al. The increasing role of percutaneous transluminal angioplasty in the primary management of critical limb ischaemia. Eur J Vasc Endovasc Surg 2002; 23(5):398–403.

Chronic Total Occlusions: Techniques and Devices

Donald L. Jacobs and Raghunandan Motaganahalli
Department of Surgery, Saint Louis University, Saint Louis, Missouri, U.S.A.

INTRODUCTION

Endovascular reconstruction of the infrainguinal arteries is increasingly utilized as an alternative to surgery in the management of critical limb ischemia. Although surgical bypass has been a well-established standard treatment for critical limb ischemia, advances in endovascular techniques have allowed for improved acute and long-term success in the treatment of these anatomically complex patients. Acceptance of these new techniques has also been driven by the inherent morbidity of open surgical bypass in the ever increasingly obese and aged patient population presenting with critical limb ischemia.

To be successful with endovascular treatment of critical limb ischemia, one must be skilled at treatment of chronic total occlusions (CTOs), as CTOs are found in a large majority of patients with critical limb ischemia and multilevel disease is the norm. In this chapter, we will discuss some of the available techniques and devices that facilitate treatment of CTOs, including devices that allow for acute success such as specific wires, catheters, laser and recanalization devices, as well as true lumen reentry devices. Reconstruction of these lesions after successful traversal will also be detailed, but additional information on the long-term outcomes with these various reconstructions is covered in other chapters.

Although it is tempting to address all occlusive diseases with endovascular means, there are factors such as the site and extent, or length of occlusion and degree of calcification that would indicate poor response to a percutaneous approach (1–4). It is important to conduct an intervention with a complete understanding of how an acute or subsequent failure of endovascular procedure might impact the options for future revascularization. As such, some aspects of patient selection will also be addressed as they relate to the choice and success of the techniques described.

CROSSING CTOs

Techniques used for crossing CTOs range from the simple to elaborate. As with most things, we start simple and escalate to the elaborate as the situation demands. We have classified the devices into wires and catheters, ablative devices, and reentry devices. It is our goal to describe the various techniques used to treat CTOs with a variety of devices, but we will not be exhaustive in discussing all of the individual wires, catheters, and devices available. Instead, the attributes of selected devices and how they are used will be described so as to provide readers the background to utilize not only these specific devices but also others with similar or varied characteristics.

The most tried and true method for crossing a CTO has been the sub-intimal dissection method of Bolia (5). The acute success noted in the early papers with this technique was 80% (6), and it has been routinely reported in later series to be near 90% (4,7,8). Technical success is higher in short noncalcified lesions and in nondiabetics (3,4,7). Some have proposed that the reconstruction after crossing the subintimal point is easier and has better long-term patency (9,10). However, the idea that crossing an occlusion is subintimal or not is unrealistic. It is proposed that with most long CTOs, there is passage of the wire in the subintimal space at some point along the occlusion in the vast majority of cases despite what technique is used.

Although the inability to reenter the true lumen distally has been the primary limitation to success in crossing CTOs (11,12), there is little to be gained by trying to avoid the subintimal space for traversal until one reaches the distal end of the occlusion and gets trapped in the subintimal space tracking beyond the occlusion. At this point, the reentry into the lumen is easily accomplished, and these techniques are discussed later.

Access

The technique for subintimal passage through a CTO is best accomplished with good supportive access. The push needed cannot be delivered in most instances without the support of a sheath of 6 or 7 Fr placed within a few centimeters of the occlusion. For iliac CTOs, retrograde access from the femoral artery is ideal for providing maximal support to cross the occlusion. For a proximal superficial femoral occlusion, a contralateral retrograde access is best with a sheath up and over into the common femoral or proximal superficial femoral artery (SFA) as close to the occlusion as possible to provide support. For a more distal SFA or popliteal occlusion, a contralateral approach can still be used, but for a resistant lesion, the antegrade ipsilateral femoral access can provide more direct support for crossing an occlusion. Tibial artery occlusions are best approached with antegrade access to provide the needed support but are often treated in conjunction with proximal disease and, in these cases, will often require treatment from the contralateral approach. Maximal support from contralateral femoral access can be provided by a braided sheath such as the 55-cm Raabe sheath (Cook, Indianapolis, Indiana, U.S.). Although most devices today can be placed via 6-Fr sheaths, a larger-diameter sheath will provide for more support to penetrate and cross an occlusion. Device options are increased as well with larger sheaths. For these reasons, we routinely use 7-Fr access for femoral-popliteal CTOs. For more distal lesions approached from contralateral access, a longer sheath such as a 90-cm Shuttle sheath (Cook) may be useful to provide additional support to cross a resistant tibial occlusion.

Ultrasound guidance for femoral access is a valuable tool to gain safe and effective access in many patients with complex arterial disease inherent in critical limb ischemia patients. Obesity is the primary indication for its use in our practice, followed by an absent pulse due to ipsilateral common iliac occlusion. It is also helpful to define locations of disease in the common femoral and adjacent vessels to allow for access in less diseased segments. Ultrasound guidance is also a key tool for gaining antegrade access in many, if not most, patients as it allows for access above the bifurcation but below the inguinal ligament. It also provides access without deformation of the soft tissue that comes with palpation of the pulse for guidance. In obese patients, the release of the compression can result in a tortuous pathway of the wire in the soft tissue that will allow for deviation and difficulty with tracking of the sheath at the time of placement into the artery.

Once access is established, the patient is anticoagulated. This prevents thrombus from forming in the subintimal plane during crossing and treatment of the occlusion. Bleeding from perforation of the vessel with early anti-coagulation was originally a concern noted by Bolia and others, but this risk now seems minimal compared with the risk of thrombosis formation in subintimal space and possible embolization once the flow is reestablished.

CTO Penetration

Penetration of the cap of the CTO is critical to any technique of crossing a CTO. For an intentional subintimal dissection, the wire is directed to the edge of the cap to facilitate entry into the subintimal space by a directional wire tip and/or an angled catheter. Our standard wire and catheter combinations are the 0.035″ angled Glidewire combined with a 4-Fr angled Glide catheter (Terumo, Somerset, New Jersey, U.S.), or combined with the 0.035″ Quick-Cross catheter (Spectranetics, Colorado Springs, Colorado, U.S.), a straight, tapered, supportive catheter designed for crossing occlusions. If there is a branch point at the top of the occlusion, the wire tends to direct into the branch rather than penetrate the occlusion. If the directional control of the wire and catheter is not sufficient to achieve the penetration, then the sheath can be positioned very close to the occlusion to provide more direct axial force with the wire and catheter. Occasionally, if additional support is needed, the sheath can be used with its dilator placed up to the fibrous cap of the occlusion to facilitate the initial penetration with the wire. This is very useful in the iliac occlusions where the sheath is easily placed up to the occlusion. A more frequent approach to a resistant femoral-popliteal occlusion is to place a small catheter at the top of the occlusion and reverse the standard support Glidewire to penetrate the cap with the stiff back end of the wire for 1 cm and then track the catheter into the occlusion for 1 cm and withdraw the wire and re-advance with the soft tip into the catheter to cross the occlusion. To minimize the risk of perforation, only a small catheter is used to follow the stiff end of the wire only a short distance into the occlusion. After advancing the catheter into the cap of the occlusion, the wire is reversed back to advance with the soft tip end. With re-advancing the soft tip end, perforation should be apparent if the wire does not follow the vessel's path. Small perforations of the vessel made by the wire or catheter during traversal of a CTO will typically not need treatment beyond prolonged balloon inflation. However, covered stents should be available if one plans to embark on treating these difficult CTOs as vessel perforation and rupture is a risk at the time of angioplasty.

CTO Traversal
0.035″ Wires and Catheters

After initial penetration of the occlusion, crossing in the subintimal plane is best accomplished with the Glidewire looped for 2 to 3 cm, with the Glide catheter used to advance the looped wire along with the catheter across the occlusion. If resistance at a point along the occlusion is felt and the loop is not advancing, then manipulation of the wire back into the catheter and redirection of the wire tip within the occlusion will then allow for further progress in crossing the

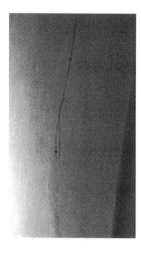

FIGURE 1 Wire looped in subintimal crossing of mid-SFA occlusion. *Abbreviation*: SFA, superficial femoral artery.

occlusion. Crossing long segments of the subintimal plane with the leading Glidewire tip not looped may be more likely to result in a perforation or in a spiraling of the wire around the core of the occlusion (Fig. 1). Subsequent angioplasty of a spiraled tract through the occlusion seems to result in more complex dissections than the non-spiraled tract of the wire with looped-tip wire crossing of the occlusion. Variations in the wires and catheters for subintimal recanalization can include straight catheters and wires; tapered supported catheters are also effective and are more a personal choice. Ideally, a wire used for subintimal crossing has a hydrophilic coating to minimize drag, particularly in longer occlusions. Hydrophilic coating on the supporting catheter is also useful to facilitate catheter traversal of the subintimal space.

With good support from a sheath, such wire and catheter techniques are successful in crossing of 90% or more of occlusions (11,13). When an occlusion cannot be crossed with the above technique, the first step is to insure that your access and catheter support is maximized. If resistance to crossing occurs after traversal of a significant length of occlusion, particularly a calcified occlusion, then angioplasty of the tract established so far may decrease the drag on the catheter and provide better force to cross the resistant segment. Advancement of the sheath closer to the resistant segment or bulking up the size of the support by adding a coaxial guide can also be useful (Fig. 2). Finally, probing the resistant point with the back end of the Glidewire as described above for penetration of the occlusion cap can allow passage, but this also carries some risk of penetration of wire outside the vessel.

After reaching the point of reconstitution of the vessel beyond the occlusion, the wire is again withdrawn into the catheter and advanced in a nonlooped fashion into the distal lumen. The angle of the Glidewire should pass without deformation along the lumen of the distal vessel, and the catheter then advanced to just below the occlusion and the wire removed to allow for injection of contrast to confirm true lumen reentry. If the wire does not pass freely into the distal true lumen, then retraction and manipulation of the wire and catheter just proximal to the end of the occlusion may afford true lumen passage. Injection of a small amount of contrast in the false lumen, taking care to inject slowly and not pressurize and dissect the vessel distally, can sometimes define a tract to the

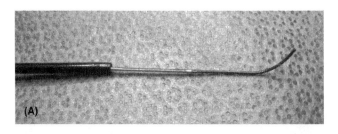

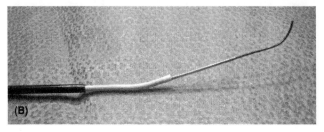

FIGURE 2 (A) Sheath and 0.035″ Quick-Cross catheter and Glidewire. (B) Coaxial arrangement of 7-Fr sheath, 6-Fr guide, 0.035″ Quick-Cross catheter and Glidewire.

true lumen and direct your wire manipulations. Balloon angioplasty of the distal occlusion may also open up a channel to the true lumen, and the wire can be centered and supported by the inflated balloon catheter to allow for manipulation through to the distal true lumen. Finally, if in a straight segment of the vessel, the use of the back end of the Glidewire to penetrate the distal aspect of the occlusion similar to the technique described above for entry to the top of an occlusion can allow for true lumen reentry. If these maneuvers fail, then use of either a true lumen reentry device or conversion to a combined retrograde recanalization (SAFARI technique) is required. These techniques are discussed later in the chapter.

0.014″ Wires and Catheters

Wires that are marketed for CTOs are all coronary wires and, as such, are all 0.014″ wires. These coronary CTO wires do not usually have hydrophilic coating. They are very useful for true lumen traversal of an occlusion, particularly in the tibial vessels, usually with the use of a 0.014″ supporting catheter. The combination of a 0.014″ wire with a supporting catheter is also a good choice for acute or chronic ischemia patients who may have acute occlusions of previously stenotic femoral-popliteal vessels, as these wires and small catheters may allow traversal more easily in the true lumen in such lesions. However, the hydrophilic 0.014″ wires are not as effective as 0.035″ wires for subintimal passage in femoral-popliteal occlusions.

Wires (0.014″) designed for crossing total occlusions have a stiff shaft and a firm nontapered tip that is effective at initiating entrance to the fibrous cap. CTO wires are particularly useful for crossing tibial artery occlusions and again are best if used with a supporting catheter. Support with either a small catheter such as the Quick-Cross 0.014″ catheter or with a low profile over the wire angioplasty balloon such as the Amphirion balloon catheter (ev3, Plymouth,

Minnesota, U.S.) is also effective and can then be tracked directly over the wire to accomplish predilation or treatment of the lesions after providing the support for wire crossing.

Our preferred 0.014" wire for crossing a CTO is the Confianza from Asahi (Abbott Vascular, Redwood City, California, U.S.). The stiff tip and supportive shaft make it able to penetrate and cross with reasonable force in a "push through" method. The tip deflection force of 9 g makes it the stiffest tip available in a 0.014" wire. The lack of hydrophilic coating and its relative lack of steerability limit the Confianza's usefulness for other purposes. The Asahi Miracle Bros (Abbott Vascular) comes in various tip stiffnesses from 3 to 6 g and is on a slightly less supportive shaft, but does provide some degree of torque and maneuverability that can allow one the ability to negotiate to get to an occlusion, though is less forceful for crossing an occlusion than the Confianza. Another wire available in the United States that has a particularly stiff tip useful for crossing an occlusion is the Persuader 9 wire (Medtronic, Santa Rosa, California, U.S.).

As noted previously, there can be an advantage of crossing some acute or subacute occlusions with a hydrophilic wire. Hydrophilic wires employ the "slip through" method to cross occlusions. Our hydrophilic 0.014" wire of choice for peripheral use is the Choice PT extra support wire (Boston Scientific, Natick, Massachusetts, U.S.). This wire offers good support and tip control and torque with excellent ability to negotiate long diffuse stenoses or occlusions of the tibial arteries with its hydrophilic coating. Alternative 0.014" wires for stenotic or occluded vessels are numerous, and again, the choice is a personal one, which has more to do with familiarity than with specific properties that allow for success. It is a general rule that the more torquable, steerable, trackable, and nontrappable the wire is, the less likely it will be able to provide force for tip penetration and pushability to allow for traversal of a chronic occlusion.

ADJUNCTIVE TOOLS FOR TRAVERSAL OF CTOs
Controlled Blunt Microdissection
Frontrunner catheter (Cordis, Miami Lakes, Florida, U.S.) is a specially designed catheter for penetration and crossing CTOs of the coronary and peripheral arteries. The end of the catheter has a small micro dissector that can spread its jaws with the repetitive movement of a pistol grip mechanism (Fig. 3). It is a low-profile device with a crossing profile of 0.039" and comes with a 4.5-Fr microguide catheter for support. With actuation, the jaws open to a maximum of 2.3-mm outer diameter. This device is mainly utilized in the coronary angioplasty; however, it may also be effective in peripheral CTOs. In a series of 44 iliac and femoral-popliteal CTOs that had failed routine catheter wire methods for crossing, micro dissection was employed, with a technical success in 40 (91%) of these lesions (14).

Controlled blunt micro dissection can facilitate penetration of the organized cap of a thrombotic CTO and allow for initiation of true lumen passage. The relatively delicate action of the Frontrunner may not be adequate to cross very fibrous or calcified lesions. The Frontrunner may be particularly useful for primary utilization for penetration of an occlusion in certain anatomic circumstances. These include the penetration of an occlusion that is flush at a branch point such as a proximal SFA occlusion where a dissection from subintimal

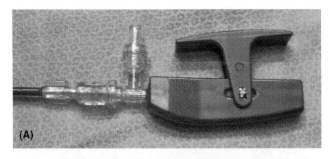

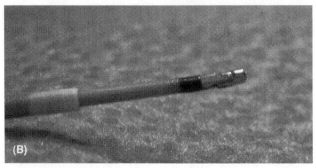

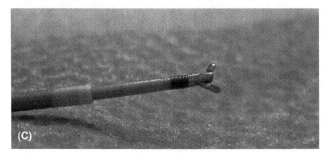

FIGURE 3 (**A**) Frontrunner catheter with trigger handle. (**B**) Dissection jaws of catheter tip closed. (**C**) Dissection jaws of catheter tip spread open.

passage at that level is undesirable. The Frontrunner may also be useful in crossing of a proximal common iliac occlusion approached from contralateral femoral access where the guiding catheter has less support to force penetration of the wire into and across the occlusion.

Radiofrequency Ablation Wire with Optical Coherence Reflectometry Guidance

The Safe-Cross system (IntraLuminal Therapeutics, Carlsbad, California, U.S.) uses a radiofrequency (RF) ablation wire combined with a fiber optic central core that can transmit light. The RF energy transducer can heat the tip of the wire to focally ablate tissue and facilitate passage of the wire through an occlusion. To guide the wire so as not to perforate outside of the vessel, near-infrared light is generated and transmitted through the wire to the tip where it is differentially absorbed, transmitted, and scattered in defined fashion by different tissues. Optical coherence reflectometry (OCR) is the principle that measures the reflectivity of near-infrared light to distinguish different tissue types. There is not an actual image of the artery reproduced by the monitor of the OCR, but rather the system gives an audible signal and a crude graphic tracing of the tissue characteristics directly in front of the tip of the catheter and warns the operator if the catheter is directed at the arterial wall. The OCR has a reported resolution of 15 μm at the catheter tip and the ability to look forward. When the system notes that the wire is directed at the wall, the operator redirects the wire so as to show a signal consistent with plaque/thrombus before activating the RF energy and advancing the wire. The reported primary limitation of the device in practice is that it is not very steerable and requires the use of an angled catheter or microguide to orient the tip. It is also reported that the redirection may often require the wire to be removed and a standard wire such as a Glidewire be used to redirect the catheter and the Safe-Cross wire then reintroduced. Use of the Safe-Cross system is reported for coronary and peripheral use in nonrandomized single-center trials. One reported series of lower extremity arterial occlusions included 17 patients with 18 peripheral lesions in whom crossing with conventional wires had previously failed; the Safe-Cross system was successful in crossing 100% of the CTOs in patients in whom conventional wire crossing had failed, whereas clinical success occurred in 94% of these patients (15).

The Safe-Cross system has not been widely utilized and remains to be studied in the peripheral interventions in a randomized controlled fashion. The ability of forward-looking OCR combined with an ablative device such as laser or directional atherectomy may have significant potential in the future in the treatment of arterial occlusions.

Excimer Laser Ablation Catheter

Excimer laser catheters have been in use for treatment of arterial occlusive disease for over 18 years but gained new impetus after the Laser-assisted Angioplasty for Critical Limb Ischemia (LACI) trial (16) as a useful tool in peripheral arterial interventions. The CLiRpath laser (Spectranetics) has cooler temperatures and shorter penetration depth than the earlier "hot tip" lasers that failed in their application to atherosclerotic disease. The excimer laser allows effective debulking of atherosclerotic lesions and has reported success in complex lower extremity interventions for critical limb ischemia (16). Use of a laser catheter as an energy source to allow for penetration and traversal of CTOs has also been reported, but with less well-defined outcomes. The "step technique" of crossing occlusions with the laser involves placing the laser catheter at the top of the occlusion without a wire extending out of the catheter. The laser is activated and the lesion penetrated for a short distance of 1 to 2 mm with the laser, the wire is then advanced out of the end of the laser catheter a short distance until resistance is met, and the laser is then activated and advanced to that point over the wire. With further ablation of the lesion at the point of resistance, the wire is again advanced to penetrate further. This sequence is repeated in a stepwise fashion to eventually traverse the entire lesion.

The limitation of the step technique is that the laser action can cause perforation. The lack of directional control of the laser catheter and the prolonged activation that may be required to ablate a resistant point in a lesion where the laser may be subintimal are likely to contribute to a perforation. The laser is also not able to ablate, penetrate, and cross some very calcified lesions that are often the point of failure when crossing a CTO with conventional catheter and wire techniques. As such, in our group's experience, there has been limited success with the laser when applied as an adjunctive device to cross a CTO after failure of conventional techniques. Although routine use of the laser as an initial device to cross CTOs before dissection with catheters and wires may allow for improved results, we have not felt the need to use it as a primary tool in crossing CTOs because of the expense and relatively rare failure to cross a CTO with conventional wires and catheters. The laser's role in definitive treatment of CTOs is discussed later in the section "Debulking of Plaque."

Ultrasound Energy Plaque Disruption Catheter

CROSSER catheter (FlowCardia, Sunnyvale, California, U.S.) is an ultrasonic energy delivery catheter that disrupts the plaque and thrombus in a CTO directly distal to the tip of the catheter, which then allows for passage of a wire through the occlusion. The peripheral application of this catheter is a 0.018" wire–based device that tracks monorail over any wire of choice. The energy is supplied by a small generator that connects to the end of the catheter. Current is then delivered to piezoelectric crystals contained within the transducer, resulting in crystal expansion and contraction propagating high-frequency mechanical vibration to the tip of the CROSSER catheter, which aids in the recanalization of a CTO. This device is in the Peripheral Approach To Recanalization In Occluded Totals (PATRIOT) trial that concluded enrollment in September 2007, and the device was released in the US in December 2007.

Image guidance with forward-looking intravascular ultrasound (IVUS) and optical coherence tomography (OCT) devices is in development. The ability to manipulate devices with magnetic guidance holds some promise in the treatment of CTOs and may eventually be coupled with image guidance from computed tomography (CT) data to allow for driving device through an occlusion. When coupled with energy-delivering technology such as laser, RF, or ultrasonic transducers at the front end of these forward-looking, image-guided devices, the systems should provide the vascular specialist with little reason not to succeed in crossing CTOs.

TRUE LUMEN REENTRY

As noted previously, failure to obtain true lumen reentry is the primary reason for acute technical failure in treatment of a CTO. Additional tools and techniques are required if one is able to cross the lesion but unable to obtain an entry back into true lumen with the standard techniques described above. In our experience, the iliac CTOs will require one of these adjunctive techniques more frequently than femoral-popliteal CTOs. The extent of calcification of the vessel frequently dictates the need for something other than standard wire catheter maneuvers. The true lumen reentry devices facilitate precise access back into the true lumen, preserve the collateral flow, and limit the extent of the dissection and subsequent stenting (13). They may reduce the fluoroscopic and procedural time required to reenter the true lumen and complete the revascularization. Most importantly, they can virtually eliminate the most common cause of technical failure of the procedure.

Fluoroscopic-Guided Needle Reentry Catheter

Catheters meant to facilitate the true lumen reentry include the Outback LTD catheter (Cordis). This is a 5-Fr catheter with retractable nitinol hypotube that has a curved needle end (Fig. 4). The needle is straight when withdrawn in the catheter and allows a single 0.014″ wire placed into the catheter tip to pass out through the nitinol hypotube to allow delivery over the wire. When the device is in place in the dissection alongside the area of true lumen reconstitution, the wire is withdrawn back into the catheter 2 to 3 cm so that it is proximal to the retracted needle tip near the distal end of the catheter. With the wire retracted, the needle can be advanced forward, allowing the precurved nitinol memory shape to point the needle tip out of a side port 1.5 cm from the distal end of the catheter and penetrate the media and intimal layer to enter the true lumen (Fig. 5). The rotational orientation of the needle deployment is provided by fluoroscopic guiding marks on the catheter (Fig. 6). Before deployment, the "L" mark is oriented to point to the true lumen, and in an orthogonal view, the "T" is oriented over the true lumen. If the needle penetrates the true lumen, then the wire freely passes. The wire can then be advanced and used to accomplish the reconstruction of the occlusion itself, or exchanged for a catheter and other wires. Occasionally, there is a need to dilate the tract of the 0.014″ wire through the plaque penetrated by the needle into true lumen with a small-diameter, low-profile balloon to facilitate the passage of other catheters, wires, or other

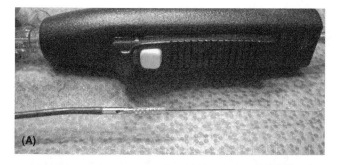

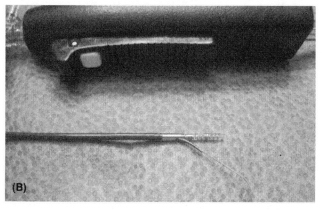

FIGURE 4 (**A**) Outback catheter handle and tip with needle retracted. (**B**) Handle with thumb slide forward and tip with needle deployed.

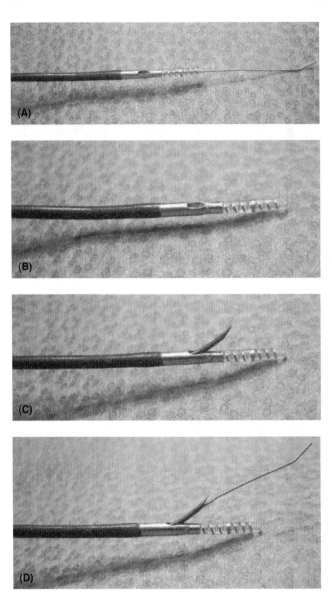

FIGURE 5 (**A**) Outback with wire out the distal tip as it would be placed in the arterial dissection. (**B**) Outback with wire retracted just proximal to the needle port. (**C**) Outback with needle
deployed after wire retracted. (**D**) Outback with wire then advanced out the curved needle.

interventional devices. Available results suggest the Outback LTD to be useful
in lesions that have failed other attempts at reentry, with a technical success rate
of 50% to 80% (17,18).

Technical tips that may improve results include using a quick throw of the
needle to penetrate the plaque rather than a slow movement that may allow the
needle to rotate off the plaque. Also, the needle can easily be deployed too far

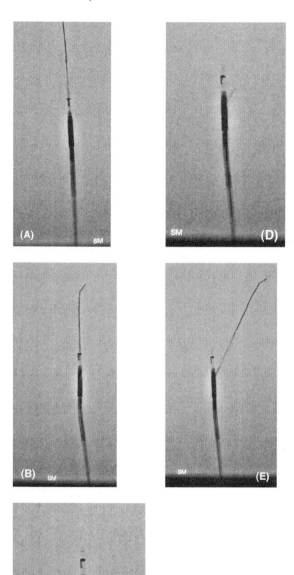

FIGURE 6 (**A**) Outback with "T" marker that indicates the needle will deploy perpendicular to the plane of view. (**B**) Outback with "L" marker alignment indicates the needle deployment in the direction the "L" is pointing. (**C**) Before deployment of the needle, the wire is retracted from the tip to the catheter to just proximal to the exit point of the curved needle. (**D**) Needle is deployed a few millimeter. (**E**) Wire is deployed out of the curved needle to gain access to true lumen.

and end up traversing the true lumen and penetrating the plaque off the opposite wall. The needle can be used in a manner similar to the classic Seldinger technique with needle penetration and then probing with the wire as the needle is withdrawn to access the lumen. Small distal target vessels of less than 4 mm are challenging to gain reentry and may not be appropriate cases for use of the Outback LTD. Likewise, tibial vessels are not adequate distal targets for the device. Calcification can limit the ability of the device to penetrate to the true lumen. Choice of a relatively calcium-free area for reentry will improve the technical success.

The Outback LTD is our primary choice for true lumen reentry in the femoral-popliteal vessels. The relatively delicate nature of the Outback LTD limits its ability to penetrate thick aortoiliac plaque. It is also more difficult to see the markings on the catheter for orientation in the aortoiliac segments because of soft tissue attenuation of the fluoroscopy. Finally, the Outback LTD typically requires multiple deployments of the needle, which raises the concern for perforation of vessels in the retroperitoneum. Though perforation is a concern when treating any CTO, the consequences of perforation in the aortoiliac segment can be severe. The ability to treat perforations with covered stents is essential when treating complex CTOs.

Intravascular Ultrasound-Guided Needle Reentry

The Pioneer catheter (Medtronic) is an intravascular ultrasound device that has a deployable needle for penetration of the dissection to allow for wire passage to the true lumen. The IVUS image provides an image of the vessel wall, the dissection, and the true lumen. There is also color flow capability of the catheter, which can show the flow in the true lumen that can help with targeting the direction of needle deployment into the true lumen. The catheter is a monorail device for delivery over a 0.014″ wire that is in place in the dissection plane near the end of the occlusion. There is a second wire lumen from the back end of the device that ends in a curved nitinol needle near the tip of the device. This nitinol hypotube with the curved needle tip is retracted upon delivery of the catheter to the site of reentry but can be deployed by sliding a portion of the handle of the catheter in a calibrated fashion to cause the needle exit a port on the side of the catheter just proximal to the IVUS transducer (Fig. 7). The port is fixed in the 12 o'clock position on the IVUS image and deploys the needle to penetrate from the dissection plane to the true lumen as the catheter is rotated to orient the true lumen at the 12 o'clock position on the IVUS image (Fig. 8). Once the needle is deployed, a 0.014″ guidewire is passed though and out of the needle into the true lumen. In the absence of a compatible IVUS console, the Pioneer catheter can be used with just fluoroscopic guidance to orient the direction of needle deployment (Fig. 9).

In our own experience, using this device to gain true lumen reentry we had 100% success in both iliac and femoral arterial segments (13). We utilized this catheter more often in iliac occlusions than in femoral arterial occlusions. True lumen reentry was successful in all cases at the level of vessel reconstitution within 2 cm of the optimal angiographically defined distal target vessel. Collateral preservation is one of the main advantages associated with this device. Reentry was possible in less than 10 minutes and routinely obtained in less than 3 minutes. Similar results have been reported from other authors (19).

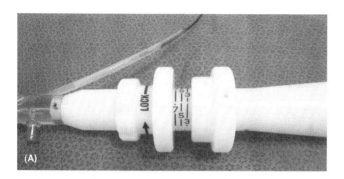

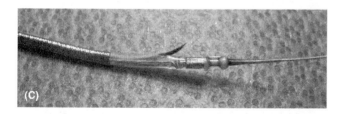

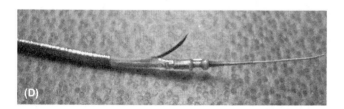

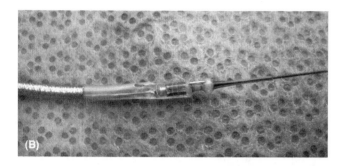

FIGURE 7 (**A**) Pioneer catheter with graduations on sliding handle to deploy needle a set depth. (**B**) Pioneer tip with needle retracted in port just proximal to the transducer at the tip. (**C**) Pioneer catheter tip with needle deployed 3 m. (**D**) Pioneer catheter with tip deployed 5 mm. (**E**) Pioneer catheter with tip deployed 7 mm. (**F**) Pioneer catheter with needle deployed and wire advanced. (*Continued*)

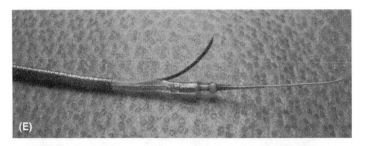

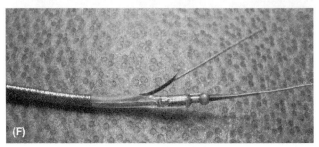

FIGURE 7 (*Continued*)

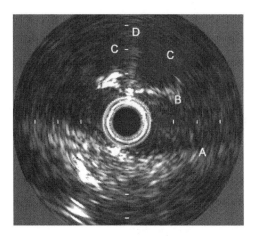

FIGURE 8 Pioneer IVUS image: (**A**) Adventitia of femoral artery. (**B**) Plaque separating dissection with catheter in place from true lumen. (**C**) Color flow denoted on IVUS image helps to delineate the true lumen for reentry. (**D**) Shadow of needle tract at 12 o'clock on the IVUS image.

The Outback LTD device utilizes fluoroscopy, while the Pioneer catheter requires the availability of the IVUS. This may limit its availability, and requires capital expense as well as additional catheter costs, as the Pioneer catheter is more expensive compared with the Outback LTD catheter. However, the IVUS guidance facilitates very accurate placement of the needle in the true lumen and better ability for penetration of calcified plaque and limits the extent of the dissection.

SAFARI Technique
Subintimal arterial flossing with antegrade-retrograde intervention (SAFARI) is a technique for subintimal recanalization of a CTO that involves proximal and distal access and wire passage from the distal to the proximal site through and

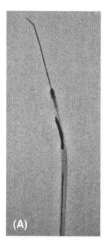

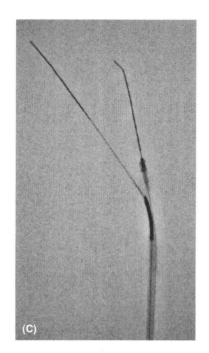

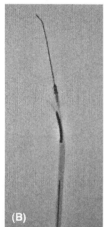

FIGURE 9 (**A**) Pioneer catheter with needle retracted, but the curve of the integral guide tube proximal to the IVUS transducer provides an indication by fluoroscopy as to what direction the needle will deploy. (**B**) Pioneer with needle deployed. (**C**) Pioneer catheter with needle and wire deployed on fluoroscopic image.

through. This technique has been described for performance of subintimal recanalization when there is failure to gain true lumen reentry from above or when there is a small diameter or limited segment of distal target artery available, making other techniques of true lumen reentry difficult. Retrograde percutaneous true lumen access is obtained with assistance of ultrasonography in the distal target artery (popliteal or tibial arteries), and a retrograde subintimal channel is created. A small catheter access is obtained retrograde in the distal artery, often with the assistance of ultrasound guidance. A retrograde dissection is made, and the wire is advanced to the proximal patent vessel or is snared in the subintimal space with a snare passed from the proximal access above down into the sub-intimal dissection. The treatment of the lesion is then done from the proximal access so as to avoid passage of large devices into the distal antegrade access.

The technique was employed after failure of conventional techniques for wire crossing of a CTO in the leg and allowed for 100% acute procedural success in 21 limbs, with limb salvage of 90% at six months with comparable results to the antegrade approach for subintimal recanalization (20). Additional studies suggest clinical improvement with no major complications related to procedure at 12-month follow-up (21). The requirement for percutaneous catheterization of a popliteal or tibial artery in a patient with significant peripheral disease risks dissection or injury to the distal site, but the limited results reported indicate no issues with the distal access site. Indeed, this technique may be most useful when an endovascular reconstruction is required for a popliteal occlusion extending into the trifurcation vessels where there was no ability to traverse from above. If a good anterior tibial or posterior tibial artery is accessible distally in a retrograde fashion from the ankle, then passage of a wire retrograde to the proximal occlusion may provide successful traversal using the SAFARI technique. This may be useful in situations where the diameter of the distally reconstituted vessel is too small to use one of the needle re-entry devices.

PATIENT SELECTION AND PROCEDURE PLANNING
Preoperative Imaging
The patency for bypass procedures is higher than that of the endovascular procedures for complex long-segment disease. However, the option of open surgical reconstruction is not available or desirable in a medically high-risk patient, or there may be no good conduit for distal reconstruction, requiring more advanced and aggressive endovascular approaches. In other patients, the open approach is available but is still less desirable, and in these patients, endovascular interventions should be conducted with the understanding that the failure of the procedure will not negate the option of an open reconstruction. Preoperative planning improves the ability to know and preserve these options.

Imaging with CT or magnetic resonance (MR) angiography can provide information regarding the complete anatomy from the aorta to the tibial arteries. The accuracy in the more distal vessels is typically less accurate, but in vessels proximal to the tibial arteries, these noninvasive tests can provide information superior to catheter-based angiography in the definition of vessel diameter, mural thrombus, calcification, and reconstitution in slow-filling segments below an occlusion. This information allows for planning to improve interventional efficiency as well as case planning to maintain surgical options. Ultrasound imaging of the femoral-popliteal vessels can be used for preoperative planning in institutions with proficiency in the technique, but is not widely practiced. The use of ultrasound to interrogate the common femoral artery as noted previously is often a critical tool to determine the best access for intervention. Guidance as to antegrade or retrograde, femoral, brachial, or open femoral access is often the most valuable information gained upon preprocedure imaging.

Iliac Occlusion in Critical Limb Ischemia
Although critical limb revascularization involves infrainguinal reconstruction in most cases, reconstruction of inflow without in-line flow to the foot is a concept well established in patients with rest pain or minimal tissue loss of the foot. If there is iliac CTO with associated severe common femoral or profunda stenosis or occlusion, then open femoral access with retrograde recanalization of iliac occlusion and open endarterectomy of significant femoral disease (treatment of two levels of occlusive disease) are definitive treatment for most patients, even in the setting of SFA or popliteal artery occlusion. Adequate revascularization for limb salvage would be expected in over 90% of such patients (22). In cases

of critical ischemia with tissue loss that requires outflow as well, the open femoral access provides retrograde iliac as well as antegrade infrainguinal endovascular reconstructions. Again, planning for reconstruction of iliofemoral occlusion can be based on CT or MR as sole imaging without catheter-based angiography.

CT and MR also provide the location and character of any calcifications and may help guide selection of options before and during the intervention such as planning primary stenting for severely calcified lesions, or planning for primary covered stents for large chronic thrombus or mild aneurysmal changes in occluded aortoiliac vessels as well as defining any aneurysmal changes in the femoral-popliteal arteries. Recanalization of moderately dilated common iliac arteries with extension of mural thrombus into the aorta in our practice is treated with iCAST PTFE covered balloon-expandable stents (Atrium Medical, Hudson, New Hampshire, U.S.), often in kissing stent fashion. If there is dilation of greater than 20 mm in the common iliac or greater than 30-mm diameter of the aorta, then the reconstruction may be best done with aortic stent grafting. We have treated eight patients with combined iliac occlusion and aortic aneurysmal disease using iliac recanalization, true lumen reentry in the abdominal aortic aneurysm (AAA), and full infrarenal aortic stent graft placement, with technical success and good long-term results to mean of 30 months in all cases (unpublished data). A retrospective series of 171 patients treated with combined iliac stenting and open common femoral endarterectomy suggests that covered stents may provide better patency than bare stents (23).

Femoral-Popliteal Occlusions

Plaque echogenicity represented by duplex ultrasonography–derived gray-scale median (GSM) can be used to predict the success of primary subintimal femoral-popliteal angioplasties (24). One can anticipate higher failures to reenter true lumen if the median GSM is more than 35. The diffuse uniform circumferential calcifications as seen in diabetic patients are less concerning than the irregular, eccentric, dense, or multisegmental calcified lesions, as these lesions are more difficult to recanalize and more often result in focal residual stenosis even after stenting, which may adversely affect long-term patency. Additionally, the success of subintimal angioplasty depends not only on the length of the lesion and calcification but also on the presence of relatively normal arterial system proximal and distal to the lesion to allow access and reentry (25).

Although lesion length is a well-accepted factor impacting the long-term results of the endovascular treatment of a CTO (4,25), what constitutes long occlusive lesion that is best treated with open surgical revascularization still remains debatable. While considering the location of the lesion, if the SFA origin is not identified upon the angiographic imaging and the common femoral artery seems to taper only to the profunda artery, then it is assumed that the occlusion of the SFA extends into the common femoral artery. With extension of the occlusion into the common femoral artery, endovascular intervention should be considered a high risk and one should favor an open surgical revascularization. If a patient has relatively acute symptoms, TPA can be administered to enhance the efforts to identify the origin of the SFA, but the cap of a chronic occlusion often does not respond effectively to TPA. Directional atherectomy catheters, such as the Turbo Booster guide for the CLiRpath laser catheter and SilverHawk

LSM atherectomy catheter (ev3), may be used to treat lesions at the origin of the SFA extending into the common femoral artery so as to reduce the chance of a sub-optimal result after PTA since stenting is not a good option at the common femoral bifurcation.

Popliteal arterial CTO is approached in the same way as an SFA occlusion, but the reconstitution by collaterals should be above the tibial origins to anticipate a reasonable chance of true lumen reentry and technical success. Popliteal stents have lower patency and may have a higher rate of fracture/deformation and recurrent stenosis and occlusion due to placement of the stents across the flexion point of the knee. The center point of the maximal flexion of the politeal artery is typically just distal to the top of the patella on a straight AP angiogram image. Therefore, the adjunctive use of plaque debulking and long balloon angioplasty to reduce the need of stenting may be warranted.

Tibial Occlusions

Tibial occlusive disease needs special mention in critical limb ischemia as it is accepted that adequate revascularization to heal significant tissue loss in the foot requires one to recanalize at least one tibial artery to ankle. If occlusions involve the origin of a tibial, the recanalization may compromise the branch points. However, repeated alternating angioplasty of the branch origins will often provide good results without the need for kissing balloons. Cutting balloon or scoring balloon treatment of the branch origins may be useful. Endovascular approach for tibial vessels is ideally suited for patients with diffuse focal stenosis or short-segment occlusions. Occasionally, multifocal high-grade tibial stenoses may appear upon angiography as a total occlusion but allows passage of a wire freely and is again ideally suited to angioplasty. Stent placement in tibial vessels with current technology should generally be avoided. To avoid the need for stent of tibial CTOs, we have used prolonged inflation angioplasty with long balloons. The long balloons seem to reduce to dissections that are seen with shorter balloons inflated sequentially. As noted previously, diffuse calcification as seen in diabetic population is not a contraindication for the endovascular approach to manage the femoral-popliteal CTO. However, recanalization of tibial occlusions can be limited by the presence of severe calcium. Long-term patency with endovascular recanalization of tibial occlusion is relatively low, but limb salvage is good. Clearly, tibial angioplasty is useful in high-risk patients who are otherwise not suitable for bypass procedures, before amputation is considered (26). Indeed, given high limb salvage rates, intervention for complex tibial disease is increasingly used as primary therapy in critical ischemia patients (27).

RECONSTRUCTION AFTER CROSSING CTOs

Restoration of the lumen after achieving wire crossing of the occlusion can be accomplished with the use of simple angioplasty or with an increasingly complex technology as the situation demands. The four primary technologies that are utilized are balloons, atherectomy, stents, and stent grafts.

Angioplasty

The use of angioplasty is the simplest and most frequently used method to restore flow after crossing CTOs. The improvements in balloon technology with lower profiles and improved trackability allow for one to get a balloon across the occlusion in nearly all cases once wire crossing is achieved. The technical aspects of angioplasty for CTOs differ little from angioplasty for stenoses. The longer balloons have improved the speed and ease of treatment of longer segments of vessel but also seem to achieve improved results with less dissection than with multiple inflations of short balloons. Positioning a long balloon to treat the occlusion as well as any adjacent stenoses simultaneously, with angioplasty of short intervening segments of relatively normal artery may improve the angiographic result and reduce the need for stenting. The goal of restoring flow with less than 50% residual stenosis or dissection can be achieved with angioplasty alone in up to 80% to 90% of femoral-popliteal arteries (28,29). Situations that increase the failure of primary angioplasty include severe calcification and longer occlusions. In our experience, the need for stenting increases with the need for true lumen reentry devices (13).

Cryoplasty in the treatment of infrainguinal disease has been reported to have good results in short lesions, but few of these were CTOs. Practical limitations in the treatment of CTOs with cryoplasty include the short balloon lengths and expense. Excellent technical results with low need for stenting have been achieved in these relatively short, mostly stenotic lesions (30). As with several other adjunctive technologies, the role of cryoplasty may be in locations like the common femoral or popliteal flexion points and bifurcations, where stenting is not a good option.

The use of cutting or scoring balloons has had little reported use in CTOs but may also have a role in focal occlusions at branch points to reduce dissections. They also have performed well in calcified lesions that are often resistant to other therapies. These balloons are all short in length, and the reports on their use have included few cases of CTOs (31,32). Use of cutting or scoring balloons in the subintimal space has a theoretical risk of increased perforation compared with standard balloon angioplasty.

Stents

When hemodynamically significant residual stenosis or dissection remains after angioplasty, the provisional use of stents is essential for improving acute and long-term results. The criterion for stenting provisionally is, typically, the presence of more than 30% to 50% residual stenosis or a flow-limiting dissection. Angiographic evaluation of the post-angioplasty vessel must be done with dynamic contrast imaging and in multiple views to insure that there is an adequate result before deciding not to stent. The "art" of this assessment is difficult, and the variation in the interpretation of the results after angioplasty as well as one's bias or inclination for or against stents can impact the decision to provisionally stent. The need for provisional stents in CTOs has ranged from 10% to 40% (28,29,33,34).

Primary stenting of extensive femoral-popliteal disease has increased recently as stent designs have improved both acute and long-term success. Several of these studies suggest that there is better patency with primary stenting of most patients, with a range of femoral-popliteal lesions from stenoses to occlusions of varying length (33,34). Some have extrapolated these findings to recommend primary stenting for all femoral-popliteal CTOs as they feel that occlusions represent the most complex level of disease. The debate of primary versus provisional stenting is still undecided and is further detailed in other chapters.

Stent Grafts

Reconstruction of CTOs with stent grafts has been proposed as an ideal therapy as it may result in less neointimal occlusion than bare metal stents. Stent grafts have recently been shown in a retrospective series to have higher patency in iliac reconstructions than bare stents (23). Series of femoral-popliteal stent grafts have reported slightly higher long-term patency rates than comparable series of bare metal stents (35,36). The difference in patency rates between covered and bare metal stents seems to be in the more complex lesions. Indeed, a more complex and costly therapy may be appropriately used in the most difficult and complex cases. In this regard, as with other technology, covered stents may be particularly well suited for treatment of the complex disease of CTOs. Currently, the cost and larger sheath sizes required for placement have limited broad use. The VIBRANT trial, a prospective randomized trial comparing Viabahn stent grafts (Gore Medical, Flagstaff, Arizona, U.S.) with bare metal stents in femoral-popliteal lesions, is currently in follow-up phase. This study will provide valuable information about patency and failure modes of these SFA treatment options and provide guidance for what role covered stents have in infrainguinal CTOs.

Debulking of Plaque

The difficulty with acute hemodynamic failures and the relatively low patency rate of stand-alone angioplasty on one hand and the difficulty of long-term recurrent stenosis when resorting to stents in the infrainguinal vessels on the other encouraged the development of atherectomy devices. The two currently available atherectomy devices are the Spectranetics excimer laser and the FoxHollow SilverHawk directional atherectomy devices. The initial studies of these devices were primarily in stenotic lesions and few CTOs. The use of the devices in CTOs was limited by a perceived high risk of perforation, particularly in subintimal recanalization. As experience grew, it was realized that there was less risk of perforation in these lesions than would be expected, even in subintimal dissections, and the use broadened. The goal to achieve lumen restoration without the need for stenting is the primary motivation in their use in CTOs. The concept that debulking with or without adjunctive angioplasty will allow for angiographic and hemodynamic results that are better than that of angioplasty alone is intuitive to their use.

SilverHawk Atherectomy

The avoidance of stretch in the arterial wall from angioplasty is a theoretical advantage of plaque excision that may reduce recurrent stenosis. In the initial studies of atherectomy with the SilverHawk in femoral-popliteal disease, the need for stenting is very low, but the lesions treated were in selected patients with primarily stenoses, and only 20% to 25% were CTOs (37–39). This compares with other contemporary studies of endovascular intervention using a range of techniques for lower extremity ischemia, with 40% to 45% of the lesions being CTOs in unselected patients and as high as 70% to 80% in critical limb ischemia patients (16,40). Subsequent studies have reported use of plaque excision in lesions of higher complexity such as occlusions of the common femoral, popliteal, and in tibial vessels where stenting is clearly less desirable (41,42). We propose that the role of the SilverHawk be limited to the treatment of relatively short CTOs and in locations that are problematic for stenting.

Excimer Laser Atherectomy

Laser atherectomy for critical limb ischemia as reported in the LACI trial included the use of the laser in patients with a 70% incidence of CTOs (16). In the overall trial, there was only a 45% incidence of a need for provisional stents in this complex level of disease. Indeed a preponderance of patients who have both diffuse stenosis and CTOs may benefit from the use of debulking of both types of lesions. The laser may be better suited for these long occlusions in diffusely diseased vessels than the SilverHawk. As noted above, the role of atherectomy in the treatment of CTOs is not clearly defined, but the desire to avoid stents, particularly in certain locations, and the difficulties in treating recurrent in-stent stenosis is the motivation for increased use of primary atherectomy in CTOs.

Embolic Protection

Traversal of CTO is rarely complicated by clinically significant distal emboli, but treatment after traversal to restore the lumen and flow with all types of techniques is associated with risks of angiographically significant embolization ranging as high as 8% to 20% (43,44). The risk as noted previously is increased with a delay in anticoagulation and formation of thrombus in the static subintimal tract created during manipulations to achieve recanalization. More importantly, there is the risk of embolization with angioplasty, atherectomy, and stenting (45). The highest rate of embolization has been reported to occur with atherectomy (45,46). We have quantified embolic debris in 33 cases of femoral-popliteal reconstructions using primarily laser and angioplasty and showed that the amount of debris captured with Spider FX embolic protection wire (ev3) ranged from 10.1 mm^3 for lesions less than 20 cm long up to 22.7 mm^3 for lesions greater that 20 cm long. It seems clear that as there is escalation in the severity of occlusive disease treated with endovascular techniques, there is escalation of the risk of embolization. Although there is no clear guidance as to what volume of embolic debris is clinically significant, we currently use embolic protection in femoral-popliteal laser or excisional atherectomy cases of TransAtlantic Inter-Society Consensus (TASC) D lesions and in cases of TASC B or greater lesions when there is compromised (e.g., single-vessel) tibial runoff.

SUMMARY

Endovascular treatment of critical limb ischemia requires one to be facile with the crossing and reconstruction of CTOs. The ability to use a range of techniques and devices is required to maximize the acute success. Key points include adequate supportive access, skill with hydrophilic wires and support catheters, and access to and familiarity with reentry devices and techniques. Adjunctive tools such as laser or RF catheters may add to the ability to cross occlusions in occasional difficult cases. Future technology that combines image guidance and energy/ablative devices may improve the ability to cross all CTOs. Reconstruction of iliac CTOs with primary stenting and in femoral-popliteal CTOs with angioplasty, atherectomy, and/or stenting affords good technical and reasonable midterm results. Reconstruction of complex long lesions with compromised tibial vessels may benefit from use of embolic protection to preserve runoff at the time of reconstruction.

REFERENCES

1. Spinosa DJ, Leung DA, Matsumoto AH, et al. Percutaneous intentional extraluminal recanalization in patients with chronic critical limb ischemia. Radiology 2002; 232: 499–507.
2. Leville CD, Kashyap VS, Claire DG, et al. Endovascular management of iliac occlusions: extending treatment to transatlantic Inter-societal classification C and D patients. J Vasc Surg 2006; 43:32–39.
3. Lazaris AM, Tsiamis AC, Fishwick G, et al. Clinical outcome of primary infrainguinal subintimal angioplasty in diabetic patients with critical lower limb ischemia. J Endovasc Ther 2004; 11:447–453.
4. Lazaris AM, Salas C, Tsiamis AC, et al. Factors affecting patency of subintimal infrainguinal angioplasty in patients with critical lower limb ischemia. Euro J Vasc Endovasc Surg 2006; 32:668–674.
5. Bolia A, Brennan J, Bell PR. Recanalisation of femoro-popliteal occlusions: improving success rate by subintimal recanalisation. Clin Radiol 1989; 40:325.
6. London NJ, Srinivasan R, Naylor AR, et al. Subintimal angioplasty of femoropopliteal artery occlusions: the long-term results. Euro J Vasc Endovasc Surg 1994; 8(2):148–155.
7. Scott EC, Biuckians A, Light RE, et al. Subintimal angioplasty for the treatment of claudication and critical limb ischemia: 3-year results. J Vasc Surg 2007; 46:959–964.
8. Markose G, Bolia A. Subintimal angioplasty in the management of lower extremity ischemia. J Cardiovasc Surg 2006; 47(4):399–406.
9. Antusevas A, Aleksynas N, Kaupas RS, et al. Comparison of results of subintimal angioplasty and percutaneous transluminal angioplasty in superficial femoral artery occlusions. Euro J Vasc Endovasc Surg 2008; 36:101–106.
10. Ko YG, Kim JS, Choi DH, et al. Improved technical success and midterm patency with subintimal angioplasty compared to intraluminal angioplasty in long femoropopliteal occlusions. J Endovasc Ther 2007; 14:374–381.
11. Lipsitz EC, Ohki T, Veith FJ, et al. Does subintimal angioplasty have a role in the treatment of severe lower extremity ischemia? J Vasc Surg 2003; 37:386–391.
12. Myers SI, Myers DJ, Ahmend A, et al. Preliminary results of subintimal angioplasty for limb salvage in lower extremities with severe chronic ischemia and limb-threatening ischemia. J Vasc Surg 2006; 44(6):1239–1246.
13. Jacobs DL, Motaganahalli R, Cox DE, et al. True lumen reentry devices facilitate subintimal angioplasty and stenting of total chronic occlusions: initial report. J Vasc Surg 2006; 43:1291–1296.
14. Mossop PJ, Amukotuwa SA, Whitbourn RJ. Controlled blunt micro dissection for percutaneous recanalization of lower limb Arterial chronic total occlusions: a single center experience. Catheter Cardiovasc Interv 2006; 68(2):304–310.
15. Kirvaitis RJ, Parr L, Kelly LM, et al. Recanalization of chronic total peripheral arterial occlusions using optical coherent reflectometry with guided radiofrequency energy: a single center experience. Catheter Cardiovasc Interv 2007; 69(4):532–540.
16. Laird JR, Zeller T, Gray BH, et al. LACI Investigators. Limb salvage following laser-assisted angioplasty for critical limb ischemia: results of the LACI multicenter trial. J Endovasc Ther 2006; 13(1):1–11.
17. Wiesinger B, Steinkamp H, König C, et al. Technical report and preliminary clinical data of a novel catheter for luminal re-entry after subintimal dissection. Invest Radiol 2005; 40(11):725–728.

18. Hausegger KA, Georgieva B, Portugaller H, et al. The outback catheter: a new device for true lumen re-entry after dissection during recanalization of arterial occlusions. Cardiovasc Intervent Radiol 2004; 27(1):26–30.
19. Saket RR, Razavi MK, Padidar A, et al. Novel intravascular ultrasound-guided method to create transintimal arterial communications: initial experience in peripheral occlusive disease and aortic dissection. J Endovasc Ther 2004; 11(3):274–280.
20. Spinosa DJ, Harthun NL, Bissonette EA, et al. Subintimal arterial flossing with antegrade-retrograde intervention (SAFARI) for subintimal recanalization to treat chronic critical limb ischemia. J Vasc Interv Radiol 2005; 16(1):37–44.
21. Gandini R, Pipitone V, Stefanini M, et al. "Safari" technique to perform difficult subintimal infragenicular vessels. Cardiovasc Intervent Radiol 2007; 30(3):469–473.
22. Savolainen H, Hansen A, Diehm N, et al. Small is beautiful: why profundaplasty should not be forgotten. World J Surg 2007; 31:2058–2061.
23. Chang RW, Goodney PP, Baek JH, et al. Long-term results of combined common femoral endarterectomy and iliac stenting/stent grafting for occlusive disease. J Vasc Surg 2008; 48(2):362–367.
24. Marks NA, Ascher E, Hingorani AP, et al. Gray-scale median of the atherosclerotic plaque can predict success of lumen re-entry during subintimal femoral-popliteal angioplasty. J Vasc Surg 2008; 47(1):109–115; discussion 115–116.
25. Norgen L, Hiatt WR, Dormandy JA, et al. Inter-society consensus for the management of peripheral arterial disease (TASC-2). J Vasc Surg 2007; 45(suppl 1):S5–S67.
26. Clair DG, Dayal R, Faries PL, et al. Tibial angioplasty as an alternative strategy in patients with limb–threatening ischemia. Ann Vasc Surg 2005; 19(1):63–68.
27. Bosiers M, Hart JP, Deloose K, et al. Endovascular therapy as the primary approach for limb salvage in patients with critical limb ischemia: experience with 443 infrapopliteal procedures. Vascular 2006; 14(2):63–69.
28. Becquemin JP, Favre JP, Marzelle J, et al. A. Systematic versus selective stent placement after superficial femoral artery balloon angioplasty: a multicenter prospective randomized study. J Vasc Surg 2003; 37:487–494.
29. Scott EC, Biuckians A, Light RE, et al. Subintimal angioplasty: our experience in the treatment of 506 infrainguinal arterial occlusions. J Vasc Surg 2008; 48(4):878–884.
30. Laird J, Jaff MR, Biamino G, et al. Cryoplasty for the treatment of femoropopliteal arterial disease: results of a prospective, multicenter registry. J Vasc Interv Radiol 2005; 16:1067–1073.
31. Ansel GM, Sample NS, Botti IC Jr., et al. Cutting balloon angioplasty of the popliteal and infrapopliteal vessels for symptomatic limb ischemia. Catheter Cardiovasc Interv 2004; 61:1–4.
32. Scheinert D, Peeters P, Bosiers M, et al. Results of the multicenter first-in-man study of a novel scoring balloon catheter for the treatment of infra-popliteal peripheral arterial disease. Catheter Cardiovasc Interv 2007; 70(7):1034–1039.
33. Krankenberg H, Schlüter M, Steinkamp HJ, et al. Nitinol stent implantation versus percutaneous transluminal angioplasty in superficial femoral artery lesions up to 10 cm in length: the femoral artery stenting trial (FAST). Circulation 2007; 116(3):285–292.
34. Schillinger M, Sabeti S, Dick P, et al. Sustained benefit at 2 years of primary femoral-popliteal stenting compared with balloon angioplasty with optional stenting. Circulation 2007; 115:2745–2749.
35. Saxon RR, Coffman JM, Gooding JM, et al. Long-term patency and clinical outcome of the Viabahn stent-graft for femoropopliteal artery obstructions. J Vasc Interv Radiol 2007; 18(11):1341–1349.
36. Alimi YS, Hakam Z, Hartung O, et al. Efficacy of Viabahn in the treatment of severe superficial femoral artery lesions: which factors influence long-term patency? Euro J Vasc Endovasc Surg 2008; 35:346–352.
37. Zeller T, Frank U, Burgelin K, et al. Initial clinical experience with percutaneous atherectomy in the infrageniculate arteries. J Endovasc Ther 2003; 10:987–993.
38. Ramaiah VG, Gammon R, Kiesz S, et al. Mid term outcomes from the TALON registry: treating peripherals with SilverHawk: outcomes collection. J Endovasc Ther 2006; 13:592–602.

39. Zeller T, Rastan A, Sixt S, et al. Long-term results after directional atherectomy of femoropopliteal lesions. J Am Coll Cardiol 2006; 48:1573–1578.
40. DeRubertis BG, Faries PL, McKinsey JF, et al. Shifting paradigms in the treatment of lower extremity vascular disease: a report of 1000 percutaneous interventions. Ann Surg 2007; 246(3):415–422; discussion 422–424.
41. Keeling WB, Shames ML, Stone PA, et al. Plaque excision with the Silverhawk catheter: early results in patients with claudication or critical limb ischemia. J Vasc Surg 2007; 45(1):25–31.
42. Zeller T, Sixt S, Schwarzwalder U, et al. Two-year results after directional atherectomy of infrapopliteal arteries with the SilverHawk device. J Endovasc Ther 2007; 14(2): 232–240.
43. Varty K, Nydahl S, Butterworth P, et al. Changes in the management of critical limb ischaemia. Br J Surg 1996; 83(7):953–956.
44. Saxon RR, Coffman JM, Gooding JM, et al. Long-term results of ePTFE stent-graft versus angioplasty in the femoropopliteal artery: single center experience from a prospective, randomized trial. J Vasc Interv Radiol 2003; 14(3):303–311.
45. Lam RC, Shah S, Faries PL, et al. Incidence and clinical significance of distal embolization during percutaneous Interventions involving the superficial femoral artery. J Vasc Surg 2007; 46(6):1155–1159.
46. Suri R, Wholey M, Postoak D, et al. Distal embolic protection during femoropoliteal atherectomy. Catheter Cardiovasc Interv 2006; 67:417–422.

9 Endovascular Strategy for Below-the-Knee Lesions

Nicolas Nelken and Peter A. Schneider
Division of Vascular Therapy, Hawaii Permanente Medical Group, Honolulu, Hawaii, U.S.A.

INTRODUCTION

Given the rapid development time of new techniques in a field as technical as this one, it is useful to separate those things that are likely to be enduring from those that are heavily device specific. Currently, endoluminal intervention is an exciting field precisely because of the rapid development of techniques and instrumentation. Therefore, a rigid hierarchy of techniques is likely to become anachronistic very quickly. A monograph on distinctions in clinical presentation is likely to be more enduring, but there is no way to write a chapter like this without a clear focus on instrumentation, at least at the level of different device "families" that have been developed with different clinical situations in mind. What follows is a series of observations and data, which help guide our personal choice of interventions in the patient with a disease below the knee.

The strategy begins with *identification* of peripheral arterial disease (PAD). PAD is common and underdiagnosed. Below-the-knee (BTK) PAD is associated with the worst risk factors and the most unfavorable outcomes. About 15% to 30% of the population over 70 years old suffers from PAD, but of this group only one patient in three is symptomatic. However, up to a third of *asymptomatic* patients have an occlusion of a major artery of the leg (1). Making matters murkier for the clinician, due to the overwhelming preponderance of very sedentary patients, progression to critical limb ischemia (CLI) is statistically independent of claudication; many frankly don't walk enough to ever develop it. Decrement in ankle brachial index (ABI) is associated with CLI, and therefore ABI is a much more sensitive screening tool than symptoms. We begin this chapter with a suggestion for regular follow-up of this easily performed and often forgotten test. Although following ABIs in patients over the long term may (and should) have little effect on first-time anatomic interventions, it has been shown to help guide the more aggressive risk factor modification, which may lead to avoidance of any intervention whatsoever (2). The term "PAD" has taken root in public perception now, and this has made our job easier. It is fascinating that a long-term patient and graduate of many interventions, both open and endoluminal, might still inquire, "Doc, do I have PAD?"

Rarely is the endoluminal solution the best solution from a pure "plumbing" perspective. It offers other benefits, including lesser degrees of pain, injury, short-term complications, and patient acceptance. As endoluminal development continues to improve, and the lay press continues to write about "miracle cures," patients are less and less likely to accept open surgery without questioning. Furthermore, the surgical literature has often ignored symptomatic side effects in studies related to open surgery (something patients intuitively understand) (3). Endoluminal interventions obviate many of the problems that used to be assumed to be the "price of doing business" in open surgery.

Endovascular long-term primary patency is generally worse than in open surgery, but sometimes all you need to do is to heal an ulcer (the metabolic energy needed to maintain healthy skin is far less than that needed to heal an injury). Patients in this cohort have an inordinately high long-term mortality rate (worse than many cancers), so this late complication propensity might not even matter in the individual patient (1). The long-term patency rate of infrageniculate angioplasty in those over 80 years has been shown to be dismal, and yet limb salvage rates are still approximately 74% at one year (4). In fact, the correlation of "clinical success rate" to "angiographic success rate" is quite poor. For example, 27% of patients with *open* vessels at one-year angiographic follow-up had poor clinical responses, compared with 55% of patients having an acceptable clinical response with known occlusion of the angioplastied vessel (5). Therefore, there is no tight relationship between patency of the treated infrageniculate segment and clinical success.

BTK interventions have been attempted for many years (6,7), but only recently has there been any real momentum in this direction. Development of 0.014" systems, low-profile balloons, and exporting of coronary devices to the periphery has been helpful in kick-starting this field in earnest. Though small platform systems are necessary to accomplish many of the more delicate procedures, some leading studies have been done with 0.035" platforms (8). The size of the vessels is very similar to those of the coronary circulation, but the flows, physiology, and extended length of the vessels and their lesions make tibial intervention substantially different from coronary intervention.

In this chapter, we describe a balanced algorithm of both open and endoluminal approaches. In brief, although we subscribe to an "endoluminal-first" approach, it is far from strict, and must be individualized to the presenting patient.

PSYCHOLOGY OF DECISIONS
There are two ways to think about what to do for a BTK clinical problem: (*i*) "What can I do?" and (*ii*) "What if it fails?"

What Can I Do?
This first question is a demonstration of relatively straightforward thinking and is what results from an unchecked acceptance of case reports and small studies that "try" various techniques. These are the studies that mostly populate the literature at this early stage. Leaders in the field need to try new things and there are plenty to try. Unfortunately, only the most successful studies are published, given the intrinsic bias for positive rather than negative data. Our results (i.e., doctor and patient together) might not be as good as what we read about. Anyone in this field who has been practicing for a decade or more has run into at least one of these divergent cycles of expectation and outcome (9). Retrospective studies generally look at patients whose procedures were chosen by the interventionists and may say more about the judgment of the interventionist than about comparisons between the techniques themselves (10).

"What can I do?" thinking is also easier to plan for and generates questions like: "What skills do I possess?"; "What inventory do I have access to?"; "What level of accreditation do I have?"; "What is the patient's anatomy?"; "What patient-specific problems might there be?"; and "What comorbidities exist?"

What if It Fails?

This thinking is less straightforward but more fruitful for complex cases. It is currently hard to back this up with statistical certainty but this is exactly why a multilevel decision tree is necessary.

This kind of thinking generates very different questions like: "What else do I have in my bag of tricks?"; "What is my endoluminal backup?"; "What is my open surgical backup?"; "What is the level of sophistication of my podiatric backup?"; "When do I give up?"; and finally, the most difficult of all, "What are my *real* capabilities in the face of impending doom?" The answers to all of these questions should ideally be available or at least accessible in any complex case before it ever gets to the suite.

OPEN SURGERY
How Do I Preserve Operative Options?

This question is probably the most important as open surgery can be considered a "mature" field at this point with more predictable outcomes. Vascular surgical societies' embrace of the Reporting Standards published in 1997 (11), combined with a 40-year head start, have placed open surgery in a position of final arbiter of limb salvage. Not all patients have an open surgical option, but to proceed without in-depth knowledge of what is possible in the individual patient can be a disaster. This knowledge involves more than just preservation of endpoints, it also requires knowledge of availability of conduit, the quality of available conduit, and basic ambulatory status of the patient.

Surgical "technique" is erroneously no longer considered an exciting topic because of the maturity of the field, and the fact is we don't do as much open surgery as we used to because of the success of many endoluminal interventions. This important fact is generating new problems. Open surgery workflows in many institutions are slowly degenerating; for example, we rarely perform once-commonplace arm-vein bypasses to the foot. Belkin's group documented a 75% reduction in open aortibifemoral bypass and axillofemoral repairs and a 30% reduction in open infrainguinal bypasses since beginning its endovascular program (12). We are now doing over 70% endovascular in our program. Continued volume is important in maintaining skills.

A List of Considerations Relating to Open Surgery

1. Conversion of an above-the-knee popliteal bypass to a BTK bypass is associated with worse clinical outcomes. Placing a stent in the above-the-knee popliteal artery does this. However, if the above-the-knee segment is very calcified, even if patent, a BTK bypass would probably have been chosen anyway. We tend to avoid very calcific segments in favor of better quality, more distal vessels.
2. Don't trash the dorsalis pedis or the distal posterior tibial (or plantar) segments. Endoluminal intervention in these segments should probably be saved for web-like lesions or truly nonsurgical candidates. Atherectomy of this very distal circulation is possible but unwise unless it occurs *distal* to the location of any possible bypass.
3. Be extra careful in situations of single-vessel runoff. This used to be a relative contraindication for endoluminal intervention but rarely stops us now.

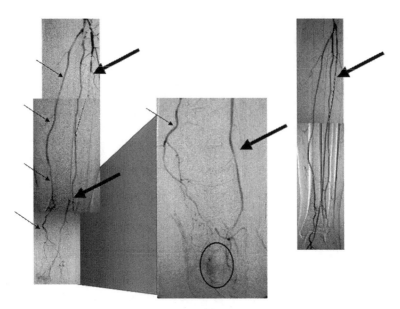

FIGURE 1   Left pane: Angiogram demonstrates open posterior tibial and peroneal artery inflow to foot with ulceration. Anterior tibial demonstrates chronic total occlusion. Normally this would be considered enough to heal the ulceration. Middle pane: Close-up of the foot demonstrates that area of ulceration fed mostly by branches of the dorsalis pedis in line with the occluded anterior tibial artery. Right pane: Balloon angioplasty of occluded anterior tibial results in more direct filling of the foot in the area of the ulceration, a demonstration of a freebie (procedure with very little risk, which greatly increases likelihood of success).

Be certain that the outflow is maintained. In more proximal interventions associated with single-vessel runoff, consider using an embolic protection device, but this can add a lot of expense to a procedure.

4. Occluded tibial segments are worth a try at recanalization as long as there is ample patent outflow. While treating the proximal end of the tibial, avoid damage to *other* tibial vessels. Buddy wires can be used in complex situations, and sometimes, "kissing" balloons are necessary in the proximal tibial vessels (13).

5. Recognize a "freebie," a situation in which the likelihood of making something worse is so low that an endoluminal success would be complete victory (Fig. 1).

    This is often found in a situation in which there is already some outflow provided by another vessel, but the microcirculation of the foot has compromised the anastomotic network or the arch. The dictum that "one open tibial vessel is enough" is not always true. To determine this, excellent biplanar angiograms of the foot are critical before intervention. Even a pedal pulse might occasionally be misleading as diabetics sometimes have pedal occlusions immediately distal to a pulsatile segment when an easily approachable lesion exists upstream from the other major artery (Fig. 2).

6. Beware of creep in the definition of a "nonoperative candidate." Before we had endoluminal options, we operated quite successfully on patients who

Pulse and Flow are not the same *especially* in Diabetics

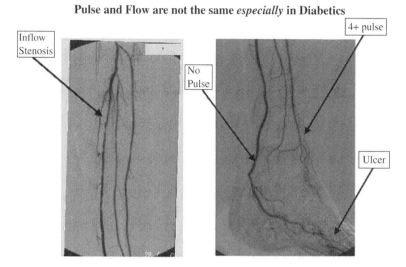

FIGURE 2 Patient with long-term nonhealing ulceration of the foot. Family physician was able to feel a distal anterior tibial pulse, and did not refer the patient because the pulse felt strong. Subsequent angiogram (more than a year later) demonstrates that the anterior tibial ends in occlusion, and the dominant artery of the foot is a nonpalpable posterior tibial distal to an easily treated stenosis. After angioplasty, lesion healed in six weeks.

are now paradoxically considered nonoperative candidates. Many creative solutions exist other than long-leg incisions, including coil embolization of tributaries in the performance of an in situ bypass, requiring only two small incisions (14). We have performed this operation with great success in difficult patients with fat legs and poor skin.

7. Any acute or simultaneous intervention above a proposed bypass graft should be stented. Although there is plenty of controversy regarding the use of stents in various beds, acutely it is critical that the inflow to a bypass be as risk-free as possible since failure of the endoluminal procedure will probably result in failure of the bypass as well. Conduit is precious.

When Do I Operate First?
Given the pressures of a patient's expectations and the lure of new technology, this question may be most difficult. The answer to this question always revolves around "What if it fails?" type thinking rather than "What can I do?" The key is that if there is almost no room for error (e.g., an isolated dorsalis pedis), surgery may be your only chance. Revascularization of pedal arteries in surgical series for CLI has resulted in limb salvage rates 100% higher than peroneal revascularization (15,16), and there is evidence to suspect that this also holds true for endoluminal cases (17–20). Preservation of in-line flow to at least *one* of these end arteries is critical. Therefore, it isn't worth "trying" and endoluminal revascularization to open a peroneal artery if a pedal artery remains isolated in a Rutherford category 6 patient. Conversely, there is almost always something endoluminal, which you can do more proximally to alleviate rest pain. Some

patients are so young that a very complex endoluminal intervention is unlikely to provide a lasting solution.

In perhaps the most dramatic statistics of the entire BTK literature, Faglia studied 420 diabetic patients with CLI who underwent infrapopliteal angioplasty. Those who had no open tibial vessels at the end of the study suffered a 62.5% amputation rate compared with a 1.7% amputation rate in patients with *at least* one open vessel to the foot (19).

ENDOLUMINAL SOLUTIONS
Anatomic Distinctions Worth Noting
Calcium

Calcium is the final frontier of endoluminal intervention. There is nothing that deals effectively with it other than bypass. Newly developed atherectomy devices have been introduced (e.g., "rock-hawk" Silverhawk atherectomy device and high-intensity excimer laser) (21), but neither of these has been released long enough for evaluation. Therefore, intervention in heavily calcified lesions should be reserved for people whose situations are not emergent and can tolerate a procedural failure without consequence or for patients who are truly not operative candidates. If a balloon will not expand, then a stent may not expand either. Irregular mechanical surfaces occur with open-cell stents (22) pushing angles of nitinol into the lumen, and this may impede safe passage of further devices.

Patients with renal failure develop medial calcinosis, which is a different anatomic entity. It is characterized by calcification of the media and may not involve endoluminal stenosis at all. Even with an open lumen, the lack of elasticity makes it impossible to feel pulses and to obtain ABIs. In fact, medial calcinosis may necessitate an endoluminal solution over open surgery because of the difficulty of creating an anastomosis in calcified segments. There is a literature of open surgical techniques for calcified arteries, and skilled surgeons are sometimes able to deal effectively with calcific segments, but there are limits. There are also limits to what can be done endoluminally for a brittle pipe. A "noncontrast arteriogram" plain film is usually good evidence that the surgical solutions may be limited. Even to the trained eye, the difference between medial calcinosis and intimal calcific atherosclerosis is often indeterminable. SFA and popliteal segments frequently contain thick atherosclerotic segments, and distal pedal and even digital vessels demonstrate calcific noncompliance. Renal failure is an independent risk factor in the failure of all sorts of vascular intervention (see below).

Sometimes, subintimal passage is the only solution (23). The subintimal plane is usually preserved in spite of massive calcification and will allow relatively easy traversal, but this is only half the battle. Reentry may not be so easy and angioplasty of the newly created subintimal channel may fail because of lack of plasticity of the calcified "rocks" at the reentry site.

Embolization of calcified debris is particularly problematic because it doesn't respond to thrombolysis or even distal excimer laser ablation. Therefore, thromboaspiration may be the only way to recanalize a segment (24). A variety of thromboaspiration catheters exist, but all are of limited size. New long 4-Fr sheaths can also be used for this purpose and have the advantage of larger lumens.

Calciphylaxis is a relative contraindication to open surgery. Cutting through calciphylactic skin patches results in nonhealing and potential exposure of the graft. Furthermore, no solution generally works with calciphylaxis, so the less injury you create, the better. There are new pharmacologic approaches that may be as successful as surgery (25), although the prognosis for patients with calciphylaxis is very poor, with up to 80% mortality (26).

Popliteal Artery

Calcification is more likely near Hunter's canal and the above-the-knee segment; BTK segments are often relatively spared. However, passing through chronic total occlusions is safer in the above-the-knee segment due to the longer outflow distance provided for gaining reentry. Reentry in the BTK segment is limited by geography and can also lead to the destruction of a potentially excellent operative target. The patency of a popliteal bypass is better than a tibial bailout procedure. If passage is attempted, it is a good idea to work off a clear road-mapped image so the reentry point is created as close to the occlusion as possible. Avoid placing stents in the popliteal artery when possible. Also, the location of the popliteal artery flexion point is not at the joint space but is usually above the knee between the joint space and Hunter's canal, which is a fixed point. This can be simply determined by performing angiography in the flexed-knee positions.

Tibioperoneal Trunk

For unknown reasons, this is often a very calcified segment. The tibioperoneal trunk is short, unforgiving, calcified, and the origin of both the posterior tibial and the peroneal arteries distally and the anterior tibial artery proximally. Buddy wire "insurance" is often worthwhile for interventions in the tibioperoneal trunk. Endpoints are very difficult to achieve. A complex lesion in this segment should always generate a "What if I fail?" question. Obliterating the bifurcation may create more trouble than you think. Before intervention, one of the two major outflow vessels often fills the other one *retrograde* via the tibioperoneal trunk's bifurcation. If the bifurcation is obliterated by a failed endoluminal intervention, the distal circulation can suffer. This situation can be best detected by looking at dynamic angiography, which will show you the *direction* of contrast flow. Static images or computed tomography (CT) angiograms fail to reveal these flow patterns. Because this artery is very rigid, because of length constraints, and also because it is relatively protected in the calf musculature high in the leg, balloon-expandable stents may be useful here.

Tibial Arteries

Reentry from the subintimal plane is easier in the tibial arteries than in the popliteal or tibioperoneal trunk. The arteries are smaller and so is the thickness of the intima in the patent segments. Reentry can be performed with a variety of methods; our current favorite is to just push through directly with a 0.014" or 0.018" Spectranetics Quick-Cross catheter (Spectranetics, Colorado Springs, Colorado, U.S.) (27). These catheters are so thick that they gravitate to the distal lumen, to be followed with the guidewire of choice. Again, anticipation of the endpoint with road mapping is critical to determine where to pull back to if reentry fails. Reentry devices like the Outback (Cordis, Miami, Florida, U.S.) are too big to use in these locations. We like to use a V-18 wire or a 0.014" Fielder wire with a hydrophilic tip. During traversal of CTOs, the ability to choose the subintimal plane versus the endoluminal plane is probably overestimated. In all likelihood, in most CTO crossings the guidewire traverses areas in all planes as it makes its way through the path of least resistance.

PHYSIOLOGIC DISTINCTIONS WORTH NOTING

Buried in a lot of the literature is risk stratification. Risk can be stratified according to clinical status (Rutherford classification, see the following text), anatomic status [TransAtlantic Inter-Society Consensus (TASC II)], and status of the outflow vessels [society of vascular surgery (SVS) outflow scale]. In fact, the differences in results according to risk stratification are far larger than the differences defined by various techniques. Early studies performed with new-generation endoluminal devices are frequently performed on patients with low risk for obvious reasons. Many studies also employ nonstandard definitions of endpoints. Therefore, formal or informal comparisons with historical controls are rarely relevant. Clinical results (survival or freedom from amputation) are always better than anatomic results (patency, target lesion revascularization, or restenosis). Clinical success with *any* intervention is generally better than 70% in one year. Therefore, distinguishing a difference with such high baseline success rates requires large studies to adequately power the statistical analysis. Very few studies in the literature are large enough to adequately do this, although many studies boast high clinical success as a justification for use of a featured device.

Rutherford classification:

0—no symptoms
1—mild claudication
2—moderate claudication
3—severe claudication
4—rest pain (CLI)
5—minor tissue loss (CLI)
6—major tissue loss (CLI)

Claudication

Performing both open and endoluminal intervention below the knee is still somewhat controversial, but not rare. Menard and Belkin reviewed the literature of open surgical bypass grafts below the knee for claudication and the outcomes were excellent, up to 80% five-year patency and single-vein bypasses (12). Claudicants comprised only 13% of total tibial bypass cases in Conte's series of open bypasses but needed to be carefully chosen (28). Nine percent of claudicants suffered major complications after vein bypass but no mortality or amputation. Excellent five-year primary (81%) and secondary (86%) patencies were noted in this study. A subset of Byrne's 1999 study included 94 tibial bypasses for claudication (3). This was a total of only 2.1% of all infrainguinal bypasses performed by their group for all causes, and 23% of their bypasses for claudication. Strangely, the primary (86%) and secondary (90%) patencies were better than both the above and BTK popliteal bypasses over four years and they suffered no 30-day mortality or long-term limb loss. These data show that good results can be obtained operatively in patients with tibial disease for claudication, but that these patients are a small minority of a vascular practice. However, careful evaluation of these retrospective studies shows a dearth of data on functional improvement, other complications and postoperative chronic lymphedema, or nerve injury. There are as yet no data comparing endoluminal versus surgical solutions for claudication due to disease below the knee (1).

Regarding endoluminal solutions, Krankenberg's group studied 78 patients with 104 endoluminal interventions of all kinds for Rutherford category 2 to 3 claudication. Initial walking distance increased from 49 to 107 m. Absolute walking distance increased from 102 to 167 m, and exercise-induced ABIs improved from 0.49 to 0.72 (all highly significant changes). One-year primary, primary assisted, and secondary patencies were 66%, 82%, and 91%, respectively. An argument can be made that since endoluminal intervention is less invasive, it should be attempted more often. This is only true if the anatomy is so favorable that there is little to be lost if things go wrong. The complication rate in Krankenberg's study was 6%, all of which were treated conservatively without severe consequence. Although this can never be guaranteed, considering the potential, downside is the most important way to strategize these cases. Consider also that the diagnosis may be wrong and sensitive to the possibility of spinal stenosis or other sources of nonvascular pain. In the TALON (Treating Peripherals with Silverhawk: Outcomes Collection) Registry, which looked at Silverhawk atherectomy results in mostly claudicants, four patients suffered acute amputation as a consequence of intervention without preprocedure tissue loss (29). The natural history of claudication demonstrates a low rate of conversion to CLI, so "preventive" interventions are not indicated. Given the significantly worse primary patency of endoluminal intervention here versus surgery, a reasonable question would be whether you pay a "penalty" for the necessary reintervention in those patients in whom restenosis occurs, over and above the cost and inconvenience of the redo procedure itself. In other words, are the results of a redo worse than the original procedure? Although not restricted to BTK procedures, DeRubertis looked at this in an analysis of 1000 endoluminal interventions in the lower extremities, and surprisingly there was *no* penalty for reintervention (Fig. 3) (30).

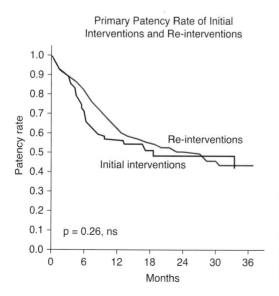

FIGURE 3 Comparison of 1000 patients with lower extremity interventions divided into those with initial interventions versus reinterventions. No significant difference in patency is noted between groups. There does not seem to be a penalty in patency associated with reintervention. *Source*: From Ref. 30.

According to the TASC II document, there is insufficient evidence to support endoluminal intervention for claudication due to infrageniculate disease; so violations of this principle must be carefully considered (1). "Patients with significant cardiopulmonary, neurologic, musculoskeletal, or other conditions likely to compromise their functional capacity or longevity would be poor candidates for reconstruction in the absence of critical ischemia (12)."

Rest Pain

Although the natural history of untreated rest pain is not benign (73% death or amputation at 1 year) (31), sometimes very simple and straightforward interventions can be enough to reverse a limb-threatening lesion. In fact, the natural history of CLI in the current era is hard to calculate since interventions are now so common. Subsets of patients who are not operative candidates and only undergo medical treatment demonstrate 40% six-month amputation rates and 20% mortality rates, but these patients had even worse risk factors than the rest of the CLI cohort (1). In one study, only 43% of CLI patients treated medically enjoyed amputation-free survival at three months post discharge (32). Treated patients have been demonstrated to have a considerably better amputation-free survival in some studies as long as five years (33). Although this is a chapter on strategy of BTK intervention, rest pain is almost always a result of multilevel disease. One of the strategies in patients with rest pain is *not* to intervene below the knee if there is an above-the-knee lesion to treat first. If an above-the-knee lesion has already been treated, question the adequacy of the previous inflow procedure before intervening below the knee. Seriously consider above-the-knee endoluminal pressure monitoring with induced hyperemia during the diagnostic angiogram before intervening. Subtle changes in pressure often solve the problem of rest pain. With respect to rest pain, generally less is more.

Ulceration and Gangrene

Conversely, gangrene requires as much blood flow to the target lesion as possible. Left alone, these patients suffer a 95% amputation rate (31). It is worth stratifying whether gangrene is simple or complex (Rutherford category 5 or 6). Small toe eschars can sometimes be treated like the rest pain described above, but any serious tissue loss will require significant improvement in blood flow. Because the metabolic requirements of healing exceed those of maintenance, the threshold pressure of CLI in gangrene is actually higher than that of rest pain (ankle pressures of 70 mmHg vs. 50 mmHg; or toe pressures of 50 vs. 30 mmHg) (17). Technical success rates of BTK endoluminal interventions in this situation approach 90%, but clinical success rates are lower at approximately 70% (1). It is interesting to note that in the largest review of BTK interventions by Bosiers, of 443 patients (661 interventions), 355 were classified Rutherford category 4, 82 category 5, and only 6 category 6 (10). This nonrandomized distribution underscores the pessimism of using endoluminal means to treat category 6 lesions. Often, you only get one chance, especially if the tissue loss is significant. Things to consider include the following:

1. Exposure of vital structures and poor intrapedal runoff are the most challenging factors to manage and endoluminal techniques are not as successful if these factors are present.

2. Toe versus heel ulcerations and their relation to the specific internal circulation of the foot.
3. How good is the circulation in the area of ulceration itself within the foot circulation?
4. What podiatric solutions exist? Put these into a hierarchy of potential interventions. An intervention may not be able to heal the lesion in question, but it may bring adequate blood flow to heal a podiatric procedure to close the wound. Primary closure is easier to heal than secondary.
5. Is there bone involvement and the predetermined need for limited amputation?
6. How sick is the patient, either from infection or unrelated disease?
7. How rapidly is the infection ascending?
8. How difficult is it going to be to achieve reasonable perfusion to the area in question, and can that be more easily achieved with a bypass? In patients with Rutherford category 6 lesions, modest gains in perfusion aren't worth it and won't complete the job.
9. Is there a role for a composite endo-open procedure?

Renal Failure

One of the worst risk factors in terms of outcome of interventions of all types is renal failure. This is probably accentuated below the knee because of extensive medial calcinosis. Aulivola studied infrapopliteal angioplasty in 79 patients with Rutherford category 5 to 6 ulceration, and the results were stratified according to renal function (34). Ulcer healing occurred in 56% of nonrenal failure patients and only 25% of renal failure patients. Similarly, "Major amputation was required in 11 (14.9%) non-ESRD and 7 (43.7%) ESRD limbs. Limb salvage was 84.4% and 80.2% in those without and 52.5% and 52.5% in those with ESRD at one and three years, respectively ($p = 0.01$)," although survival did *not* differ between the two groups. They reasonably question the utility of infrapopliteal intervention in this group. Finnish registry data in 5575 endoluminal interventions demonstrate clearly the worse prognosis in patients with renal failure and diabetes (35). Although "Primary technical success reached 97%, hemodynamic improvement was obtained in only 50% (19/38) of the limbs treated. The pedal arteries were severely diseased in all, and complete occlusion of the pedal arch was found in 58% (18/31) of limbs on completion angiography (36)." A 27% one-year amputation rate was noted, but Leers' series demonstrated rates as high as 44%. About 40% of *these* amputations were performed with *open* bypasses, and *no* patient with heel gangrene healed (37). In Söder's study of infrapopliteal angioplasty, only elevated creatinine and poor angiographic outcome severely affected clinical success independently by stepwise multiple logistic regression analysis compared with a long list of other unrelated variables (5). In spite of these depressing data, we do aggressively treat lesions in patients with renal failure but also experience very mixed outcomes.

SPECIFIC TECHNIQUES

You will almost never find a good enough comparative study between techniques or equipment to make up your mind on the basis of the literature alone. As far as BTK interventions, you have to evaluate the studies and compare raw success data, knowing of course that there is little statistical support for this practice. This is a product of design. The number of patients required for a study

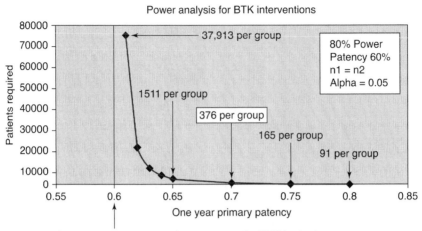

Power analysis for BTK interventions

FIGURE 4   Power calculations showing number needed per group to demonstrate a statistically significant difference in patency. Assuming the control group patency to be 60%, it would require 376 patients per group (752 per study) to demonstrate a 10% difference in patency between devices assuming an improvement in patency to 70%. Smaller differences require far more patients as demonstrated by the curve.

powered to discern clear differences between different techniques would be vast. As an example, the figure below demonstrates the number of patients per group needed to prove a difference in primary patency from the estimated 60% primary patency of plain old balloon angioplasty (POBA). To prove a 10% improvement in one device would require a study of about 750 patients (Fig. 4).

What follows is a technique-by-technique discussion of our BTK strategy as honed by experience and as much of the literature as we can safely analyze.

Diagnostic Angiography

Please visit chapter 5 on diagnostic techniques earlier in this book, our comments are meant only to augment this. First decide on antegrade versus retrograde access. Tall patients may be too long to use 135 cm devices, and sometimes it is worth going antegrade under ultrasonic guidance in an overweight patient rather than run out of catheter length. Some devices are 110, 120, 135, and 150 cm in length. Whatever portion of your sheath sticks out of the patient also has to be subtracted from these lengths. There is nothing more frustrating than having to give up on a case because the devices aren't long enough. Antegrade access can be tricky. Just to get into the SFA requires a first-order selective catheterization, but the stability gained for more distal interventions is often extremely helpful and can make the difference between a successful and an unsuccessful case. Deciding which patients would benefit from antegrade puncture also requires an excellent preprocedure duplex or a CT angiography. If there is a proximal SFA lesion, go up and over.

Intervention below the knee in the contralateral limb should be performed through as long a sheath as possible to increase pushability and also to allow detailed angiography through the sheath placed close to the site of intervention (10).

Make liberal use of pressure measurements, although keep in mind that the catheter itself may affect the results you are seeing in an antegrade catheterization. Make certain that you have good biplanar views of the foot before and at least one good view after any intervention to make certain that there has been no embolization, and that tarsal and plantar anatomies are well understood. Next, decide on contrast agent. Renal insufficiency and renal failure is very common in the population requiring BTK treatment. We make liberal use of CO_2 but also use diluted Visipaqe (sometimes to as low a concentration as 1:5, we call it "cheap stuff") for almost all cases. It is possible to do a complex case with ~20 cc of contrast. We almost never use full strength contrast for anything. The aortogram is performed with CO_2, especially if the initial duplex shows good biphasic inflow. CO_2 is used to evaluate the diseased segments with the catheter placed directly into the leg arteries. When the amount of occlusive disease is severe, CO_2 is less effective and dilute liquid contrast is used. Ascher and colleagues published an article on ultrasound-guided infrapopliteal angioplasty, which makes use of contrast optional except for completion studies. Although possible, it is probably more work than necessary since once the anatomy is understood, a lot can be done with fluoroscopy alone (38). Although multidetector CT angiography has been touted as a quantum leap in technology, large doses of iodinated contrast are necessary (80–180 cc), which may limit its usefulness in high-risk patients (39). The use of magnetic resonance angiography has been limited in this population by the risk of nephrogenic systemic fibrosis.

Medications

Almost every patient in our service is on aspirin for many reasons, which don't need to be articulated here. Although we are still waiting for a good randomized study in the periphery, standard of practice now indicates preloading patients with clopidogrel before engaging in peripheral angioplasty. Most of the data have been inferred from the cardiology literature (CAPRIE STUDY). The more distal and smaller the vessels, the more important this is perceived to be. We pretreat for five days if possible with standard doses, or load with 300 mg on the morning of the procedure. The only time this is not performed is if the likelihood of open surgery is high, in which case, the effects of plavix can be very tedious, especially in redo operations. It is important to realize that there are really no data to support these practices in the periphery.

Doses of anticoagulants during the cases have also not been standardized. When there are particularly worrisome characteristics of the case, such as poor runoff or the need for an embolic protection device, we use full anticoagulating doses of heparin and achieve an activated clotting time (ACT) more than 250 seconds.

Facility with thrombolytic agents and percutaneous thrombectomy devices is advised, and access to thrombectomy catheters like the "export" catheter is important. Acute intraprocedural thrombi in small vessels may be well treated with simple aspiration, considerably easier than in larger vessels like the popliteal or femoral arteries.

Spastic vessels can be treated with injections of nitroglycerine 100 to 200 µg especially in situations where flow is very slow. Some practitioners pretreat patients with nifedipine 10 mg (5).

POBA

POBA has now become the standard intervention for comparison with all other endoluminal interventions. Advantages include availability, simplicity, and cost. Superb balloons are now available in 0.014" platform, multiple sizes, and lengths up to 150 mm, which can angioplast half the length of a tibial artery in one inflation. Balloons have become so low in profile that many operators are using the balloon angioplasty catheter as a recanalization catheter for tibial occlusions. If more than one balloon inflation is required, we recommend doing the more distal inflation first in a long lesion since the balloon's profile changes significantly after the first inflation and may not be able to be subsequently advanced. Compliant and noncompliant designs are also available.

In a comparison of results for above versus BTK angioplasty in patients with CLI (Rutherford categories 4–6), a total of 180 patients underwent 198 angioplasties. Primary cumulative patency, limb salvage, and survival for femoropopliteal angioplasty ($n = 166$) at two years were 75%, 90%, and 88%, respectively, and 60%, 76%, and 82% for infrapopliteal angioplasty ($n = 32$) (40). There was a very similar restenosis rate (defined as >50% recurrent stenosis) of 68% and 65% at two years for the femoropopliteal and infrapopliteal angioplasty groups, respectively. In the same study, there was a comparison with primarily performed surgical bypass. A total of 153 comparative control patients underwent 162 bypass procedures during the same period. Primary cumulative patency, limb salvage, and survival for femoropopliteal bypass ($n = 80$) at two years were 69%, 87%, and 76%, respectively, and were 53%, 57%, and 64% for infrapopliteal bypass ($n = 82$). Although the raw success rates are better here for endoluminal therapy, this was not a prospective study and the rates cannot be compared, since there were undoubtedly biases in patient choice. Nevertheless, these results fuel an endoluminal-first policy (Table 1).

In an earlier paper, Dorros studied 111 patients with infrapopliteal angioplasty; 47% were claudicants. Forty percent recurrence was noted at nine months, two-thirds of which were in sites *separate* from the treated lesion and represented progression of disease instead. Even back in 1990, the severe complication rate was only 3% and anatomic success was 99% in stenotic and 65% in occluded vessels (41). The high population of claudicants probably contributed to the high initial success rate.

Dorros published a second article in 1998 of 417 tibial angioplasties, which stands as the largest series thus far. Acute success was 95% in stenotic lesions and an acceptable 77% in occluded lesions (42). This is especially notable, given

TABLE 1 Data Demonstrating Slightly Better Two-Year Outcomes with Angioplasty Vs. Bypass in a Nonrandomized Study

Two-year data	Primary patency (%)	Limb salvage (%)	Survival (%)
Fem-pop percutaneous transluminal angioplasty (PTA)	75	90	88
Fem-pop bypass	69	87	76
Below-knee PTA	60	76	82
Below-knee bypass	53	57	64

Although no conclusions can be reached about the superiority of angioplasty in this situation, the fact that the numbers do not demonstrate worse outcomes is encouraging to an endoluminal-first policy.
Source: From Ref. 40.

the equipment available at the time of intervention, the last case having been performed in 1997. Technically speaking, the standard for successful angioplasty is defined as less than 30% residual stenosis (5), but this standard is frequently violated in reports.

Unfortunately, follow-up of these patients was not provided, but the article gives a good idea of what is possible in the short term. A list of sub-trifurcation angioplasty publications was compiled by Rastogi and gives an idea of both the expected outcomes and also the variability in the literature (43,44).

The legend in Table 2 is as important as the table itself. There is no uniformity in the data reported in these studies. Attempts have been made to create crossover endoluminal standards derived from the SVS-recommended reporting

TABLE 2 Data Showing Total Lack of Adoption of Standards Between All Papers Reporting Subtrifurcation Angioplasty Over a 13-Year Period.

Author	Year	Number of limbs	Technical success (%)	Clinical result (%)
Schwarten and Cutliff	1988	114	97	83[a]
Brown et al.	1988	11	75	48[b]
Bakal et al.	1990	53	78	53[c]
Horvath et al.	1990	71	96	75[a]
Dorros et al.	1990	111	90	40[d]
Flueckiger et al.	1992	91	91	64[e]
Saab et al.	1992	14	100	71[f]
Bull et al.	1992	168	77	62[a]
Wagner et al.	1993	158	95	88[g]
Buckenham et al.	1993	14	100	85[c]
Matsi et al.	1993	84	83	49[a]
Brown et al.	1993	55	95	53[a]
Durham et al.	1994	14	100	77[g]
Sivanathan et al.	1994	41	96	58[h]
Bolia et al.	1994	24	86	NR
Varty et al.	1995	40	98	79[a]
Lofberg et al.	1996	86	88	75[a]
Hauser et al.	1996	47	80	77[a]
Gross et al.	1996	43	79	NR
Madera et al.	1997	25	84	75[i]
Dorros et al.	1998	417	96	NR
Boyer et al.	2000	49	92	87[j]
Soder et al.	2000	72	76	63[k]
Dorros et al.	2001	284	95	91[l]

The most interesting part of this table is the legend, which details conditions in various reports. No comparison is possible between reports.
NR, not reported.
[a]Limb salvage at two years.
[b]Limb salvage at eight months.
[c]Early clinical response.
[d]Maintained clinical benefit at nine months.
[e]Patency at three years.
[f]Limb salvage at 19 months.
[g]Limb salvage at 17 months.
[h]Maintained clinical benefit at 21 months.
[i]Maintained clinical benefit longer than 30 days (mean 20 months).
[j]Limb salvage at three years.
[k]Rutherford–Becker category of the limb improved at least one grade.
[l]Limb-salvage rate at five years (8% of group had surgical bypass).
Source: From Refs. 43 and 44.

standards for open surgery (45), but few studies have followed the recommendations.

Technical success for infrapopliteal interventions in patients selected for CLI by comparison is not as impressive as more general populations. Soder's CLI paper demonstrated only 84% immediate technical success for stenotic lesions versus 61% for occluded tibial vessels in a prospective study. Restenosis was 32% in 10 months for stenotic vessels and 52% for occlusions (5).

The best, randomized prospective comparison of surgery versus angioplasty is the BASIL trial (Bypass Versus Angioplasty in Severe Ischemia of the Leg) (46). This trial was restricted to patients with CLI. Although not restricted to patients with BTK lesions, it is a true randomized trial of surgery versus angioplasty. The patients were randomized after identifying a group of patients "who on diagnostic imaging had a pattern of disease which, in their joint opinions, could equally well be treated by either infrainguinal bypass surgery or balloon angioplasty." Ninety-five percent of patients had diagnostic angiography before randomization, something that now would be practically impossible since decisions are clinically made on the table for the most part. Primary outcomes were amputation-free survival or death. The first part of the trial was an audit in 6 of the 27 participating hospitals. In this portion, 456 CLI patients presented with infrainguinal disease, about half were treated without revascularization, 236 were left of which only 29% were suitable for randomization (70 total). Of this diminishing number, 31% refused randomization, so really only 48 were randomized. (That is only a little more than 10% of the total who presented, so this demonstrates that this is a highly selected trial in spite of its attempt at randomization.) A full third of the nonrandomized patients were thought *not* to be revascularizable at all by *either* method underscoring the complexity of this particular patient group. In the follow-up trial as a whole (nonaudited segment) 452 patients enrolled in the study from an unreported denominator. Mortality was the same between groups. Complication rate was high for both groups; 56% of the open surgery and 41% of the angioplasty patients had at least one complication within 30 days ($p < 0.05$ in favor of angioplasty). Angioplasty demonstrated a very high technical failure rate of 20% immediately. Only about a third of the interventions were to the crural arteries, which is our focus in this chapter. Unfortunately, separate analyses were not performed on this subgroup, but 62% of angioplasty patients had at least part of their procedure distal to the SFA. Clinical success over 12 months was noted in 50% of angioplasty and 56% of bypass patients. The reintervention rate was 18% for surgery and 26% for angioplasty, and this difference was significant. There was, however, no significant difference in primary endpoints at one year or three years, *but* there was a trend toward better result with angioplasty in the first six months and toward a good result with surgery after six months. This became significant *after* two years in favor of surgery (Fig. 5). It is hard to read too much into this, but it may support the bias that for the CLI patient with a longer life expectancy, surgery may be a better option. HRQL (health-related quality-of-life measure) scores were really no different between groups, which is surprising. Cost was about a third higher for surgery. Importantly, there was "no suggestion that a clinically failed angioplasty prejudiced the results of any subsequent surgical intervention...." This is an important statement, given the fear of some that endoluminal intervention makes subsequent surgery harder. The bottom line is that it doesn't matter too much what you do, the results in

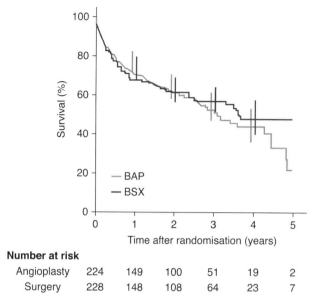

FIGURE 5 Results from the BASIL trial that show similar results of angioplasty versus surgery in spite of numerous statistical challenges in the study. *Source*: From Ref. 46.

CLI patients are poor! It supports our bias for an endoluminal-first policy for reasons of cost and patient acceptability alone.

Subintimal Angioplasty
The subintimal plane is the path of least resistance, and sometimes it greatly facilitates traversal and occlusion. Bolia demonstrated a very high success rate with SFA lesions in the early 1990s. The original concept was anti-intuitive. Pushing into the subintimal plane used to be considered a complication and there is a long learning curve for this procedure. In 2002, a study of subintimal angioplasty in *isolated* infragenicular vessels was performed; technical failure was only 14% (47). Limb salvage was 94% and freedom from CLI 84%, all at 36 months, which is longer follow-up than most studies. This was a very aggressive study, and the excellent results were probably due to the fact that in 36% of patients, all three tibial vessels were opened with a technical success rate of 86%. Seven percent of the patients were perforated, but only half of these required coil embolization and the other half were self-limited. Limb salvage and freedom from CLI were associated with nondiabetics, though diabetes was not associated with technical failure. Ninety-one percent of the patients in the study had CLI. Only 3% of patients developed acute ischemia as a complication of the procedure.

In the tibial vessels we perform subintimal traversal either with guide-wires (V18 or 0.014″ platforms) or directly with a CTO catheter, such as the Spectranetics Quick-Cross catheter. It is often impossible to know how much is subintimal and how much is endoluminal. It probably doesn't make much difference. As mentioned above, reentry is less difficult than in the popliteal segment. However, if the guidewire gets outside of the artery profile (and likely

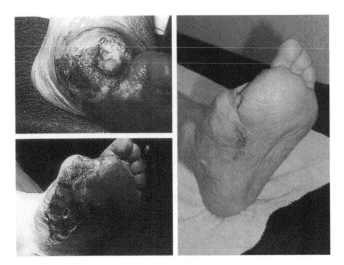

FIGURE 6 Slide from Vraux demonstrating excellent result in a patient with combination of dorsalis pedis conventional angioplasty and posterior tibial subintimal angioplasty. *Source*: From Ref. 49.

outside the adventitia as well), it is almost impossible to get back into the subintimal space (Fig. 6).

Cryoplasty

Encouraged by in vitro studies that show apoptosis associated with cold injury in vascular smooth muscle cells, a nitrous oxide powered angioplasty balloon that inflates at -20°C has been developed. Sold by Boston Scientific as "Polar-Cath," potential advantages of cryoplasty include the following: (*i*) it weakens the plaque, which promotes uniform dilation and results in less vessel trauma; (*ii*) it reduces vessel wall recoil; and (*iii*) it induces apoptosis of the smooth muscle cells, limiting a potent stimulus for neointima formation. In a recent study entitled "below-the-knee chill study" (48), Das et al. reported six-month outcomes using infrapopliteal cryoplasty in CLI patients from 16 centers. This study is limited in scope, and although it includes 111 limbs, it only reports acute technical success rate (97.3%), a very low rate of clinically significant dissection (0.9%), 6.3% minor dissection, and only two residual stenoses of greater than 50%. This compares favorably to historical controls across multiple studies, which have ranges of procedural success from 82% to 100% with POBA (5,18,33,34,36,49–55). Clinical outcomes were similar to other studies.

Seven retrospective series are available, and only the one mentioned above pertains to infrapopliteal vessels. Technical success in these studies is encouraging but is not a basis for distinguishing cryoplasty from POBA. One reason to select cryoplasty over traditional balloon angioplasty is if you are concerned that there is an increased likelihood of dissection in your target vessel. The clinical induction of apoptosis is less clearly shown. Karthik studied 10 patients with *restenotic* lesions. Restenotic lesions were chosen to test whether the apoptosis proposed to be associated with cryoplasty might specifically prevent neointimal hyperplasia in these already hyperplastic lesions. Technical success was 100%. However, 50% failed in six months and all 12 procedures failed by one year.

Only two patients remained asymptomatic at the end of the follow-up period and both of these had hemodynamically significant restenotic lesions as well. This study clearly does not support the idea that cryoplasty decreases neo-intimal hyperplasia in restenotic lesions. Picking these patients to test the theory of increased apoptosis associated with cryoplasty may have had the unintended consequence of the opposite effect: picking patients who are more likely to restenose. As a result of these preliminary results, the study was cut short.

Stents

The first report of stent deployment in the infrapopliteal arteries was published in 1993 by Dorros. This was done for an angioplasty-related dissection. Bosiers performed a study in patients with infrapopliteal lesions with Rutherford categories 4, 5, and 6 CLI and demonstrated that overall patency was slightly higher with stents in the tibial arteries than with angioplasty alone. This was not a randomized trial (10). Seventy-nine patients received BTK angioplasty versus 300 patients with angioplasty and stenting. All manner of stents were used, including balloon-expandable, self-expanding, and absorbable metal stents. One-year primary patency rates were 68.6% for PTA and 75.5% for stenting (NS); limb salvage rates were 96.7% and 98.6% (NS). Only 30% of the stents were performed for inadequate angioplasty leaving 70%, which were placed "within the context of the trial," in other words, surgeon choice (Fig. 7).

In a later study of infrapopliteal stenting using the Xpert stent (Abbott Vascular, Illinois, U.S.), Bosiers showed a binary restenosis rate at one year of 20.45% (>50% threshold). One-year primary patency and limb salvage rates were 76.3% and 95.9%, respectively. It is interesting to note that the limb salvage

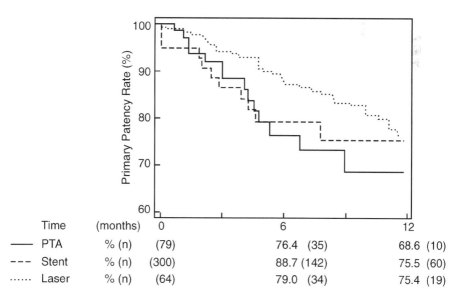

Time	(months)	0	6	12
—— PTA	% (n)	(79)	76.4 (35)	68.6 (10)
– – – Stent	% (n)	(300)	88.7 (142)	75.5 (60)
⋯⋯⋯ Laser	% (n)	(64)	79.0 (34)	75.4 (19)

FIGURE 7 Data from Bosiers demonstrating somewhat better results from stenting in the infrapopliteal region versus either angioplasty or laser. Since data were not randomized, no definitive conclusions can be drawn, although clearly stents did not result in inferior patency. *Source*: From Ref. 10.

rate was significantly better in patients with proximal BTK lesions, than in those with midsection or distal lesions (100% vs. 81.8%; $p = 0.0071$) (56).

In 2006, Rand performed a study that compared carbon-coated stents with PTA in the infrapopliteal region with an improvement in the stented group (8). Two thresholds of stenosis were examined (50% and 70%) by either re-angiography or CT angiogram. At six months, there was statistical superiority in the stented group at both thresholds (83% versus 61% for a 70% threshold stenosis and 80% vs. 46% at the 50% threshold $p < 0.05$).

Drug-eluting stents do not appear to be a panacea in this vascular bed. Siablis et al. (57) performed a study with paclitaxel-eluting stents in the tibial circulation (57). All patients had CLI, and drug-eluting stents were only placed after unsuccessful angioplasty (>30% residual stenosis or dissection). Follow-up was angiographic at six months and one year. Technical success was an impressive 100%; however, the patients were only enrolled if they had failed angioplasty, implying that lesion traversal had already been accomplished. In spite of the high technical success rate, the one-year outcome was quite poor. In-stent primary patency was only 30% and the restenosis rate was 77.4%. Clinical results were acceptable as a limb salvage rate was 88.5%. Nonetheless, there is nothing about this study to suggest that drug-eluting stents yet have a place in BTK interventions. Bosiers also studied sirolimus-eluting stents in infrapopliteal vessels in 20 patients with CLI. Survival and limb salvage rates were excellent, but technical results did not differ from historical controls. In a later study, Siablis et al. (57) reported one-year angiographic and clinical outcomes and the comparison study of sirolimus versus bare-metal stents. Again, stenting was used as a bailout procedure. There were 29 patients in each group. In this study, after six months and one year, there *was* a statistically significant improvement with sirolimus-eluting stents compared with bare-metal stents. Primary patency, in-stent restenosis, and in-segment restenosis were all noted to be better at the $p = 0.001$ level. Reinterventions were significantly decreased as well (26.2% bare vs. 9.1% drug eluting). Clinical endpoints, however, did not show any difference. Given the cost, further work is necessary before a recommendation can be made to use drug-eluting stents.

A conservative recommendation from these data might be that residual stenosis of 30% or clinically significant dissection after primary tibial angioplasty would suggest the use of either stents or other intervention to improve the bad technical result. But the often-quoted fear that stents probably *worsen* long-term results is not born out by the studies (58) (Fig. 8). There is however some evidence that the balloon-expandable stents may be more easily deformed in the mid to distal leg. The leg not only undergoes numerous stresses but is also less protected than the thigh. We use balloon-expandable stents only in the very proximal leg for this reason, and then only occasionally. Self-expanding stents are used for everything else.

Silverhawk Atherectomy

One atherectomy device commonly used in the infrapopliteal region is the Silverhawk atherectomy catheter from Foxhollow-EV3 (59). The device consists of a rotating carbide blade within a catheter housing, which flexes to push the blade against the arterial wall in a directionally controlled fashion. The blade revolves at 8000 rpm and captures intimal "shavings" in a hollow nosecone at the tip of the device. Generally between 5 and 10 passes are necessary to properly atherectomize lesions (Fig. 9).

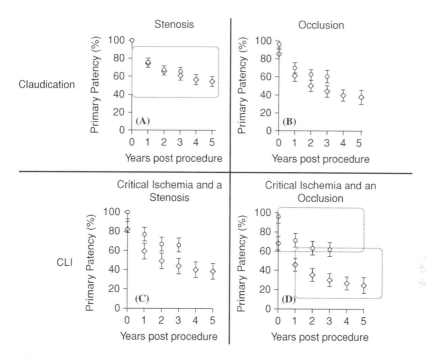

FIGURE 8 Data from a meta-analysis of Muradin comparing 923 balloon angioplasties with 423 stents in the lower extremities stratified in one dimension by claudication versus CLI, and in the other by stenosis versus occlusion. Upper left lesions are less severe than lower right lesions. A trend is seen demonstrating the superiority of stents over angioplasty in the more severe lesions, but no difference in the less severe lesions. *Source*: From Ref. 58.

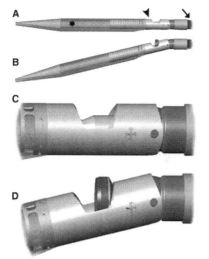

FIGURE 9 Diagram taken from Zeller demonstrating housing and function of the Silverhawk atherectomy device. *Source*: From Ref. 59.

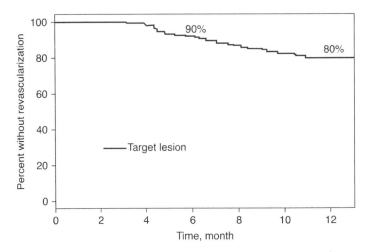

FIGURE 10 Data from the TALON registry of Silverhawk atherectomy demonstrating excellent results in freedom from target lesion revascularization. Data were not stratified, and most patients in the study had low Rutherford scores. Compare these data with Figure 11 in which stratification of data were performed with a different patient subset. *Source*: From Ref. 29

The statistics surrounding atherectomy are a good demonstration of how different data sets can affect results. The data on strictly BTK interventions are sparse, but larger studies on all lower extremity interventions are illustrative of the effects of risk pools on outcomes. Keeling demonstrated a strong decrement in the outcomes of patients with worsening Rutherford category and also worsening TASC II lesion classification (60). The TALON registry by contrast is the largest lower extremity atherectomy study to date (*not* restricted to BTK lesions) with a total of 1258 lesions treated (29). This was a community-based study, so the patient mix was far less diseased than in Keeling's study. In fact, 11% of the patients in the TALON registry had either no symptoms at all or mild claudication (Rutherford score 0–1) and only 30% had CLI (Rutherford scores 4–6) of whom less than 1% were Rutherford score 6. The clinical results parallel Keeling's *low*-grade stratified patients fared better than the high-grade patients. The TALON registry is by far the largest study to date, but blind adherence to its data might be misleading in higher-risk patients (Figs. 10 and 11).

A short-term investigation of 52 *infrapopliteal* lesions demonstrated 96% technical success and 14% restenosis within three months and 26% after six months (defined as >70% luminal reduction) (61). The total average number of passes of the atherectomy catheter to achieve these results was seven. Infrapopliteal atherectomy in CLI patients has been shown to have an event-free clinical success rate of 58% at one year and 43% at two years (62). Primary and secondary patencies in 49 lesions at one year are 67% and 91%, and at two years 60% and 80%. These patients were taken from a group of Rutherford category 4 and 5 patients but *no* patients in category 6 were represented. Amputation rate was not reported, nor was healing of ulcerations. Although these statistics are acceptable, they are not substantially different than other interventions in this cohort.

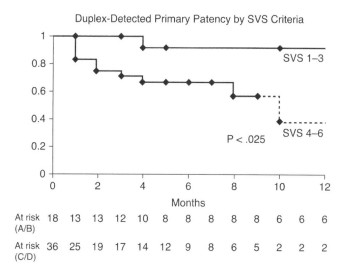

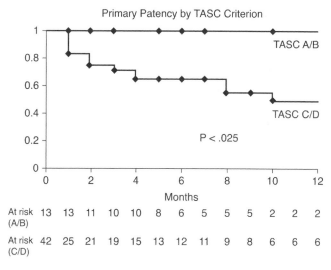

FIGURE 11 Stratified data in outcomes for Silverhawk atherectomy demonstrate inferior results in patients with worse SVS and Rutherford scales. Risk stratification is important to the outcome. *Source*: From Ref. 60.

Regarding technique, about one-third of patients underwent pre-atherectomy angioplasty and two-thirds underwent primary atherectomy. The recommendation of the manufacturer is to perform atherectomy without pre-atherectomy angioplasty though there are few data to back this up. The lesion is a more stable target for the device if it is done primarily.

Our personal recommendations for atherectomy are as follows:

1. It is probably the best device for eccentric lesions. Eccentric lesions don't respond well to angioplasty because the more elastic segment is the healthy

portion of the artery, which recoils back to its original shape whereas the plaque remains undisturbed. The directional nature of the atherectomy device allows it to specifically target this eccentric plaque.

2. Atherectomy may also be better than angioplasty for in-stent restenosis because of the restricted volume defined by the previously placed stent. However, it can also cut into the stent and even get stuck within the tines of the nitinol. In this, laser atherectomy may also be useful (see below). Data also show that directional atherectomy is very effective in vein graft stenoses (63).

3. Less than 1% of the patients in the TALON registry suffered distal embolization (29). This has neither been our experience nor that of Suri's group in whose study *all 10* studied cases had recoverable embolic material in an embolic protection device (64). We now use distal protection in any femoral or popliteal atherectomy case with large plaque burden, poor runoff, or in any claudicants.

Excimer Laser

The excimer laser is a higher energy and different spectrum (ultraviolet as opposed to infrared) than the old "hot-tipped" laser. Its penetration distance is approximately 50 μ instead of up to 1 mm for the old lasers. It works by three different mechanisms.

1. It breaks carbon-carbon (C–C) bonds through resonant frequency instead of heating up water. Each photon can break a single C–C bond with an efficiency of about 2%. This decreases heat transfer, and allows laser to work not only against plaque, but also thrombus. Therefore the excimer laser is useful for chasing embolized particles created during a procedure in addition to treating the primary lesion. This includes particles which are non-thrombotic in origin and therefore do not respond to thrombolytics.

2. There is agitation surrounding the 50-μ vaporization zone. Each pulse vaporizes approximately 10 μ of tissue The laser is pulsed between 25 and 80 times/sec in extremely short (20 billionths of a second) bursts, which greatly decreases heat transfer due to the heat-sink effect of the surrounding blood (65). For this reason there appears to be almost no heat transfer to the surrounding vessel wall, which was thought to be responsible for the very high rates of neointimal hyperplasia in the previous generation of *hot*-tipped lasers.

3. Steam expansion explodes cells vaporization zone.

Probably the most important difference between laser and most other forms of intervention is its ablative capacity; instead of compressing a lesion, laser produces a true atherectomy. Strategies for lesion expansion versus atherectomy have yet to be fully optimized.

Another mechanical feature is that the device works primarily from the tip of the catheter instead of from the side. It is really the only device to do so, and this unique feature may be one of the most helpful parameters of its design. Laser can be used for "decapping" chronic total occlusions by resting the tip against the end of an occlusion and delivering laser energy (66). This can begin the process of penetration within the luminal plane as opposed to the subintimal plane. Often, a chronic thrombus cap covers the occluded segment. In essence, this is a cul-de-sac of thrombus, which is fairly easily penetrated by laser energy. If it is not possible to pass a guidewire through the occlusion, a "step-by-step" approach has been described in which the laser tip was advanced a couple of millimeters followed by a guidewire in the back and forth type maneuver to penetrate a lesion that is otherwise not penetrable with the guidewire alone. The end-on action also allows it to be used for embolized particles.

The PELA study included 251 patients randomized between excimer laser angioplasty and stenting versus angioplasty and stenting alone. It demonstrated little improvement with laser in superficial femoral artery occlusions in patients with claudication. The only real meaningful difference between the groups was a decrease in the number of stents deployed in the laser group versus the simple angioplasty group. I suspect that the decision whether or not to use laser will ultimately be based on more subtle criteria than simply occlusion.

At higher fluencies, it actually is able to penetrate calcified plaque (67). The newest generation of fibers, though very small, has been designed to accommodate these larger focused deliveries of laser energy.

Technical keys to successful laser deployment include the following:

1. Very slow advancement, 1 mm/sec or less. Faster traversal results in less atherectomy.
2. Be certain that all iodinated contrast is removed in the area being lased, as contrast absorbs some laser energy, boils and is unpredictable.
3. Saline infusion improves specificity and control by removing the energy absorption of blood.
4. A device called a "turbo-booster" offsets the laser tip around an axis, which can be rotated to increase the diameter of atherectomy. Multiple passes can be performed with the tip in different orientations. Similar to Silverhawk atherectomy, the degree of rotation can be controlled manually under fluoroscopy. This technique may be the best therapy for in-stent restenosis.
5. The laser atherectomy is often not sufficient on its own to complete the procedure. Subsequent angioplasty or other intervention is almost always needed.
6. For the step-by-step procedure, initiation of traversal of a chronic total occlusion should begin approximately 1 to 2 mm proximal to the occlusion. Very slow advancement should be attempted in the hopes that the cavitation bubble slowly affects the cap of the occlusion before direct contact is made.
7. When traversal of an extremely difficult occlusion is attempted, it is advantageous to use the smallest fiber possible. The 0.9 mm fiber is perfect for this use for two reasons.
   a. If it penetrates the wall of the vessel, such a small puncture is well tolerated. This can be considered a "pilot hole" (68).
   b. There is more concentration of laser energy, focused on the calcific elements.
8. Multiple passes improve tissue obliteration. One should plan on doing more than a single pass.

Whether the long-term results of excimer laser will justify its expense is as yet unknown. We use it preferentially in situations in which there is more calcium, and to traverse more difficult chronic total occlusions. It is also useful in situations where tissue ablation is more important. It may turn out to be one of the best treatment modalities for in-stent restenosis where the volume of the repair is constrained by the stent (68).

SUMMARY

The introduction of exciting new technology suitable for intervention in the BTK segments produces far more choices than can be adequately assessed using the current literature. Review of this literature demonstrates that success is associated more with risk groups and degree of clinical presentation and ischemia than with technique. Conversely, the BTK atherosclerosis selects for patients with more physiologic risk factors associated with failure. Differences between techniques have never been adequately compared, and these comparisons have been selected against by the marketplace. In assessing patients with BTK lesions, renal failure, calcium, and Rutherford category 6 present unusual challenges. It is often helpful to plan for failure in preference to planning for success to make certain that all contingencies are considered before embarking on a case. Open surgical options should be spared and sometimes utilized first in spite of our predilection for an endoluminal-first policy. It is usually better to start simply and more economically with angioplasty unless there is an unusual feature that strongly implies the use of a more complex device. Each particular device generally has a feature that holds more promise with respect to promoting *acute* procedural success rather than long-term clinical success. Getting to know the differences and quirks between different devices is a complex task and very expensive.

With all this in mind, the following algorithm is proposed (Fig. 12).

1. First, determine whether or not the patient has CLI. If the patient is a claudicant, decide whether the patient "needs" the intervention. This is always really a negotiation of sorts, but if the decision is to proceed then whether to utilize endoluminal versus open solutions is based on anatomic risks. Patients with unstable-looking lesions and those with limited outflow should undergo surgery. Those with obesity, poor conduit, poor skin, or other surgical risk factors, and those with fairly straightforward endoluminal solutions can be treated with catheters. The risks are low, the successes are good, and you don't lose much by reintervening knowing the primary patency is often worse than surgery. Don't proceed with endoluminal intervention for claudication if there is a good chance of destroying operative targets.

2. If the patient *does* have CLI (and something which needs more complex management than a simple fix for rest pain), then the most important question to answer first is whether to operate on the patient. Patients with significant tissue loss in whom you can't open a direct line to the foot should be operated upon unless there are confounding surgical risks. Additionally, if you are worried that outflow is limited and you can't be certain that you won't make the anatomy worse (e.g., very tenuous pedal outflow or very embologenic lesion) then surgery is also favored.

3. If the decision is made to proceed by endoluminal means, there are really almost no data to help you make a decision based on long-term outcomes. Failing that, then the decision is based on acute procedural success, something we know a little more about. In simple cases angioplasty is just fine. It is less expensive and there are very few convincing data to assume that anything else is much better. Although there is controversy over whether stents improve outcomes, the critical fact here is that it looks as if stenting doesn't *penalize* you much in terms of outcomes. This means that although

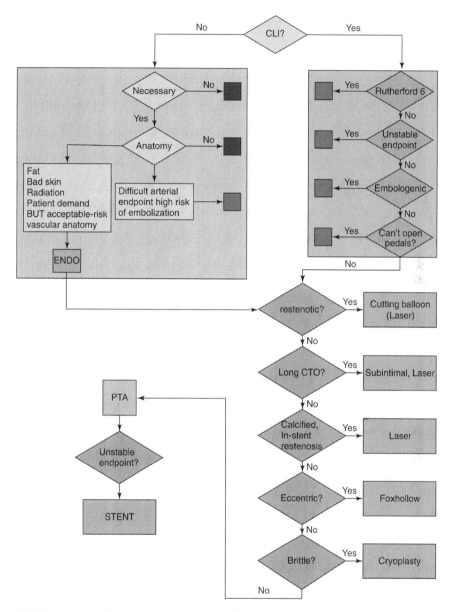

FIGURE 12 Algorithm; small black squares indicate abort procedure and continue with medial management. Small grey squares indicate patient should be referred for open surgery. Refer to detailed algorithm on page 174.

there is no reason to spend the extra money on a stent in the average case, if there is a dissection or a residual more than 30% stenosis, then you can place a stent to improve the immediate outcome without worrying too much that it will worsen the long-term results. All that is left then is to decide when to use the expensive and specialized devices. On the basis of current knowledge and personal prejudices, we recommend

a. for restenotic lesions or calcific short rings: cutting balloon;
b. for eccentric lesions: directional atherectomy catheter (consider embolic protection);
c. for long CTOs: either subintimal technique or laser atherectomy;
d. for severe calcification: laser atherectomy, possibly rotational atherectomy (consider embolic protection);
e. for in-stent restenosis: laser atherectomy with eccentric turbo-booster platform;
f. for lesions that appear brittle or unstable: cryoplasty may improve the stability of the acute result; and
g. for inadequate posttreatment results: stent placement.

REFERENCES

1. Norgren L, Hiatt WR, Dormandy JA, et al. Inter-Society Consensus for the Management of Peripheral Arterial Disease (TASC II). J Vasc Surg 2007; 45(suppl S):S5–S67.
2. Ballard JL, Mazeroll R, Weitzman R, et al. Medical benefits of a peripheral vascular screening program. Ann Vasc Surg 2007; 21(2):159–162.
3. Byrne J, Darling RC 3rd, Chang BB, et al. Infrainguinal arterial reconstruction for claudication: is it worth the risk? An analysis of 409 procedures. J Vasc Surg 1999; 29(2): 259–267; discussion 267–269.
4. Atar E, Siegel Y, Avrahami R, et al. Balloon angioplasty of popliteal and crural arteries in elderly with critical chronic limb ischemia. Eur J Radiol 2005; 53(2):287–292.
5. Soder HK, Manninen HI, Jaakkola P, et al. Prospective trial of infrapopliteal artery balloon angioplasty for critical limb ischemia: angiographic and clinical results. J Vasc Interv Radiol 2000; 11(8):1021–1031.
6. Dotter CT, Judkins MP. Transluminal treatment of arteriosclerotic obstruction. Description of a new technic and a preliminary report of its application. Circulation 1964; 30:654–670.
7. Sprayregen S, Sniderman KW, Sos TA, et al. Popliteal artery branches: percutaneous transluminal angioplasty. AJR Am J Roentgenol 1980; 135(5):945–950.
8. Rand T, Basile A, Cejna M, et al. PTA versus carbofilm-coated stents in infrapopliteal arteries: pilot study. Cardiovasc Intervent Radiol 2006; 29(1):29–38.
9. Seeger J, Abela GS. Current status of laser angioplasty. Surg Annu 1990; 22:299–315.
10. Bosiers M, Hart JP, Deloose K, et al. Endovascular therapy as the primary approach for limb salvage in patients with critical limb ischemia: experience with 443 infrapopliteal procedures. Vascular 2006; 14(2):63–69.
11. Rutherford RB, Baker JD, Ernst C, et al. Recommended standards for reports dealing with lower extremity ischemia: revised version. J Vasc Surg 1997; 26(3):517–538.
12. Menard MT, Belkin M. Infrapopliteal intervention for the treatment of the claudicant. Semin Vasc Surg 2007; 20(1):42–53.
13. Mewissen MW, Beres RA, Bessette JC, et al. Kissing-balloon technique for angioplasty of the popliteal artery trifurcation. AJR Am J Roentgenol 1991; 156(4):823–824.
14. Wittens CH, van Dijk LC, du Bois NA, et al. A new "closed" in situ vein bypass technique. Eur J Vasc Surg 1994; 8(2):166–170.
15. Robinson J, Cross MA, Brothers TE, et al. Do results justify an aggressive strategy targeting the pedal arteries for limb salvage? J Surg Res 1995; 59(4):450–454.
16. Andros G, Harris RW, Salles-Cunha SX, et al. Lateral plantar artery bypass grafting: defining the limits of foot revascularization. J Vasc Surg 1989; 10(5):511–519; discussion 520–521.
17. Bakal CW, Sprayregen S, Scheinbaum K, et al. Percutaneous transluminal angioplasty of the infrapopliteal arteries: results in 53 patients. AJR Am J Roentgenol 1990; 154(1):171–174.

18. Alfke H, Vannucchi A, Froelich JJ, et al. [Long-term results after balloon angioplasty of the crural artery.] Rofo 2007; 179(8):811–817.
19. Faglia E, Clerici G, Clerissi J, et al. When is a technically successful peripheral angioplasty effective in preventing above-the-ankle amputation in diabetic patients with critical limb ischaemia? Diabet Med 2007; 24(8):823–829.
20. Stoner MC, deFreitas DJ, Phade SV, et al. Mid-term results with laser atherectomy in the treatment of infrainguinal occlusive disease. J Vasc Surg 2007; 46(2):289–295.
21. Shafique S, Nachreiner RD, Murphy MP, et al. Recanalization of infrainguinal vessels: Silverhawk, laser, and the remote superficial femoral artery endarterectomy. Semin Vasc Surg 2007; 20(1):29–36.
22. Nelken N, Schneider PA. Advances in stent technology and drug-eluting stents. Surg Clin North Am 2004; 84(5):1203–1236, v.
23. Bolia A. Subintimal angioplasty in lower limb ischaemia. J Cardiovasc Surg (Torino) 2005; 46(4):385–394.
24. Starck EE, McDermott JC, Crummy AB, et al. Percutaneous aspiration thromboembolectomy. Radiology 1985; 156(1):61–66.
25. Velasco N, MacGregor MS, Innes A, et al. Successful treatment of calciphylaxis with cinacalcet-an alternative to parathyroidectomy? Nephrol Dial Transplant 2006; 21(7): 1999–2004.
26. Meissner M, Gille J, Kaufmann R. Calciphylaxis: no therapeutic concepts for a poorly understood syndrome? Dtsch Dermatol Ges 2006; 4(12):1037–1044.
27. Golzar JA, Belur A, Carter LI, et al. Contemporary percutaneous treatment of infrapopliteal arterial disease: a practical approach. J Interv Cardiol 2007; 20(3): 222–230.
28. Conte MS, Belkin M, Donaldson MC, et al. Femorotibial bypass for claudication: do results justify an aggressive approach? J Vasc Surg 1995; 21(6):873–880; discussion 880–881.
29. Ramaiah V, Gammon R, Kiesz S, et al. Midterm outcomes from the TALON Registry: treating peripherals with SilverHawk: outcomes collection. J Endovasc Ther 2006; 13(5): 592–602.
30. DeRubertis BG, Faries PL, McKinsey JF, et al. Shifting paradigms in the treatment of lower extremity vascular disease: a report of 1000 percutaneous interventions. Ann Surg 2007; 246(3):415–422; discussion 422–424.
31. Wolfe JH, Wyatt MG. Critical and subcritical ischaemia. Eur J Vasc Endovasc Surg 1997; 13(6):578–582.
32. ICAI-Group. A prospective epidemiological survey of the natural history of chronic critical leg ischaemia. The I.C.A.I. Group (gruppo di studio dell'ischemia cronica critica degli arti inferiori). Eur J Vasc Endovasc Surg 1996; 11(1):112–120.
33. Dorros G, Jaff MR, Dorros AM, et al. Tibioperoneal (outflow lesion) angioplasty can be used as primary treatment in 235 patients with critical limb ischemia: five-year follow-up. Circulation 2001; 104(17):2057–2062.
34. Aulivola B, Gargiulo M, Bessoni M, et al. Infrapopliteal angioplasty for limb salvage in the setting of renal failure: do results justify its use? Ann Vasc Surg 2005; 19(6):762–768.
35. Vainio E, Salenius JP, Lepäntalo M, et al. Endovascular surgery for chronic limb ischaemia. Factors predicting immediate outcome on the basis of a nationwide vascular registry. Ann Chir Gynaecol 2001; 90(2):86–91.
36. Brosi P, Baumgartner I, Silvestro A, et al. Below-the-knee angioplasty in patients with end-stage renal disease. J Endovasc Ther 2005; 12(6):704–713.
37. Leers SA, Reifsnyder T, Delmonte R, et al. Realistic expectations for pedal bypass grafts in patients with end-stage renal disease. J Vasc Surg 1998; 28(6):976–980; discussion 981–983.
38. Ascher E, Marks NA, Hingorani AP, et al. Duplex-guided balloon angioplasty and subintimal dissection of infrapopliteal arteries: early results with a new approach to avoid radiation exposure and contrast material. J Vasc Surg 2005; 42(6):1114–1121.
39. Willmann JK, Baumert B, Schertler T, et al. Aortoiliac and lower extremity arteries assessed with 16-detector row CT angiography: prospective comparison with digital subtraction angiography. Radiology 2005; 236(3):1083–1093.

40. Haider SN, Kavanagh EG, Forlee M, et al. Two-year outcome with preferential use of infrainguinal angioplasty for critical ischemia. J Vasc Surg 2006; 43(3):504–512.
41. Dorros G, Lewin RF, Jamnadas P, et al. Below-the-knee angioplasty: tibioperoneal vessels, the acute outcome. Cathet Cardiovasc Diagn 1990; 19(3):170–178.
42. Dorros G, Jaff MR, Murphy KJ, et al. The acute outcome of tibioperoneal vessel angioplasty in 417 cases with claudication and critical limb ischemia. Cathet Cardiovasc Diagn 1998; 45(3):251–256.
43. Rastogi S, Stavropoulos SW. Infrapopliteal angioplasty. Tech Vasc Interv Radiol 2004; 7(1):33–39.
44. Cooper S, Bakal C. Subtrifurcation angioplasty: techniques and results. In: Darcy M, Vedantham S, Kaufman J, eds. Peripheral Vascular Interventions. 2nd ed. Fairfax, CA: Society of Cardiovascular and Interventional Radiology, 2001:309–317.
45. Rutherford RB. Reporting standards for endovascular surgery: should existing standards be modified for newer procedures? Semin Vasc Surg 1997; 10(4):197–205.
46. Adam DJ, Beard JD, Cleveland T, et al. Bypass versus angioplasty in severe ischaemia of the leg (BASIL): multicentre, randomised controlled trial. Lancet 2005; 366(9501):1925–1934.
47. Ingle H, Nasim A, Bolia A, et al. Subintimal angioplasty of isolated infragenicular vessels in lower limb ischemia: long-term results. J Endovasc Ther 2002; 9(4):411–416.
48. Das T, McNamara T, Gray B, et al. Cryoplasty therapy for limb salvage in patients with critical limb ischemia. J Endovasc Ther 2007; 14(6):753–762.
49. Vraux H, Bertoncello N. Subintimal angioplasty of tibial vessel occlusions in critical limb ischaemia: a good opportunity? Eur J Vasc Endovasc Surg 2006; 32(6):663–667.
50. Kandarpa K, Becker GJ, Hunink MG, et al. Transcatheter interventions for the treatment of peripheral atherosclerotic lesions: part I. J Vasc Interv Radiol 2001; 12(6): 683–695.
51. Tartari S, Zattoni L, Rolma G, et al. Subintimal angioplasty of infrapopliteal artery occlusions in the treatment of critical limb ischaemia. Short-term results. Radiol Med (Torino) 2004; 108(3):265–274.
52. Sigala F, Menenakos Ch, Sigalas P, et al. Transluminal angioplasty of isolated crural arterial lesions in diabetics with critical limb ischemia. Vasa 2005; 34(3):186–191.
53. Krankenberg H, Sorge I, Zeller T, et al. Percutaneous transluminal angioplasty of infrapopliteal arteries in patients with intermittent claudication: acute and one-year results. Catheter Cardiovasc Interv 2005; 64(1):12–17.
54. Bosiers M, Deloose K, Verbist J, et al. Percutaneous transluminal angioplasty for treatment of "below-the-knee" critical limb ischemia: early outcomes following the use of sirolimus-eluting stents. J Cardiovasc Surg (Torino) 2006; 47(2):171–176.
55. Salas CA, Adam DJ, Papavassiliou VG, et al. Percutaneous transluminal angioplasty for critical limb ischaemia in octogenarians and nonagenarians. Eur J Vasc Endovasc Surg 2004; 28(2):142–145.
56. Bosiers M, Deloose K, Verbist J, et al. Nitinol stenting for treatment of "below-the-knee" critical limb ischemia: 1-year angiographic outcome after Xpert stent implantation. J Cardiovasc Surg (Torino) 2007; 48(4):455–461.
57. Siablis D, Kraniotis P, Karnabatidis D, et al. Sirolimus-eluting versus bare stents for bailout after suboptimal infrapopliteal angioplasty for critical limb ischemia: 6-month angiographic results from a nonrandomized prospective single-center study. J Endovasc Ther 2005; 12:685–695.
58. Muradin GS, Bosch JL, Stijnen T, et al. Balloon dilation and stent implantation for treatment of femoropopliteal arterial disease: meta-analysis. Radiology 2001; 221(1): 137–145.
59. Zeller T, Frank U, Bürgelin K, et al. Initial clinical experience with percutaneous atherectomy in the infragenicular arteries. J Endovasc Ther 2003; 10(5):987–993.
60. Keeling, WB, Shames ML, Stone PA, et al. Plaque excision with the Silverhawk catheter: early results in patients with claudication or critical limb ischemia. J Vasc Surg 2007; 45(1):25–31.

61. Zeller T, Rastan A, Schwarzwälder U, et al. Midterm results after atherectomy-assisted angioplasty of below-knee arteries with use of the Silverhawk device. J Vasc Interv Radiol 2004; 15(12):1391–1397.
62. Zeller T, Sixt S, Schwarzwälder U, et al. Two-year results after directional atherectomy of infrapopliteal arteries with the SilverHawk device. J Endovasc Ther 2007; 14(2): 232–240.
63. Porter DH, Rosen MP, Skillman JJ, et al. Mid-term and long-term results with directional atherectomy of vein graft stenoses. J Vasc Surg 1996; 23(4):554–567.
64. Suri R, Wholey MH, Postoak D, et al. Distal embolic protection during femoropopliteal atherectomy. Catheter Cardiovasc Interv 2006; 67(3):417–422.
65. Biamino G. The excimer laser: science fiction fantasy or practical tool? J Endovasc Ther 2004; 11(suppl 2):II207–II222.
66. Garnic JD, Hurwitz AS. Endovascular excimer laser atherectomy techniques to treat complex peripheral vascular disease: an orderly process. Tech Vasc Interv Radiol 2005; 8(4):150–159.
67. Taylor K, Reiser C. Next generation catheters for excimer laser coronary angioplasty. Lasers Med Sci 2001; 16(2):133–140.
68. Fretz EB, Smith P, Hilton JD. Initial experience with a low profile, high energy excimer laser catheter for heavily calcified coronary lesion debulking: parameters and results of first seven human case experiences. J Interv Cardiol 2001; 14(4):433–437.

10 Results for Infrapopliteal Endovascular Interventions: Angioplasty, Stenting, and Atherectomy

Marc Bosiers and Koen Deloose
Department of Vascular Surgery, AZ St-Blasius, Dendermonde, Belgium

Jürgen Verbist and Patrick Peeters
Department of Cardiovascular and Thoracic Surgery, Imelda Hospital, Bonheiden, Belgium

INTRODUCTION

The application of percutaneous techniques for the treatment of peripheral arterial occlusive disease (PAOD) has gained widespread interest over the last decade. Together with the development of new endovascular tools and with an increasing operator experience, the minimal invasive percutaneous therapy became first-line therapy at many institutions.

Patients with critical limb ischemia (CLI) due to infrapopliteal lesions are often no good candidates for infrageniculate bypass surgery (IBS), as they often present with prohibitive comorbidities, inadequate conduit, and lack of suitable distal targets for revascularization. Therefore, CLI patients due to blockage of below-the-knee (BTK) arteries are in benefit of the endovascular approach: it offers the advantages of local anesthesia, potentially reduced costs (even anticipating the need for reintervention in many patients), and shorter hospital stays. The current article provides an overview of the diagnosis and endovascular treatment strategies for infrapopliteal lesions in patients with CLI and gives recommendations for future infrapopliteal device technology advancements.

ANGIOPLASTY
Percutaneous Transluminal Angioplasty

The current TransAtlantic Inter-Society Consensus (TASC) recommendation states there is increasing evidence to support a recommendation for angioplasty in patients with CLI and infrapopliteal artery occlusion where in-line flow to the foot can be reestablished and where there is medical comorbidity (1). Infrapopliteal percutaneous transluminal angioplasty (PTA) became feasible with the introduction of low-profile peripheral balloon systems and the use of coronary balloons. In our center, after successful lesion passage, we standardly insert a multipurpose guiding catheter into the popliteal artery. This provides sufficient support for the balloon catheter to pass the lesion and is particularly important with the rapid exchange catheters. The diameter of the native infrapopliteal vessel and/or the dimension of the proximal and distal reference segment determine the selection of the PTA balloon. Oversizing should be avoided to prevent dissection. Mostly we opt for a hydrophilic-coated balloon catheter with a diameter range from 2.5 to 4.0 mm and a length chosen according to the lesion length. To avoid any further vessel wall damage, we preferably select a balloon that is shorter than the target lesion.

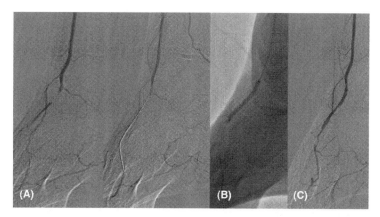

FIGURE 1 Short focal lesion of the distal anterior tibial artery (**A**) before and (**B**) after wire passage and (**C**) during and after PTA-alone strategy with a 2.0 × 30 mm Fox SV balloon (Abbott Vascular).

The Bypass Versus Angioplasty in Severe Ischaemia of the Leg (BASIL) trial participants recently published the outcome of their randomized controlled trial (RCT) comparing the outcome of PTA versus bypass surgery in patients presenting with CLI. They found that in the short term, PTA is cheaper than surgery and that there are similar outcomes in terms of 12-month amputation-free survival for a bypass surgery–first and a balloon angioplasty–first strategies being 68% and 71%, respectively (2).

This excellent limb salvage rate after PTA is confirmed by other earlier publications giving limb salvage rates of above 90% (3–6). The published primary patency rates are less uniform and vary from 15% to 70% (4–7).

The treatment of longer lesions is often more complex and has a worse prognosis than the treatment of short lesions. A long segment stenosis is best treated with a gentle PTA using a low-pressure balloon with sizes ranging from 8 to 10 cm in length and 2.5 to 3.5 mm in diameter. A perfect angiographic result is rarely achievable in this circumstance; therefore, an arteriographic evaluation of the flow through the vessel is extremely important (Fig. 1).

Cutting or Scoring Balloon
The mechanism of action of peripheral cutting or scoring balloons has been referred to as atherotomy. With these advanced PTA technique either atherotomes are mounted on the surface of a noncompliant balloon as with the Peripheral Cutting Balloon (Boston Scientific, Natick, Massachusetts, U.S.) or a nitinol scoring element encircles a minimally compliant balloon as with AngioSculpt (AngioScore Inc., Fremont, California, U.S.) device. This technique decreases vessel elastic recoil and perivascular injury by a focal concentration of the dilating force. Preliminary data described that these devices appear to lower the need for infrapopliteal stents (8,9). Our personal experience using the AngioSculpt in 31 CLI patients endovascularly treated for severe infrapopliteal disease has been published recently. The device was used to treat in total 36 complex, tibioperoneal, atherosclerotic lesions. Eleven patients (35.5%)

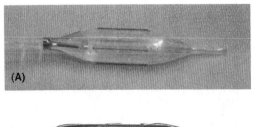

(A)

(B)

FIGURE 2 **(A)** Inflated peripheral cutting; **(B)** Inflated AngioSculpt.

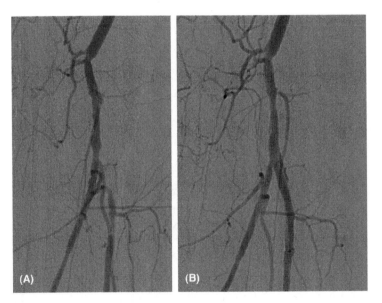

FIGURE 3 Restenotic lesion at the level of the tibiofibular trunk **(A)** before and **(B)** after scoring with the AngioSculpt device.

required additional stenting for minor dissections or suboptimal stenosis reduction. One-year survival and limb salvage were 83.9% and 86.3%, respectively (Figs. 2 and 3) (10).

Cryoplasty

With the cryoplasty technique, the treated vessel wall is simultaneously dilated and quickly cooled to -10°C. The cooling of the vessel wall reduces the vessel elasticity, which uniforms the dilatation over the vessels and limits medial injury and dissection. Animal studies have shown an apoptosis of the smooth muscle cells and reduction of neointimal hyperplasia. The PolarCath (Boston

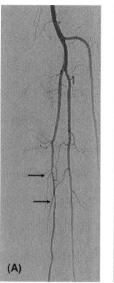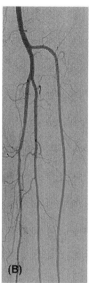

(A) **(B)**

FIGURE 4 Tandem lesion on midsegment posterior tibial artery (**A**) before and (**B**) after cryoplasty with the 2.5 × 40 mm PolarCath.

Scientific) may have a role in infrapopliteal interventions by reducing the risk of flow-limiting dissection compared with traditional angioplasty, and thereby reducing the need for stent implantation (11). Joye demonstrated in his initial experience with infrapopliteal cryoplasty in 20 CLI patients a 95% technical success rate and 95% freedom from amputation at six months (12). In Belgium, the investigators of the CLIMB registry are including 100 CLI patients treated with the PolarCath device to validate the safety and efficacy of the technique in the infrapopliteal vasculature (Fig. 4).

Subintimal Angioplasty
In some centers subintimal angioplasty (SIA) is gaining popularity for long segment occlusions below the knee. The concept of passing a wire into the subintimal space and inflating a balloon to create a channel for blood flow violates many of the traditional endovascular principles and is somewhat counterintuitive. However, the group of Bolia has reported their technical and clinical success rates of, respectively, 86% and 80% in a consecutive series of 67 patients. Limb salvage rates of 94% and freedom of CLI of 84% were reported after 36 months (13–15). Nydahl et al. investigated the use of subintimal PTA for restoring blood flow in the infrapopliteal vessels. After one year they reported a limb salvage rate of 85%, even though the subintimal canal was hemodynamically patent in only 53% of the cases (16). Vraux et al. found comparable low 12-month primary patency rates (56%) with a remarkably better 81% limb salvage rate (17).

STENTING
The TASC II guidelines do not mention implantations of stents in the infrapopliteal bed (1). Although the use of stents is common in other peripheral vessels, their application in the BTK vessels remains highly controversial. The fear that

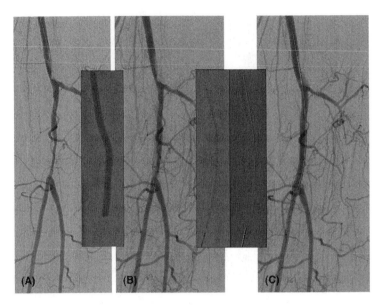

FIGURE 5 Stenting currently remains reserved for suboptimal PTA. (**A**) Preoperative angiographic imaging shows lesion at the level of the tibiofibular trunk, which is (**B**) suboptimally treated with PTA followed by (**C**) successful stenting with Chromis Deep. *Abbreviation*: PTA, percutaneous transluminal angioplasty.

early thrombosis and late luminal loss due to intimal hyperplasia formation potentially leads to insufficient long-term patency rates can explain the reluctance on implanting stents in these small diameter vessels. Therefore, infrapopliteal stent implantation is generally reserved for cases with a suboptimal outcome after PTA (i.e., >50% residual stenosis, flow-limiting dissection). It is only recently that evidence starts to build favoring the use of stenting in the tibial area. Because of the diameter similarities with coronary arteries, the first stents applied in the infrapopliteal vessels were all coronary devices. Since the feasibility of the stenting approach with these coronary products was shown, device manufacturers started to develop a dedicated infrapopliteal product range (Fig. 5).

Bare-Metal Balloon-Expandable Stents
The MULTI-LINK VISION (Abbott Vascular, Redwood City, California, U.S.) is a premounted bare-metal balloon-expandable stent L-605 cobalt chromium (CoCr) alloy coronary stent with radial strength and fluoroscopic visibility superior to stainless steel stents. A recent publication of our group described our experience with this type of stent in a cohort of 50 patients with CLI who were all diagnosed with infragenicular occlusive arterial disease. After one year, a limb salvage rate of 89.3% was calculated with a duplex-derived primary patency of the treated vessel of only 62.8% (18). Other studies using bare-metal stents (BMSs) supported our findings. Scheinert et al. found a 6-month binary restenosis rate of 39.1%, using the Bx SONIC (Cordis, Miami, Florida, U.S.) stent (19), while Siablis et al. reported 12-month binary in-stent restenosis on

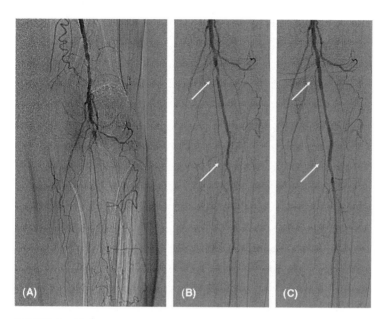

FIGURE 6 (**A**) Preoperative angiographic imaging showing total occlusion of the infragenicular vascular bed treated by (**B**) PTA, resulting in flow-limiting dissection and (**C**) optimized by the implantation of two MULTI-LINK VISION stents.

angiography of 78.6%, with a remarkable 100% limb salvage rate after having used a range of commercially available uncoated coronary BMSs (20). Although satisfactory limb salvage rates are observed using coronary BMSs in the lower leg, the longer-term vessel patency seems to be too low to guarantee sustained interventional success (Fig. 6).

The company Invatec was the first to develop a dedicated infrapopliteal CoCr BMS, the Chromis Deep (Invatec, Roncadelle, Italy). The stent is available in longer lengths (up to 78 mm) and has a higher radial force as coronary-derived BMSs, and because of its closed cell design it offers homogeneous scaffolding of the vessel wall. Furthermore, the stent struts have a low thickness, which provides the stent with a better flexibility as the coronary ones. Our group has enrolled 50 BTK stenting cases in patients undergoing angioplasty followed by insertion of 58 Chromis Deep stents. Interim analysis with limited number of patients reaching the primary study endpoint revealed six-month primary patency and limb salvage of 74.2% and 93.2%, respectively (Fig. 7).

Passive-Coated Balloon-Expandable Stents
A first attempt to optimize the outcome of infrapopliteal stenting is application of passive stent coatings (carbon or silicon carbide), which inhibit the deposition of thrombocytes and erythrocytes on the stent surface, preventing early thrombosis and intimal hyperplasia due to thrombus formation.

Peeters et al. presented our unpublished first infrapopliteal experience using the silicon carbide–coated Lekton (Biotronik AG, Bülach, Switzerland) at the Transcatheter Cardiovascular Therapeutics (TCT) 2003. Our series of

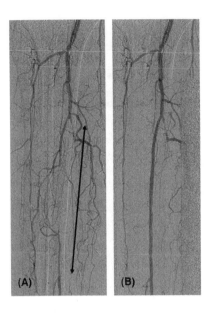

FIGURE 7 (**A**) Preoperative and (**B**) postoperative view of long occlusion of posterior tibial artery treated with a long dedicated infrapopliteal Chromis Deep stent.

50 consecutive patients treated with Lekton stent implants in infrapopliteal lesions showed a six-month primary patency rate of 91.1% on duplex, a limb salvage rate of 100%.

More important was the RCT of the Vienna group: they were the first to prove that the angiographic outcome after stenting, using a stent with a passive coating, is superior to PTA alone in infrapopliteal vessels. Fifty-one patients presenting with CLI due to infrapopliteal lesions were randomized for treatment by PTA (53 lesions in 27 patients) or stent application (42 lesions in 24 patients). Patients in the stent arm all received the coronary balloon-expandable carbon-coated InPeria Carbostent (Sorin, Biomedica, Italy). For the stent group, the cumulative primary patency at six months was 83.7% at the 70% restenosis threshold, and 79.7% at the 50% restenosis threshold. For PTA, the primary patency at six months was 61.1% at the 70% restenosis threshold and 45.6% at the 50% restenosis threshold. Both results were statistically significant ($p < 0.05$) (21).

Drug-Eluting Balloon-Expandable Stents

To further improve infrapopliteal stent outcome, another coronary stent technique was transferred to the infrapopliteal vascular bed: the use of drug-eluting stents (DES). An active stent coating (sirolimus or paclitaxel) inhibits the inflammatory response and smooth muscle cell proliferation in the vessel wall during a certain period, but in fact merely delays the process of intimal hyperplasia as demonstrated by the two-year results of the SIROCCO study (22).

Feiring et al. were the first to demonstrate the safety and utility of using coronary DES in the tibial vessels and paved the way for a more widespread application of DES for treating infrapopliteal disease (23).

On the basis of the outcome of four independent investigator-initiated studies, the Cypher sirolimus-eluting stent (SES) (Cordis) has been CE marked for the below knee (BK) indication (19,24–26). Our own study published in 2006 evaluating the Cypher stent for BK applications in 18 CLI patients (Rutherford categories 4 and 5), resulted in a six-month limb salvage rate of 94.4%, with an angiographic late lumen loss of only 0.38 mm in the surviving patients (25). Commeau et al. used SES to treat 30 consecutive patients with CLI, (Rutherford categories 3–6) and a minimum of two diseased infrapopliteal vessels. A limb salvage rate of 100% was achieved at a mean follow-up of 7.7 months, and all surviving patients treated with Cypher stents had marked clinical improvement, with 97% primary patency as measured by target lesion revascularization (26). Siablis et al. compared the outcome of 29 CLI patients treated with the sirolimus-eluting Cypher stent with another 29 CLI patients receiving a BMS for infrapopliteal revascularization. The six-month primary patency rate was significantly higher in the Cypher group compared with the BMS group (92.0% and 68.1%, respectively, $p < 0.002$). Angiographic follow-up six months post index intervention revealed a binary in-stent restenosis of only 4.0% after Cypher stent implantation, while the rate was as high as 55.3% after BMS implantion ($p < 0.001$) (24). Siablis et al. also published their one-year follow-up results showing 86.4% primary patency in patients with DES, whereas patients with BMS had primary patency of 40.5% ($p < 0.001$). Likewise, the binary in-stent restenosis was better with DES, 36.7% in the Cypher stent group and 78.6% in the BMS group ($p < 0.001$) (20). The same highly significant difference in six-month angiographic outcome between the Cypher and the non-drug-eluting Bx SONIC stent was confirmed by Scheinert et al. in a nonrandomized study. The study evaluated 60 consecutive patients presenting with infrapopliteal lesions. The binary restenosis rate was found to be 0% in the Cypher arm and 56.5% in the control BMS arm ($p < 0.001$) (19).

Feiring and Wesolowski recently proposed a new technique for combining antegrade popliteal arterial access with tibial DES implantation in patients with occluded SFA occlusions. Five patients scheduled for BK amputations successfully received overlapping infrapopliteal DES via this approach. After a mean follow-up period of 29 months, no deaths, no amputations, and no target limb revascularization (TLR) were recorded (27).

To date, there is one publication on the use of paclitaxel-eluting stents (PESs) in the given indication. Siablis et al. reported the one-year angiographic and clinical outcomes of their prospective study investigating the infrapopliteal use of the TAXUS PES (Boston Scientific, Natick, Massachusetts, U.S.) in a group of 29 CLI patients (32 limbs, 50 lesions, 62 PESs). At one year after index intervention, the limb salvage rate was 88.5%. The published angiographic in-stent primary patency rate was only 30.0%; with an in-stent binary (>50%) restenosis was 77.4%. The one-year incidence of clinically driven repeat interventions was 30.5%. From their first experience with infrapopliteal PES, they concluded to have reached acceptable clinical results, even though PES implantation failed to inhibit vascular restenosis and decrease the need for repeat interventions (28).

Although evidence currently indicates that the implantation of DES in the infrapopliteal vasculature leads to favorable outcomes with high midterm primary patency and limb salvages rates, further support for the use of DES in patients with CLI and BK lesions will be gained from well-designed RCT. Such trials are about to start in conjunction with industry support. Another concern using DES in the infrapopliteal arteries is the delayed endothelialization around the stent struts as seen in coronaries, which makes the stent more susceptible to

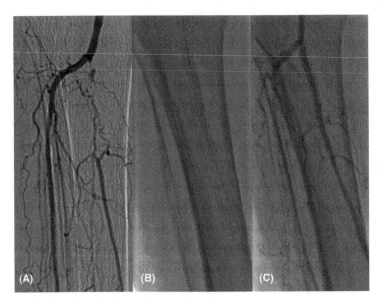

FIGURE 8 (**A**) Preoperative and (**B,C**) postoperative angiographic control of stenting with a sirolimus-eluting Cypher stent of a short focal infrapopliteal occlusion.

thrombosis. Despite the fact that DES thrombosis in the peripheral circulation has not the lethal consequences as in coronaries, dual antiplatelet therapy after DES is also warranted for PAOD to guarantee optimal stent performance and patient clinical well-being. Nevertheless, the use of dual antiplatelet therapy is related with an increased incidence (1–2% per annum) of major bleeding complications and is expensive (29,30). The duration of treatment with dual antiplatelet therapy after both coronary and peripheral implantation of DES remains a subject of ongoing debate. On the basis of emerging evidence, many cardiologists are recommending a minimum of 12 months of aspirin and clopidogrel, but some are advocating indefinite use of dual antiplatelet therapy after DES implantation (31). One year of clopidogrel costs approximately US$1000.00. This expense is in addition to the cost already incurred by using a DES, which is usually fourfold greater than the bare-metal equivalent; one coronary BMS costs US$800.00, while one DES costs up to US$2500.00 (Fig. 8) (32).

Nitinol Self-Expanding Stents

Despite these good outcomes in published trials, balloon-expandable stents are prone to fractures, as was recently documented by Schwarzmaier-D'Assie et al. (33). Keeping in mind the findings in the superficial femoral artery, where Scheinert et al. found a direct link between stent fractures and lesion reocclusions, the fracture-prone nature of balloon-expandable stainless steel could potentially lead to less encouraging long-term outcomes (34). Therefore it has been opted to develop self-expanding nitinol stents for the infrapopliteal vessels. The potential advantage of nitinol could probably be explained by the crush-resistant, highly flexible nature of the alloy. Moreover, the design of dedicated small vessel nitinol stents such as Xpert (Abbott Vascular), Maris Deep (Invatec),

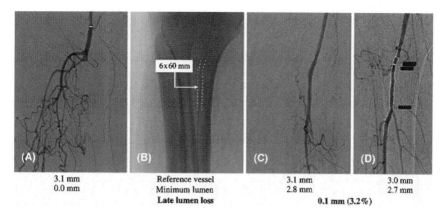

3.1 mm	Reference vessel	3.1 mm	3.0 mm
0.0 mm	Minimum lumen	2.8 mm	2.7 mm
	Late lumen loss		
		0.1 mm (3.2%)	

FIGURE 9 QVA analysis of patient treated with 6 × 60 Xpert nitinol stent for a total occlusion of the TFT. (**A**) Preprocedural image showing total occlusion of the TFT; (**B**) location of stent implantation; (**C**) immediate postoperative image showing less than 10% residual stenosis; (**D**) one-year angiographical control showed a LLL of only 0.1 mm (LLL index 3.2%). *Abbreviations*: TFT, tibiofibular trunk; LLL, late lumen loss.

and Astron Pulsar (Biotronik AG) intends to improve results by a reduced strut profile, lowering the wall coverage up to 20%, independent of the stent diameter. The rationale behind is that optimal maintenance of flow dynamics in the infrapopliteal arteries lowers lumen loss and improves patency rates.

Kickuth et al. were first to present their initial experience with the Xpert nitinol stent in the given indication with good clinical outcome after six months (35). Our group published the one-year angiographic outcome of 47 CLI patients that received 67 Xpert stents for the treatment of 58 infrapopliteal lesions in 51 limbs. Quantitative vascular analysis (QVA) after one year showed a binary restenosis rate of 20.45%. Kaplan-Meier analysis reported one-year primary patency and limb salvage rates of 76.3% and 95.9%, respectively (Fig. 9) (36).

Absorbable Stents

With all of presented stent types, target lesion revascularization remains required on a certain percentage of patients to guarantee limb salvage. The permanent presence of an artificial implant is believed to be the potential trigger for late restenosis. Recently the stenting technology has moved toward the development of temporary implants composed of biocompatible materials, which mechanically support the vessel during the period of high risk for recoil and then completely degrade on the long-term perspective (31,37–39). Therefore, bioabsorbable stents are discussed as a means to combine a mechanical prevention of vessel recoil with various advantages of the long-term perspective compared with permanent implants, including the possibility for late outward vessel remodeling, and improved reintervention options (38). The bioabsorbable magnesium alloy stent (Biotronik AG) was the first of its kind to be proved that it could be implanted safely in human arteries and that it absorbed in a time frame as it was intended to (37,38). In the absorbable metal stent (AMS) BTK study, clinical results using AMS stents for treatment of infrapopliteal lesions in 20 patients

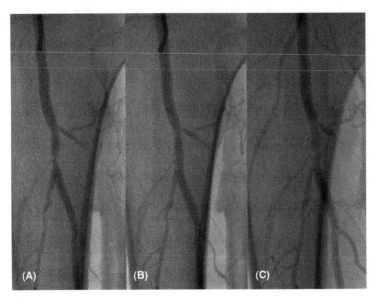

FIGURE 10 Angiographic control of an (**A**) 80% stenosis of the tibiofibular trunk, (**B**) with 5% residual stenosis after AMS (Biotronik AG) implantation, and (**C**) 36% in-stent restenosis at six months after index procedure.

with CLI were presented. After 12 months, the resulting values for primary clinical patency and limb salvage were 73.3% and 94.7%, respectively (40). On the basis of these findings, the AMS INSIGHT-1 RCT was set up to give further proof of the AMS safety and efficacy. The AMS INSIGHT-1 investigators have enrolled 117 CLI patients with BTK 149 lesions; the patients were randomized to implantation of an AMS (60 patients, 74 lesions) or stand-alone PTA (57 patients, 75 lesions). Seven PTA-group patients "crossed over" to AMS stenting. The 30-day complication rate (primary safety endpoint and defined as absence of major amputation and/or death within 30 days after index intervention) was 5.3% (3/57) and 5.0% (3/60) in patients randomized for PTA alone and PTA followed by AMS implantation, respectively. The six-month angiographic patency rate (primary efficacy endpoint, intention-to-treat based core-laboratory analysis) was significantly inferior ($p = 0.013$), for the lesions treated with AMS (31.8%) was significantly inferior ($p = 0.013$) to those treated with PTA (58.0%) (Fig. 10) (41).

ATHERECTOMY
The main idea of atherectomy is the physical removal of the plaque from the artery. This can be done either by fragmentation of the atheroma into small particles (i.e., ablative atherectomy) or by collection and removal of the athe-rosclerotic material (i.e., excisional atherectomy).

Ablative Atherectomy
The Excimer laser (Spectranetics Corporation, Colorado Springs, Colorado, U.S.) cannot only be used to create an initial lesion but also as a clear atherectomy device. It debulks and ablates tissue (thrombus or plaque) without damaging surrounding tissue, thus minimizing restenosis. The Excimer laser employs

exact energy control (shallow tissue penetration) and safer wavelengths, thereby decreasing perforation and thermal injury to the treated vessels. It is a cold-tipped laser that delivers bursts of ultraviolet/xenon energy (308 nm) in short pulse durations, which ablates on a photochemical, rather than a thermal, level. The ultraviolet light provides a direct lytic action that ablates 5 µm of tissue on contact without a rise in surrounding tissue temperature (42–44). A conventional mechanical guidewire is used to cross the entire occlusion up to the distal vessel beyond the target lesion. Next, the occlusion or stenosis can be treated with two different techniques: (*i*) a 0.9 or 1.4 laser catheter is used to debulk the vessel to ease PTA catheter delivery and to improve PTA results; (*ii*) a 1.7 or 2.0 laser catheter is used to ablate enough tissue so that the sole use of the laser results in an acceptable intraluminal diameter and flow.

Our own experience with 64 consecutive excimer laser cases for tibial occlusive disease results in a one-year primary patency of 75.4% and a limb salvage rate of 87.9% (4).

Ablation can also be performed with high-speed rotational devices, such as the Rotablator. Early research has indicated, although high initial technical success rate can be achieved using the Rotablator in the treatment of infrapopliteal lesions, they lead to very poor six-month results. Jahnke et al. published their experience treating 19 infrapopliteal lesion in 15 patients and reported that at six months angiographic control only 1 out of 12 treated vessels (8.3%), which were investigated, remained patent without presenting a hemodynamically relevant restenosis (45).

Other rotational ablative atherectomy devices are currently under investigation. The CSI Orbital Atherectomy device (Cardiovascular Systems Inc., St. Paul, Minnesota, U.S.) utilizes an eccentrically shaped wire coil and diamond-coated abrasive crown, unlike the symmetric rotating burr of traditional rotational atherectomy. Another technology is the rotational aspirating atherectomy device (Pathway Medical Technologies, Redmond, Washington, U.S.). It combines the two actions of aspiration with differential plaque removal and may be useful in calcified lesions.

Excisional Atherectomy

The SilverHawk Plaque Excision System shaves atherosclerotic plaque and contains it in a distal storage chamber. The device self-apposes the atheroma through a hinge system and contains a carbide cutter with variable height depending on the device used, which rotates at speeds up to 8000 rpm. Zeller et al. have reported their outcomes using the SilverHawk for infrapopliteal lesions. In total, 36 patients with both claudication and CLI received excisional atherectomy for the treatment of 49 infrapopliteal lesions. In 33 (67%) of the lesions, primary atherectomy was performed, while 16 (33%) received PTA before SilverHawk atherectomy. The 12- and 24-month primary patencies as estimated by Kaplan-Meier analysis were 58% and 46%, respectively (46).

CONCLUSIONS

Limb preservation should be the goal in patients with CLI due to tibial occlusive disease. With a prompt diagnosis, treatment can be started early and serious consequences may be avoided. Any type of revascularization that can prevent amputation must be applied to overall treatment strategy (47).

Since the publication of the BASIL RCT (2), it needs no more debate, that endovascular interventions should be considered the primary approach in this group of patients (4). The PTA-first strategy gave as good clinical results as the surgery-first approach in CLI and the endovascular approach showed to be cheaper on at least the short run. Moreover endovascular interventions do not prohibit future bypass or additional treatments.

Taking into account the findings of this literature review and the theory on the different stent designs, the authors believe that the future of infrapopliteal stents might lay in the development of small vessel sirolimus-eluting, self-expanding nitinol stents or of sirolimus-eluting absorbable stents.

To date, the PTA-first strategy remains the standard of care as it gives an acceptable clinical outcome at a low procedural cost. In case of suboptimal PTA, stent implantation with dedicated BTK stents improves both the clinical outcome and decreases the need for TLR. For short focal lesions, current single-center studies indicate that primary BTK stenting can be a viable option in the infragenicular bed, but we will have to await future RCTs comparing stenting versus PTA to tell whether the current or future stent improvements will be able to change the idea about the optimal endovascular strategy.

ACKNOWLEDGMENT
The authors take great pleasure in thanking the staff of Flanders Medical Research Program (www.fmrp.be), with special regard to Koen De Meester for performing the systematic review of the literature and providing substantial support to the data analysis and the writing of the article.

REFERENCES
1. Norgren L, Hiatt WR, Dormandy JA, et al. Inter-society consensus for the management of peripheral arterial disease (TASC II). J Vasc Surg 2007; 45(suppl S):S5–S67.
2. Adam D, Beard J, Cleveland T, et al. Bypass versus angioplasty in severe ischaemia of the leg (BASIL): multicentre, randomised controlled trial. Lancet 2005; 366:1925–1934.
3. Faglia E, Clerici G, Clerissi J, et al. When is a technically successful peripheral angioplasty effective in preventing above-the-ankle amputation in diabetic patients with critical limb ischaemia? Diabet Med 2007; 24:823–829.
4. Bosiers M, Hart JP, Deloose K, et al. Endovascular therapy as the primary approach for limb salvage in patients with critical limb ischemia: experience with 443 infrapopliteal procedures. Vascular 2006; 14:63–69.
5. Dorros G, Jaff MR, Dorros AM, et al. Tibioperoneal (outflow lesion) angioplasty can be used as primary treatment in 235 patients with critical limb ischemia: five-year follow-up. Circulation 2001; 104:2057–2062.
6. Hanna GP, Fujise K, Kjellgren O, et al. Infrapopliteal transcatheter interventions for limb salvage in diabetic patients: importance of aggressive interventional approach and role of transcutaneous oximetry. J Am Coll Cardiol 1997; 30:664–669.
7. Parsons R, Suggs W, Lee J, et al. Percutaneous transluminal angioplasty for the treatment of limb threatening ischemia: do the results justify an attempt before bypass grafting? J Vasc Surg 1998; 28:1066–1071.
8. Ansel G, George B, Botti C Jr., et al. Infrapopliteal endovascular techniques: indications, techniques, and results. Curr Interv Cardiol Rep 2001; 3:100–108.
9. Scheinert D, Graziani L, Peeters P, et al. Results from the multi-center registry of the novel angiosculpt scoring balloon catheter for the treatment of infra-popliteal disease. Cardiovasc Revasc Med 2006; 17:113.
10. Bosiers M, Cagiannos C, Deloose K, et al. The use of the angiosculpt scoring balloon for infrapopliteal lesions in patients with critical limb ischemia: one year outcome. Vascular 2009; 17(1):29–35.

11. Laird JR, Biamino G, McNamara T, et al. Cryoplasty for the treatment of femoropopliteal arterial disease: extended follow-up results. J Endovasc Ther 2006; 13(suppl 2):52–59.
12. Joye J. Overview of cryoplasty. Endovasc Today 2004; 3:54–56.
13. Bolia A, Sayers RD, Thompson MM, et al. Subintimal and intraluminal recanalisation of occluded crural arteries by percutaneous balloon angioplasty. Eur J Vasc Surg 1994; 8:214–219.
14. Ingle H, Nasim A, Bolia A, et al. Subintimal angioplasty of isolated infragenicular vessels in lower limb ischemia: long-term results. J Endovasc Ther 2002; 9:411–416.
15. Bolia A. Subintimal angioplasty: which cases to choose, how to avoid pitfalls and technical tips. VEITH Symposium 2003:8.1–8.3
16. Nydahl S, Hartshorne T, Bell P, et al. Subintimal angioplasty of infrapopliteal occlusions in critically ischaemic limbs. Eur J Vasc Endovasc Surg 1997; 14:212–216.
17. Vraux H, Hammer F, Verhelst R, et al. Subintimal angioplasty of tibial vessel occlusions in the treatment of critical limb ischaemia: mid-term results. Eur J Vasc Endovasc Surg 2000; 20:441–446.
18. Bosiers M, Kallakuri S, Deloose K, et al. Infragenicular angioplasty and stenting in the management of critical limb ischaemia: one year outcome following the use of the MULTI-LINK VISION stent. EuroIntervention 2007; 3:470–474.
19. Scheinert D, Ulrich M, Scheinert S, et al. Comparison of sirolimus-eluting vs. bare-metal stents for the treatment of infrapopliteal obstructions. EuroIntervention 2006; 2:169–174.
20. Siablis D, Karnabatidis D, Katsanos K, et al. Sirolimus-eluting versus bare stents after suboptimal infrapopliteal angioplasty for critical limb ischemia: enduring 1-year angiographic and clinical benefit. J Endovasc Ther 2007; 14:241–250.
21. Rand T, Basile A, Cejna M, et al. PTA versus carbofilm-coated stents in infrapopliteal arteries: pilot study. Cardiovasc Intervent Radiol 2006; 29:29–38.
22. Duda S, Bosiers M, Lammer J. Drug-eluting and bare nitinol stents for the treatment of atherosclerotic lesions in the superficial femoral artery: long-term results from the SIROCCO trial. J Endovasc Ther 2006; 13:701–710.
23. Feiring A, Wesolowski A, Lade S. Primary stent-supported angioplasty for treatment of below-knee critical limb ischemia and severe claudication: early and one-year outcomes. J Am Coll Cardiol 2004; 44:2307–2314.
24. Siablis D, Kraniotis P, Karnabatidis D, et al. Sirolimus-eluting versus bare stents for bailout after suboptimal infrapopliteal angioplasty for critical limb ischemia: 6-month angiographic results from a nonrandomized prospective single-center study. J Endovasc Ther 2005; 12:685–695.
25. Bosiers M, Deloose K, Verbist J, et al. Percutaneous transluminal angioplasty for treatment of "below-the-knee" critical limb ischemia: early outcomes following the use of sirolimus-eluting stents. J Cardiovasc Surg (Torino) 2006; 47:171–176.
26. Commeau P, Barragan P, Roquebert P. Sirolimus for below the knee lesions: mid-term results of SiroBTK study. Catheter Cardiovasc Interv 2006; 68:793–798.
27. Feiring A, Wesolowski A. Antegrade popliteal artery approach for the treatment of critical limb ischemia in patients with occluded superficial femoral arteries. Catheter Cardiovasc Interv 2007; 69:665–670.
28. Siablis D, Karnabatidis D, Katsanos K, et al. Infrapopliteal application of paclitaxel-eluting stents for critical limb ischemia: midterm angiographic and clinical results. J Vasc Interv Radiol 2007; 18:1351–1361.
29. Diener HC, Bogousslavsky J, Brass LM, et al. Aspirin and clopidogrel compared with clopidogrel alone after recent ischaemic stroke or transient ischaemic attack in high-risk patients (MATCH): randomised, double-blind, placebo-controlled trial. Lancet 2004; 364:331–337.
30. Eisenstein E, Anstrom K, Kong D, et al. Clopidogrel use and long-term clinical outcomes after drug-eluting stent implantation. JAMA 2007; 297:159–168.
31. Waksman R. Update on bioabsorbable stents: from bench to clinical. J Interv Cardiol 2006; 19:414–421.
32. Harper R. Drug-eluting stents coronary stents—a note of caution. Med J Aust 2007; 186: 253–255.

33. Schwarzmaier-D'Assie A, Karnik R, Bonner G, et al. Fracture of a drug-eluting stent in the tibioperoneal trunk following bifurcation stenting. J Endovasc Ther 2007; 14:106–109.
34. Scheinert D, Scheinert S, Sax J, et al. Prevalence and clinical impact of stent fractures after femoropopliteal stenting. J Am Coll Cardiol 2005; 45:312–315.
35. Kickuth R, Keo H, Triller J, et al. Initial clinical experience with the 4-F self-expanding XPERT stent system for infrapopliteal treatment of patients with severe claudication and critical limb ischemia. J Vasc Interv Radiol 2007; 18:703–708.
36. Romiti M, Albers M, Brochado-Neto F, et al. Meta-analysis of infrapopliteal angioplasty for chronic critical limb ischemia. J Vasc Surg 2008; 47:975–981.
37. Di Mario C, Griffiths H, Goktekin O, et al. Drug-eluting bioabsorbable magnesium stent. J Interv Cardiol 2004; 17:391–395.
38. Peeters P, Bosiers M, Verbist J, et al. Preliminary results after application of absorbable metal stents in patients with critical limb ischemia. J Endovasc Ther 2005; 12:1–5.
39. Bosiers M, Deloose K, Verbist J, et al. Will absorbable metal stent technology change our practice? J Cardiovasc Surg (Torino) 2006; 47:393–397.
40. Bosiers M, Deloose K, Verbist J, et al. First clinical application of absorbable metal stents in the treatment of critical limb ischemia: 12-month results. Vasc Dis Manage 2005; 2:86–91.
41. Bosiers M, Peeters P, D'Archambeau O, et al. AMS INSIGHT: absorbable metal stent implantation for treatment of 'below-the-knee' critical limb ischemia: 6-month analysis. Cardiovasc Intervent Radiol 2009 Mar 17; [Epub ahead of print].
42. Das T. Percutaneous peripheral revascularisation with excimer laser: equipment, technique and results. Lasers Med Sci 2001; 16:101–107.
43. Bosiers M, Peeters P, Deloose K, et al. Excimer laser revascularisation for critical limb ischemia—has a solution been found? Technology & Services. Business Briefing: Global Surgery 2003:1–4.
44. Tan JW, Yeo KK, Laird JR. Excimer laser assisted angioplasty for complex infrainguinal peripheral artery disease: a 2008 update. J Cardiovasc Surg (Torino) 2008; 49: 329–340.
45. Jahnke T, Link J, Muller-Hulsbeck S, et al. Treatment of infrapopliteal occlusive disease by high-speed rotational atherectomy: initial and mid-term results. J Vasc Interv Radiol 2001; 12:221–226.
46. Zeller T, Sixt S, Schwarzwälder U, et al. Two-year results after directional atherectomy of infrapopliteal arteries with the SilverHawk device. J Endovasc Ther 2007; 14:232–240.
47. Allie D, Hebert C, Lirtzman M, et al. Critical Limb ischemia: a global epidemic. A Critical analysis of current treatment unmasks the clinical and economic costs of CLI. EuroIntervention 2005; 1:75–84.

11 Surgical Options for Critical Limb Ischemia

Frank J. Veith
Department of Surgery, Cleveland Clinic Foundation, Cleveland, Ohio, and Department of Surgery, New York University Medical Center, New York, New York, U.S.A.

Neal S. Cayne
Department of Surgery, New York University Medical Center, New York, New York, U.S.A.

Nicholas J. Gargiulo III
Department of Surgery, Montefiore Medical Center, New York, New York, U.S.A.

Enrico Ascher
Department of Surgery, Maimonides Medical Center, New York, New York, U.S.A.

Evan C. Lipsitz
Department of Surgery, Montefiore Medical Center, New York, New York, U.S.A.

INTRODUCTION

This chapter discusses open surgical options for critical lower limb ischemia, which may be defined as sufficiently poor arterial blood supply to pose a threat to the viability of the lower extremity. Manifestations of critical ischemia are rest pain, ulceration, and gangrene. These manifestations typically occur because of arteriosclerotic occlusive disease of large, medium-sized, and/or small arteries, although other etiologies may produce or contribute to these manifestations. For example, several nonvascular etiologies may cause rest pain, infection may cause or contribute to gangrene, and trauma and decreased sensation may produce ulceration. Although thromboembolism and other etiologies can produce acute critical limb ischemia, this chapter only deals with chronic lower extremity ischemia due to obliterative arteriosclerosis. Over the last three decades, it has become increasingly apparent that limbs that are threatened by this process almost always have multilevel occlusive disease, which often includes occlusions of arteries in the leg and foot (1).

Surgical options for chronic, critical lower limb ischemia include local amputations of toes and other portions of the foot, a variety of debriding procedures including open amputations of portions of the foot to control infection, and a variety of traditional surgical revascularization procedures, primarily vein and prosthetic arterial bypasses above or below the inguinal ligament. These may, on occasion, be supplemented with localized endarterectomies or patch angioplasties. However, endarterectomy alone is rarely enough to save a severely ischemic limb.

TOE AND FOOT AMPUTATIONS, DEBRIDEMENTS, AND CONSERVATIVE TREATMENT

Although a detailed description of these procedures is beyond the scope of this chapter, certain principles should be emphasized. Gangrenous and infected toes can be successfully amputated by closed or open techniques in patients with good circulation. Extensive debridements and partial foot amputations will also usually heal in such patients if all infected and necrotic tissue is excised. Such procedures will result in patients regaining an effective walking status. Amputation of one or more gangrenous or ulcerated toes or limited debridements may also sometimes result in a healed foot in patients without distal pulses and substantial arterial occlusive disease [e.g., an occluded superficial femoral artery (SFA)]. Determination of moderately good collateral circulation by ankle-brachial indices or pulse volume recordings may be helpful in predicting such healing, but sometimes in patients with borderline circulation, a trial of such local procedures is warranted before proceeding with a major effort at revascularization. If healing is not thereby achieved, the revascularization is clearly justified.

In addition, some patients with critical ischemia as manifest by mild ischemic rest pain and/or limited gangrene or ulceration can be successfully managed conservatively with good foot care, antibiotics, analgesics, and limited ambulation (2). A trial of such conservative treatment is particularly indicated in patients who might not tolerate revascularization procedures because of major comorbidities. Long periods of palliation and occasional healing of small ulcerations and patches of gangrene may take place in a limited proportion of such patients with critical ischemia (2).

HISTORY OF AGGRESSIVE APPROACH TO LIMB SALVAGE IN PATIENTS WITH CRITICAL ISCHEMIA DUE TO ARTERIOSCLEROSIS AND EVOLUTION OF THE RELATIONSHIP BETWEEN OPEN BYPASS SURGERY AND ANGIOGRAPHIC TECHNIQUES AND ENDOVASCULAR TREATMENTS

In the 1960s and 1970s, major below-knee or above-knee amputation was regarded as the safest and best treatment for gangrene and ulceration from arteriosclerotic occlusive disease below the inguinal ligament (3), despite the effectiveness of reconstructive arterial surgery (bypass and endarterectomy) for aortoiliac occlusive disease and despite some occasional positive results from femoropopliteal and even femorotibial bypasses. Because we had access to unusually good arteriography, which visualized all the arteries in the leg and foot (Fig. 1), we developed and espoused an aggressive approach to salvage threatened limbs including those with extensive gangrene (4). Over 96% of patients with threatened limbs were subjected to an effort to save the limb. Only 4%, those with severe dementia or gangrene extending beyond the mid-foot, were excluded. Only 6% of all patients with threatened limbs, when examined by this extensive arteriography, had no patent artery in the leg or foot, which could serve as an outflow site for a bypass (4). With improvements in technique, which we and others developed, this proportion of patients with arteries unsuitable for a bypass fell to 1% to 2% (1,5–11). Successful foot salvage was achieved in 81% to 95% of patients in whom bypasses were performed for the period that they lived up to five years (1,4). However, 52% of these limb salvage patients had much medical comorbidity and died, usually from cardiac causes, within the first five years after their initial bypass (4). More than two-thirds of the patients who lived beyond five years retained a useable limb and were able to ambulate beyond the five-year time point (4). However, to maintain limb salvage, many of these patients required some form of reoperation or reintervention because they developed a failed (thrombosed) or failing (threatened but patent) graft from a lesion in their graft or its inflow or outflow

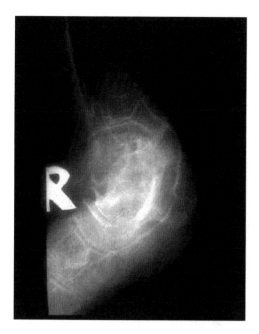

FIGURE 1 An 83-year old diabetic presented with a gangrenous great toe. Vein bypass to the posterior tibial artery resulted in limb salvage and this arteriogram was obtained 10 years after the limb-threatening event.

tract (1,4,5). These worthwhile limb salvage results were in part achieved because of a myriad of improvements in the surgical techniques (1,4–11), development of methods to facilitate the many reoperations these patients required (12–14), and importantly, because of improved anesthetic and intensive care management of these limb salvage patients who often had advanced cardiorespiratory disease, poor kidney function, and diabetes. Collectively, these improvements made possible attempts at limb salvage in almost every patient with a threatened limb and intact brain functions (1,4,9), and many vascular centers throughout the world adopted these policies and were able to achieve equally good results.

EARLY USE OF ENDOVASCULAR TECHNIQUES
(ANGIOPLASTY AND STENTING) WITH BYPASS SURGERY

In the mid-1970s, we and some other centers embraced the use of percutaneous transluminal angioplasty (PTA) to treat these old, sick patients with threatened lower limbs (4). At the outset, PTA was used to correct hemodynamically significant iliac artery stenosis. In most instances, this was combined with some form of infrainguinal bypass. However, as PTA techniques improved, balloon angioplasty was used to treat short iliac occlusions and some SFA lesions as well. Approximately 19% of patients with a threatened limb could be treated by PTA alone without an adjunctive bypass, while another 14% required some form of open surgical revascularization along with their PTA (1). These percentages increased further, and results improved with the introduction of iliac stents. As technical improvements in endovascular technology were developed, our group was one of the first to use popliteal, infrapopliteal, and tibial PTA to facilitate the treatment of these limb salvage patients, to manage them less invasively and to avoid some of the systemic and local complications of the lengthy and sometimes difficult distal operations in these old, sick patients (15–17). We also used and advocated these endovascular techniques, where possible, to help in the

treatment of patients with failed or failing bypasses, since reoperative procedures were often more difficult than primary bypass operations (1,4,18,19).
Sometimes (in approximately 20% of patients) PTA eliminated the need for
a secondary bypass; more often it made the secondary bypass simpler. In
addition, we developed a number of unusual approaches to lower extremity
arteries to facilitate reoperations by eliminating the need to redissect previously
dissected arteries (6,12–14,20).

CURRENT AND FUTURE RELATIONSHIP BETWEEN ENDOVASCULAR TREATMENTS AND OPEN BYPASS SURGERY

Recent improvements in catheter, guidewire, stent, and stent-graft technology
have transformed the treatment of critical lower limb ischemia from a primarily
open surgical (bypass) modality supplemented by some catheter-based treatments to a primarily endovascular modality. Most who treat critical ischemia
today regard endovascular treatments as the first option to save limbs threatened
by chronic obstructive arteriosclerosis at all levels including disease in the leg and
foot, and most of this volume is devoted to a discussion of improved endovascular techniques for doing so. Indeed, there are some endovascular enthusiasts
who mistakenly believe they have originated the limb salvage concept, and some
who go even further and maintain that, if a limb cannot be salvaged by endovascular treatment, the next option should be a major amputation.

While we are also endovascular enthusiasts and also believe that endovascular treatment should be the first therapeutic option to revascularize a critically
ischemic limb in almost all patients, we still believe that some patients whose leg
and foot cannot be saved by some form of endovascular treatment can undergo an
open surgical bypass procedure or a partially open removal of a resistant clot with
a successful salvage of the foot. The remainder of this chapter will be devoted to a
description of these open operative procedures and when they are indicated.

Although almost all experts will agree that there are still some indications
for open surgical bypasses for limb threatening ischemia, there is wide variation
in opinions about the proportion of patients with critical ischemia who will
require an open bypass at some point in their disease process. We currently
believe that at least 20% to 30% of patients with critical ischemia will require open
surgery at some point in the course of their disease, although we acknowledge
that endovascular techniques continue to improve so that this proportion may
decrease in the future. We also believe that such procedures will usually be
indicated after failures of one, or usually more, endovascular treatments, although
there are rare patients with very long occlusions, limited target outflow arteries,
and a good greater saphenous vein in whom a bypass should be considered as a
primary option from the outset. To some extent, such an option will depend on
many factors such as the age and health of the patient, the pattern of disease, and
the skills of the involved interventionalist and surgeon. One real concern is that,
as fewer bypasses will be required, fewer surgeons will be skilled in these
demanding bypass techniques, particularly in the difficult circumstances in which
they will be required. Perhaps referral centers for such bypasses should be
established for the same reasons that such centers have been recommended for
the few patients who require open thoracoabdominal aneurysm repair.

It has been recognized for many years that repetitive or redo procedures
are an important component of care for patients with critical ischemia (1,4,5).

Endovascular procedures may be used to salvage limbs after failed or failing open surgical bypasses (1,18,19). This tendency will increase as technology improves. Similarly, bypass operations or partially open thrombectomy will be required after early or late failure of endovascular treatment or prior bypasses in patients in whom no further endovascular options are available. We believe most of the 20% to 30% of critical ischemia patients who will require an open surgical bypass or thrombectomy will require it in such a setting.

There are certain principles and precautions that those performing endo-vascular interventions for critical ischemia should observe. These interventions should be used in a way that preserves at least one good target outflow artery, thereby leaving the option of an open surgical rescue if the intervention fails. In addition, care must be taken not to render initially patent arterial segments unusable, thereby necessitating a more distal bypass than would have been required prior to the endovascular procedure. Moreover, key collateral vessels should be preserved so that the patient will not be worse off than the original presentation if the endovascular intervention fails. This is particularly important to avoid the need for some reinterventions if ulcerated or gangrenous lesions have healed.

SPECIFIC OPEN SURGICAL REVASCULARIZATION PROCEDURES

These fall under two major headings: bypass procedures and revision of failed (thrombosed) prior bypasses that cannot be reopened by endovascular means. The latter circumstance is usually associated with an organized fibrinous plug that cannot be lysed, dilated, or removed at either the proximal or distal anastomosis of a prosthetic bypass.

Aortoiliac Occlusive Disease

Almost all aortoiliac occlusive disease can be treated with endovascular techniques. Exceptions might be juxtarenal aortic occlusions and failed stents resistant to endovascular recanalization. Aortofemoral prosthetic bypass may be indicated in such circumstances. With juxtarenal aortic occlusions, suprarenal or supraceliac aortic control is advisable. The technical steps to gain supraceliac or suprarenal aortic control with vessel loop or clamp control of the renal arteries to prevent renal embolization have been described (21,22). With such control the infrarenal aorta, which is generally free of serious atherosclerotic involvement, is divided and thrombectomized to serve as the origin for the bypass. In such patients with scarred abdomens and multiple comorbidities, axillobifemoral bypass may be indicated if aortoiliac PTA and stenting cannot be performed. In most patients with critical ischemia and aortoiliac occlusions, revascularizing the common or deep femoral arteries will be sufficient to relieve the critical ischemia. However, in patients with extensive foot gangrene, some form of infrainguinal PTA or bypass may also be required to save the limb. These may be carried out as part of a one- or two-staged procedure.

SFA and Above-Knee Popliteal Occlusive Disease

With the introduction of improved total occlusion crossing techniques, sub-intimal or intraluminal PTA can be used to treat most occlusions of the SFA and above-knee popliteal artery. Nitinol self-expanding stents and stent-grafts

(Viabahn) can be used as adjuncts to these procedures (23–25). When performing these procedures, care must be taken not to violate the principles and precautions outlined above and to preserve important collateral vessels. In the unusual instance when these endovascular interventions fail and cannot be restored to patency or when technical difficulty is encountered, a femoropopliteal bypass can be performed to the below-knee popliteal artery or tibioperoneal trunk via standard medial approaches (26). This is best performed with a reversed greater saphenous vein harvested via skip incisions, although endoscopic vein harvest has been described (27). However, this technique requires special equipment and technical expertise. In situ vein bypass offers no advantage in the femoropopliteal position. If the groin is heavily scarred or infected, the distal two-thirds of the deep femoral artery can be accessed directly in the thigh and used for bypass inflow (or outflow if a bypass ends in the groin) (13). In circumstances in which the medial approaches to the popliteal artery are rendered difficult or impossible because of scarring or infection, both the above-knee and the below-knee popliteal artery can be accessed via lateral approaches and used for bypass outflow (14). If this is done, the graft can be tunneled laterally in a subcutaneous plane. If patients do not have a saphenous vein or arm vein or if their veins are too small (<3.5 mm in distended diameter) or involved with preexisting disease (28) and they require a femoropopliteal bypass, a 6-mm polytetrafluoroethylene (PTFE) conduit may be used (29). If this is done or even if a vein is used, duplex surveillance is warranted, and reintervention is justified for a failing (threatened) graft. However, if the graft has failed (thrombosed), reintervention is only indicated if critical ischemia recurs, which only occurs in about 65% of cases (12).

Tibial and Peroneal Artery Bypasses

These may be indicated after multiple failures of endovascular treatments. Some also believe they are indicated when long segments of all three crural vessels and the below-knee popliteal or tibioperoneal trunk are occluded. In this circumstance, some believe long segment tibial subintimal PTA is effective (30). However, we have not been able to duplicate professor Bolia's tibial artery results despite our enthusiasm for subintimal PTA in the femoral and popliteal arteries (31).

For tibial and peroneal bypasses, autologous vein is the graft of choice, provided it is disease free (28). The source of the superficial vein can be from any limb or site, and the vein can be used in either the reversed or in situ configuration. Our own randomized comparison of reversed and in situ vein grafts to crural arteries demonstrated no significant patency or limb salvage differences except for veins less than 3 mm in distended diameter (32). In this circumstance, in situ grafts performed better, but the difference was not statistically significant. To facilitate the use of vein as the conduit, the grafts should be as short as possible and the SFA, the popliteal, and even tibial arteries have proven to be effective sites of origin for these distal bypasses when there is no important proximal disease (6–8,10) (Figs. 2–4). If there is proximal disease, it can often be treated by PTA, enabling a distal short vein graft without compromising patency (33). Moreover, if there is a patent popliteal blind or isolated segment (without tibial or peroneal outflow) and limited lengths of autologous vein, a composite sequential bypass may be performed with the distal component being a vein graft from the isolated popliteal to a patent tibial artery and the proximal component being a PTFE graft from a femoral artery to the proximal end of the

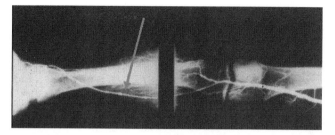

FIGURE 2 This arteriogram shows a vein bypass from the below-knee popliteal artery to the dorsalis pedis artery that was patent for more than 10 years.

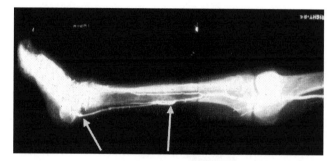

FIGURE 3 This tibio-tibial bypass was performed utilizing reversed vein as was patent 12 years later.

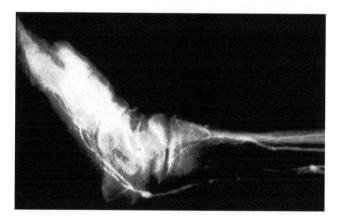

FIGURE 4 This is a magnified arteriographic view of the foot from the patient shown in Figure 3. Long-term limb salvage was achieved despite an incomplete plantar arch.

vein graft (34). If a critical ischemia patient is faced with an imminent amputation and is totally without satisfactory autologous vein, a PTFE tibial bypass is in our opinion an acceptable option, and over the years we have obtained good secondary patency and limb salvage results (43% 5-year secondary patency and 66% 5-year limb salvage) in this setting (29,35) (Figs. 5 and 6). Although some

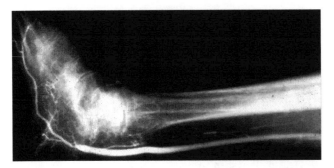

FIGURE 5 This prosthetic bypass (PTFE) to the posterior tibial artery was performed for limb salvage. The arteriogram shown was performed four years postoperatively. Patency was maintained for six years. *Abbreviation*: PTFE, polytetrafluoroethylene.

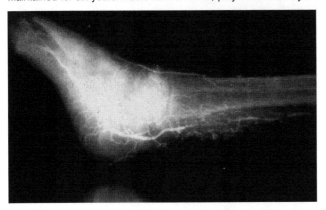

FIGURE 6 The arteriogram of this patient with great toe gangrene shows only an isolated posterior tibial segment. There is no autologous vein available for bypass.

advocate the use of a distal vein patch or cuff to improve patency (36), we have not been convinced that any of these adjunctive procedures improve patency results more than a carefully constructed distal PTFE graft anastomosis. We have also reviewed our recent experience with PTFE bypasses to leg arteries and are convinced that they have a role in achieving and maintaining limb salvage when other options are not available (37). The graft must, however, be implanted into a leg artery that has luminal continuity to its normal terminal branches and preferably richly supplies the foot, and the surgeon must be willing to do a secondary or redo prosthetic tibial bypass if the original graft fails (37). We also acknowledge that many groups have not been able to duplicate our results although some have (38,39).

Bypasses to Foot Arteries and Their Branches
In the late 1970s and early 1980s, we realized that many patients who were thought to have patterns of arteriosclerosis totally unsuited for revascularization actually had patent named arteries in their feet that could be used as outflow sites for distal bypasses (1,4,7,10) (Fig. 7). By performing bypasses to these

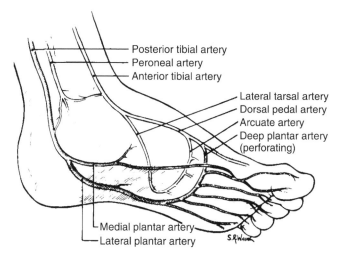

FIGURE 7 Diagram showing important pedal vasculature that is used in strategic planning for limb salvage revascularization.

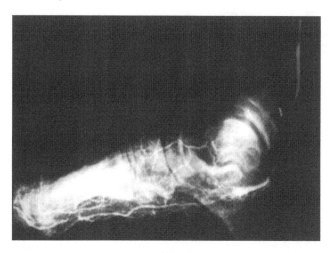

FIGURE 8 This arteriogram was performed four years after reversed vein bypass to the lateral plantar artery.

vessels, we could substantially increase the number of critical ischemia patients who could have their threatened limbs saved (1,7,10) (Figs. 8 and 9). Many other groups subsequently confirmed our initial results.

These very distal grafts can only be performed with vein as a conduit. However, many of these very distal grafts can originate from the below-knee popliteal artery or even from patent proximal tibial arteries (1,6,7,10) (Figs. 2–4). As with all infrainguinal bypass grafts, and especially those to crural arteries, the procedures must be performed with care and technical perfection. Any technical error in graft preparation, tunneling, or anastomotic construction will result in failure. Good lighting (headlight), a dry field, and patience are essential. Magnification and microsurgical instruments are often required, and care

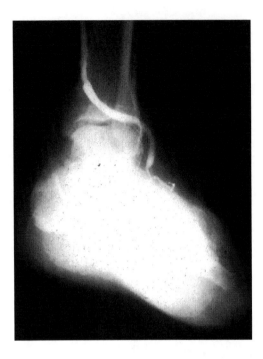

FIGURE 9 A 12-year-old who underwent reversed vein bypass to the lateral
tarsal artery.

must be taken to treat outflow arteries atraumatically and to preserve all outflow
branches, even those small ones that are unnamed. Completion arteriography is
also essential, as with all infrapopliteal bypasses to assure good anastomotic
configuration and bypass flow rates. If spasm or decreased flow is noted, vasodilators (nitroglycerin, papaverine) may be helpful (40). Further technical
details and illustrations are provided in a recent textbook chapter, which goes
beyond the scope of this chapter (26).

Although these foot artery procedures were developed before endovascular approaches existed to revascularize these very distal arteries, foot artery
bypasses still have a role today. We acknowledge that the use of 014″ guidewire-
based systems, coronary balloons, and stents are now being used to revascularize patent arteries in the lower leg and even the foot. How well these techniques will work, and how their results will compare to those of bypass
operations remain to be determined. We embrace and use these newer techniques and are optimistic that they will work. However, that remains to be shown,
and we believe there will always be a place for these very distal bypasses when
an endovascular option is not available—provided there are surgeons trained
and willing to do them.

NEWER TECHNIQUES FOR REDO PROCEDURES AFTER
FAILED BYPASSES: THROMBECTOMY AND TOTAL OR
PARTIAL RESCUE OF A FAILED PTFE BYPASS OR TOTALLY
NEW BYPASSES

It is well known that infrainguinal revascularization procedures, both endovascular and open, are associated with specific failure rates, with the potential
for diminished luminal caliber followed by thrombosis. This is due to both

intimal hyperplasia, largely a reaction to vascular injury, and progression of the arteriosclerotic process. When bypasses that have been performed for critical ischemia fail after a patency interval of six months or longer, the originally threatened limb is only rethreatened in about 65% of patients. This may be due to healing of the original gangrenous or ulcerated lesion and the fact that greater blood flow is required to achieve healing than to maintain it. Alternatively, the maintenance of a healed foot after bypass failure may be due to improved collateral blood flow or absence of the trauma or infection, which contributed to the gangrene or ulceration in the first place.

Whatever the reason, management strategies for patients with failed revascularization procedures should be influenced by the fact that critical ischemia may not recur. Only if it does, should a secondary intervention be undertaken since such secondary procedures are generally more difficult and have worse results than primary procedures. Thus, redo procedures are not indicated to prevent critical ischemia from developing. The one exception is when a primary procedure is determined by physical examination, symptoms, or noninvasive testing to be in the failing state, which is threatened by the development of a new or recurrent lesion that reduces flow but without thrombosis of the revascularization. In this case, there are many relatively straightforward procedures that may be employed to prevent graft failure.

A full description of all possible redo procedures that are indicated when a primary bypass, with a vein or prosthetic, fails is beyond the scope of this chapter and is available elsewhere (12) Nevertheless, some principles, in addition to those already mentioned, deserve emphasis. First, endovascular interventions should always be considered the first option in patients requiring a redo procedure even if the original revascularization was a bypass. Improved technology that was previously unavailable may be effective and may provide sufficient increased blood flow to maintain foot viability.

Second, redissection of previously dissected arteries, particularly in the groin, should be avoided since they are difficult and prone to a fivefold increased risk of infection. If a totally new bypass is required, as is usually the case when a failed vein graft cannot be freed of clot, alternate or new approaches to patent arteries should be used, and these have been well described (12–14,20).

Third, complete preprocedural arteriography should precede any reoperative attempt. Planning can only be optimized when the surgeon or interventionalist is fully aware of the location and extent of all occlusive and stenotic arterial disease throughout the iliac system and the entire lower extremity.

Fourth, if the failed bypass is a prosthetic conduit, an effort should be made to restore patency percutaneously, using mechanical thrombectomy devices and lytic agents. This is often facilitated if the proximal anastomotic hood of the original graft can be seen angiographically to facilitate guidewire passage. Only if interventional procedures fail, should reoperation be undertaken. This is generally required when the proximal or distal organized thrombotic plug cannot be lysed or removed by percutaneous means. In this circumstance, the PTFE graft is approached at its most accessible mid-portion, usually in a subcutaneous position and remote from any anastomosis. The graft is opened longitudinally and the liquified clot gently removed with balloon catheters. Then, using fluoroscopic guidance, guidewires and catheters are gently used to traverse the anastomosis. Fluoroscopy with contrast injections is used to identify any inflow or anastomotic lesions and similarly any outflow lesions. A double lumen balloon catheter is then passed over the guidewire across the anastomosis, the balloon is inflated with dilute contrast, and under fluoroscopic control the balloon is gently withdrawn to remove free clot. By observing the distortion of the balloon, hyperplastic and arteriosclerotic lesions can be observed and corrected by PTA without or with stent placement (41,42). Balloon distortion within the proximal graft indicates the presence of an organized gelatinous or fibrinous plug, which cannot usually be removed with a balloon catheter. In that case and because loose clot has been removed, there may often be some flow in the opened graft presenting a problem with hemostasis. If so, a 9-Fr hemostatic sheath is placed into the graft, and bleeding around the sheath is controlled with doubled vessel loops. The sheath and its dilator are passed over the wire across the anastomosis. The dilator is removed and an adherent clot removal catheter (Edwards Lifesciences) is passed within the sheath under fluoroscopic control. The sheath is retracted and the wires of the clot removal catheter are deployed only within the graft under fluoroscopic control to engage the adherent plug and remove it without injuring the adjacent artery. Angiography is used to demonstrate absence of residual luminal defects. A similar procedure is then carried out distally. If unobstructed distal flow cannot be obtained after PTA and stent placement, the proximal graft now with unobstructed inflow is transected and used as the origin for a partially new bypass to another patent distal artery accessed via a virginal approach (14,20). After completion, contrast fluoroscopy demonstrates an adequate lumen without defects and unimpeded flow, and the procedure is terminated.

MULTIPLE REDO PROCEDURES

Some patients are subject to repetitive failure of lower extremity revascularization procedures including bypasses. Some believe that patients who have failure of two or more bypasses in the same lower extremity should, if they redevelop critical ischemia, undergo a major amputation. We do not agree with this concept and have recently demonstrated the value of repetitive redo bypasses, usually performed over several years (up to 15), in preserving the limb and lifestyle of these patients (43). We observed the duration of patency following more than three bypasses was substantial and resulted in more than three years of extended limb salvage in more than 50% of the patients who would otherwise have required an amputation (43). These beneficial results were only obtained when the repetitive bypasses were performed according to the principles already outlined in this chapter. Moreover, repetitive bypasses should only be performed when the patient would otherwise require an immediate major amputation.

CONCLUSIONS

The bottom line of all these treatment efforts for critical ischemia is that everything possible should be done to salvage the threatened foot in these elderly, sick patients who do not walk well after one major amputation and certainly do not do so after bilateral amputations, which 25% of this population may otherwise require at some point in their course. Although the methods needed to save limbs initially and maintain this salvage may be time consuming and technically demanding, and although they require continuing commitment on the part of the surgeon-caregiver, they are gratifying to those that carry them out effectively and are rewarding in maintaining an acceptable life style in this group of patients with advanced atherosclerosis.

REFERENCES

1. Veith FJ, Gupta SK, Wengerter KR, et al. Changing arteriosclerotic disease patterns and management strategies in lower limb threatening ischemia. Ann Surg 1990; 212:402–414.
2. Rivers SP, Veith FJ, Ascer E, et al. Successful conservative therapy of severe limb-threatening ischemia: the value of nonsympathectomy. Surgery 1986; 99:759–763.
3. Stoney RJ. Ultimate salvage for the patient with limb-threatening ischemia: realistic goals and surgical considerations. Am J Surg 1978; 136:228–233.
4. Veith FJ, Gupta SK, Samson RH, et al. Progress in limb salvage by reconstructive arterial surgery combined with new or improved adjunctive procedures. Ann Surg 1981; 194:386–401.
5. Veith FJ, Weiser RK, Gupta SK, et al. Diagnosis and management of failing lower extremity arterial reconstructions prior to graft occlusion. J Cardiovasc Surg 1984; 25:381–384.
6. Veith FJ, Gupta SK, Samson RH, et al. The superficial femoral and popliteal arteries as inflow sites for distal bypasses. Surgery 1981; 90:980–991.
7. Ascer E, Veith FJ, Gupta SK. Bypasses to plantar arteries and other tibial branches: an extended approach to limb salvage. J Vasc Surg 1988; 8:434–441.
8. Ascer E, Veith FJ, Gupta SK, et al. Short vein grafts: a superior option for arterial reconstruction to poor or compromised outflow tracts. J Vasc Surg 1988; 7:370–377.
9. Leather RP, Shah DM, Chang BB, et al. Resurrection of the in situ vein bypass: 1000 cases later. Ann Surg 1988; 205:435.
10. Veith FJ, Ascer E, Gupta SK, et al. Tibiotibial vein bypass grafts: a new operation for limb salvage. J Vasc Surg 1985; 2:552–557.
11. Ascer E, Veith FJ, White-Flores SA. Infrapopliteal bypasses to heavily calcified rock-like arteries. Management and results. Am J Surg 1986; 152:220–223.
12. Veith FJ, Gupta SK, Ascer E, et al. Improved strategies for secondary operations on infrainguinal arteries. Ann Vasc Surg 1990; 4:85–93.
13. Veith FJ, Nunez A, Gupta SK, et al. Direct approaches to the middle and distal portions of the deep femoral artery for use as sites of origin or termination for secondary bypasses. Perspect Vasc Surg 1988; 1:94–102.
14. Veith FJ, Ascer E, Gupta SK, et al. Lateral approach to the popliteal artery. J Vasc Surg 1987; 6:119–123.
15. Sprayregen S, Sniderman HW, Sos TA, et al. Popliteal artery branches: percutaneous transluminal angioplasty. Am J Roentgenol 1980; 135:945–951.
16. Bakal CW, Sprayregen S, Scheinbaum K, et al. Percutaneous transluminal angioplasty of the infrapopliteal arteries: results in 53 patients. Am J Roentgenol 1990; 154:171–174.
17. Veith FJ, Gupta SK, Wengerter KR, et al. Impact of nonoperative therapy on the clinical management of peripheral arterial disease. Circulation 1991; 83:137–142.
18. Sanchez L, Gupta SK, Veith FJ, et al. A ten-year experience with one hundred fifty failing or threatened vein and polytetrafluoroethylene arterial bypass grafts. J Vasc Surg 1991; 14:729–738.
19. Sanchez LA, Suggs WD, Marin ML, et al. Is percutaneous balloon angioplasty appropriate in the treatment of graft and anastomotic lesions responsible for failing vein bypasses? Am J Surg 1994; 168:97–101.
20. Dardik H, Dardik I, Veith FJ. Exposure of the tibial-peroneal arteries by a single lateral approach. Surgery 1974; 75:337.
21. Veith FJ, Gupta S, Daly V. Technique for occluding the supraceliac aorta through the abdomen. Surg Gynecol Obstet 1980; 151:426–428.
22. Gupta FJ, Veith FJ. Management of juxtarenal aortic occlusions: technique for suprarenal clamp placement. Ann Vasc Surg 1992; 6:306–312.

23. Schillinger M, Sabeti S, Loewe C, et al. Balloon angioplasty versus implantation of Nitonol stents in the superficial femoral artery. N Engl J Med 2006; 354:1879–1888.
24. Lammer J, Dake MD, Bleyn J, et al. Peripheral arterial obstruction: prospective study of treatment with a transluminally placed self-expanding stent graft. Radiology 2000; 217:95–104.
25. Fischer M, Schwabe C, Schulte K-L. Value of the Hemobahn/Viabahn endoprosthesis in the treatment of long chronic lesions of the superficial femoral artery: 6 years of experience. J Endovasc Ther 2006; 13:281–290.
26. Veith FJ, Lipsitz EC. Femoral-popliteal-tibial occlusive disease. In: Hobson RW, Wilson SE, eds. Vascular Surgery: Principles and Practice. New York: Marcel Dekker, 2004:455–484.
27. Jordan WD Jr, Alcocer F, Voellinger DC, et al. The durability of endoscopic saphenous vein grafts: a 5-year observational study. J Vasc Surg 2001; 34:434–439.
28. Panetta TF, Marin ML, Veith, FJ, et al. Unsuspected pre-existing saphenous vein disease: an unrecognized cause of vein bypass failure. J Vasc Surg 1992; 15:102–112.
29. Veith FJ, Gupta SK, Ascer E, et al. Six-year prospective multicenter randomized comparison of autologous saphenous vein and expanded polytetrafluoroethylene grafts in infrainguinal arterial reconstructions. J Vasc Surg 1986; 3:104–115.
30. Bolia A. Subintimal angioplasty in lower limb ischaemia. J Cardiovasc Surg 2005; 46 (4):385–394.
31. Lipsitz EC, Ohki T, Veith FJ, et al. Does subintimal angioplasty have a role in the treatment of severe lower extremity ischemia? J Vasc Surg 2003; 37:386–391.
32. Harris PL, Veith FJ, Shanik GD, et al. Prospective randomized comparison of in-situ and reversed infrapopliteal vein grafts. Br J Surg 1993; 80:173–176.
33. Wengerter KR, Yang PM, Veith FJ, et al. A twelve-year experience with the popliteal-to-distal artery bypass: the significance and management of proximal disease. J Vasc Surg 1992; 15:143–151.
34. Gargiulo NJ, Veith FJ, Lipsitz, EC, et al. Experience with a modified composite sequential bypass technique for limb threatening ischemia. Ann Vasc Surg 2008 (manuscript submitted).
35. Parsons RE, Suggs WD, Veith FJ, et al. Polytetrafluoroethylene bypasses to infrapopliteal arteries without cuffs or patches: A better option than amputation in patients without autologous vein. J Vasc Surg 1996; 23:347–456.
36. Neville RF, Tempesta B, Sidway AN. Tibial bypass for limb salvage using polytetrafluoroethylene and a distal vein patch. J Vasc Surg 2001; 33(2):266–271.
37. Gargiulo NJ, Veith FJ, Lipsitz EC, et al. Polytetrafluoroethylene bypasses to infrapopliteal arteries without cuffs, patches or other adjunctive procedures: a 20-year experience (manuscript in preparation).
38. Schweiger H, Klein P, Lang W. Tibial bypass grafting for limb salvage with ringed polytetrafluoroethylene prostheses: results of primary and secondary procedures. J Vasc Surg 1993; 18 (5):867–874.
39. Klinkert P, van Dijk PJ, Breslau PJ. Polytetrafluoroethylene femorotibial bypass grafting: 5-year patency and limb savage. Ann Vasc Surg 2003; 17(5):486–491.
40. Gargiulo NJ III, Veith FJ, Lipsitz EC, et al. Pseudodefects in completion arteriography and their management by less invasive means (manuscript in preparation).
41. Parsons RE, Marin ML, Veith FJ, et al. Fluoroscopically assisted thromboembolectomy: An improved method for treating acute arterial occlusions. Ann Vasc Surg 1996; 10:201–210.
42. Cayne NS, Veith FJ, Lipsitz EC, et al. Improved technique for reoperations on failed PTFE grafts (manuscript in preparation).
43. Lipsitz EC, Veith FJ, Cayne NS, et al. Multiple reoperations are effective for limb salvage (manuscript in preparation).

Management of Acute Lower Extremity Ischemia

George H. Meier

Division of Vascular Surgery, University of Cincinnati College of Medicine, Cincinnati, Ohio, U.S.A.

INTRODUCTION

The absence of adequate blood flow to the lower extremity presents in many different ways depending on the acuity of the events leading to presentation. In the setting of chronic ischemia, the leg may be a nuisance, with disabling claudication, but little else. At the other extreme, the pain associated with acute arterial embolus is undeniable, often leading to urgent presentation to the nearest source of medical care within minutes of its onset. Thus, while the absence of nutrient perfusion to the lower extremity is a continuum, in its most acute presentation, the afflicted individual seeks emergency care because of the severity of the symptoms. With each passing minute, the biochemical derangements in the extremity increase, ultimately leading to irreversible ischemia. While the underlying cause of the ischemia is related to the presentation, there is no one way for patients with lower extremity ischemia to present.

While many definitions of acute ischemia exist, for the purposes of this chapter, it will be arbitrarily defined as that of less than 14 days duration. While some patients with acute ischemia may present after 14-day symptom duration, these patients are an exception and are relatively uncommon.

With acute ischemia, ulcers or gangrene are rare changes until the stage of irreversible ischemia has been reached. Typically, the changes in the extremity reflect the traditional five Ps: pain, pallor, paresthesias, pulselessness, and paralysis. These symptoms are related to the severity of the acute ischemia and represent an extremity that will progress to irreversible ischemia if left untreated. Typically, the viability of the extremity is related to the preservation of sensation and motor function. When physicians refer to the extremity as "viable," the implication is that sensation and motor activity are present. In the presence of abnormal sensation or motion, the urgency of revascularization increases to avoid irreversible ischemia.

Objective criteria have been proposed by several authors to define the level of acute ischemia at presentation. Perhaps the most widely used is that first proposed by Rutherford in 1997 (1). In this scheme, limbs are divided into viable, threatened, or irreversible ischemia on the basis of sensory loss, muscle weakness, and arterial and venous Doppler signals (Table 1). The use of such objective criteria allows the literature to compare patients and treatment strategies, an important adjunct if evidence-based treatments are the goal. Nonetheless, these criteria are, by necessity, somewhat arbitrary and do not necessarily allow for an individual patient to be easily classified. Objective criteria for data comparisons nonetheless remain useful when reporting data on acute ischemia.

TABLE 1   Rutherford Classification of Acute Limb Ischemia

		Findings		Doppler signals	
Category	Description/ prognosis	Sensory loss	Muscle weakness	Arterial	Venous
I, viable	Not immediately threatened	None	None	Audible	Audible
IIa, threatened marginally	Salvageable if treated	Minimal (toes) or none	None	Inaudible	Audible
IIb, threatened immediately	Salvageable with immediate revascularization	More than toes, associated with rest pain	Mild, moderate	Inaudible	Audible
III, irreversible	Major tissue loss or permanent nerve damage	Profound, anesthetic	Profound, paralysis (rigor)	Inaudible	Inaudible

PATHOPHYSIOLOGY

Underlying all ischemia, whether acute or chronic, is a lack of oxygen delivery to the tissues. In chronic ischemia, this represents a lack of nutrient flow causing tissue damage, such as ulcers or gangrene, or symptoms, such as claudication or rest pain. In acute ischemia, however, the ultimate change in the extremity is similar, with a lack of sensation and motor function in the final common pathway. The main difference between patients with acute ischemia has to do with the underlying cause for the ischemia and the duration of the ischemia.

Tissue tolerance to ischemia is specific to the type of tissue involved. In an extremity, skin, nerve, muscle, bone, and connective tissue are all exposed to the ischemia, but their metabolic demands vary from tissue to tissue. Their sensitivity to oxygen deprivation is proportional to their metabolic rate. As in the brain, nerve tissue is most sensitive to hypoxia, with bone at the other extreme. Muscle is intermediate, but is much of the bulk of the tissue in the extremity. For this reason, muscle tolerance to ischemia determines much of the extremity's sensitivity to hypoxia. Generally, the "six-hour rule" of acute ischemia applies, meaning that reperfusion is generally successful when accomplished within this time window. While there are numerous factors that influence the tolerance of the extremity to ischemia, the main contributor to tolerance is prior ischemic conditioning by chronic vascular disease, allowing biochemical adaptation as well as collateral formation to occur (2,3). In the setting of chronic arterial insufficiency, the presentation of the patient with superimposed acute arterial occlusion may be significantly delayed and much better tolerated, to the point of presenting as a chronic condition rather than an acute one. While ultimately every stenosis that leads to occlusion obstructs acutely, the underlying chronic disease may allow the acute event to pass unnoticed, leading the patient to chronic disease.

An additional issue associated with acute ischemia is the potential for irreversibility. If the biochemical derangements persist for a critical duration, then irreversible injury can occur. This is commonly referred to as ischemia-reperfusion injury. In ischemia-reperfusion injury, the derangements accumulate with time, ultimately resulting in the irreversible injury. Nonetheless, many factors interact to lead to the extreme of irreversible ischemia. While an exhaustive discussion of ischemia-reperfusion injury is beyond the scope of this chapter, it is important that the reader has a firm grasp of the elements responsible to allow optimum treatment of the patient with acute ischemia (4–10). Fundamentally, oxygen, while essential for human survival, is a toxic agent that easily and commonly forms free radicals, which can then lead to tissue damage. The generation of these free radicals is related to a number of elements, but current thought centers on the xanthine oxidase/xanthine dehydrogenase enzyme systems as the major sources of free radical generation in acute ischemia (11–16).

For years, medical students were taught that xanthine oxidase is the major enzyme system for xanthine and hypoxanthine metabolism, important intermediaries in purine metabolism. It was only several years later that it was discovered that xanthine oxidase does not occur in normal living humans. Postmortem, under hypoxic conditions, xanthine dehydrogenase is converted to xanthine oxidase. Why is this important? With reoxygenation, xanthine oxidase generates oxygen free radicals as the enzyme is converted back to xanthine dehydrogenase under normal oxygenation. These free radicals rapidly overwhelm the natural scavenging systems for free radicals, specifically glutathione and superoxide dismutase. The free radicals are then released into the circulation where injury to the vessel can occur.

With free radical injury to the endothelium, white blood cells adhere to the vessel lumen, ultimately obstructing the lumen of the arterioles and capillaries. Thus, the final step in the irreversibility of ischemia-reperfusion injury is secondary to luminal obstruction by white blood cells, preventing flow to the tissues. This is referred to as the "no-reflow" phenomenon. Often this is seen after a short period of hyperemic flow with resultant reoxygenation, followed by recurrent permanent ischemia.

First and foremost, treating this complex process is by pharmacologic manipulation to allow recovery of flow and avoidance of free radical injury. There are two basic strategies for these pharmacologic approaches to prevent free radical injury: prevention of free radical production and quenching of free radicals once generated. Since most of the oxygen free radicals are generated from the xanthine oxidase/xanthine dehydrogenase enzyme system, one option is to inhibit these enzymes in an effort to avoid free radical production with reoxygenation. In fact, allopurinol, a relatively nontoxic medicine developed in the 1950s for the treatment of gout, effectively inhibits xanthine oxidase–derived free radical generation (13,14,17–19). By administration of allopurinol, up to 95% of oxygen free radicals can be prevented in ischemia-reperfusion and the damage caused can be significantly diminished. Unfortunately, allopurinol is only available as an oral medication, requiring administration to a conscious patient early enough to allow absorption of the drug from the gastrointestinal tract and adequate distribution of the drug to the underperfused tissues. In many emergency settings like that seen with acute lower extremity ischemia, it may be impossible to administer the drug in a timely fashion prior to reoxygenation. Moreover, the distribution of the drug is by perfusion of the tissues, leading to limited early phase levels of drug in ischemic tissues. Therefore, early administration of allopurinol in acute ischemia is critical to drug distribution to the tissues where it will be needed.

As an alternative to inhibiting free radical production is quenching of free radicals once formed. While the body has endogenous free radical quenching systems utilizing glutathione and superoxide dismutase, as noted above, these natural mechanisms are rapidly overwhelmed in the setting of reperfusion. Therefore, exogenous quenching substrates may be beneficial to treat the free radicals generated. Again, delivery to the ischemic tissues is critical to success. One of the most effective exogenous free radical quenchers is mannitol, a six-carbon sugar initially used as an osmotic diuretic. In the 1960s, mannitol became common in both cardiac and vascular surgeries, reaching the point of routine use in aortic and open-heart surgeries. Only in the 1980s did its free radical quenching properties become apparent (18,20,21). In reperfusion, oxygen free radicals interact with the mannitol molecule, generating a mannitol free radical. This mannitol free radical interacts with another mannitol molecule, preferentially generating a mannitol dimer and avoiding tissue injury. The mannitol dimer is then safely excreted by the kidney. Mannitol remains inexpensive, readily available in most operating rooms, and effective for quenching free radicals associated with reoxygenation, independent of their source. Typically, mannitol is given intravenously at a dose of 0.25 to 1 g/kg of body weight; while it can be administered systemically, some prefer to deliver this intra-arterially to the involved extremity to allow direct free radical quenching to occur at the point of reperfusion. In either case, the important aspect is the delivery prior to reoxygenation of the involved extremity, in adequate doses to allow effective quenching of free radicals to occur.

ETIOLOGY OF ACUTE ISCHEMIA

While acute ischemia obviously involves the sudden irreparable restriction of blood flow to the involved extremity, the underlying causes can be any of a number of etiologies. Perhaps the most classic paradigm for acute ischemia is that of acute arterial embolism. In embolism, a preformed clot from other locations breaks free and travels to the lower extremity where the clot lodges in the blood vessel, suddenly obstructing limb blood flow. Most of the time, the patient can remember the exact moment when this occurs, since the restriction of blood flow is sudden and unrelenting. The patient immediately becomes symptomatic, with progressive worsening of symptoms. Usually, the patient seeks medical attention because of the sudden persistent symptoms that result.

The most common source for arterial emboli is the heart (22–25). Patients may form clots within the heart under a number of situations, but perhaps the most common is in the setting of atrial arrhythmias. A patient with intermittent atrial fibrillation or flutter may form a clot in the left atrium when the heart is beating irregularly; with restoration of a regular sinus rhythm, atrial contraction may lead to ejection of the clot thus formed, leading to embolization. This clot may have been formed days or weeks earlier in the atrium, thus making it refractory to endogenous lysis and breakdown. These emboli typically travel through the arterial circulation until the caliber of the artery decreases sufficiently to prevent further passage (Fig. 1). Most commonly, this occurs just below a branch point in the artery. While fresh clots may lyse spontaneously, chronic clot is typically resistant to any endogenous breakdown. Distally in the artery, intact endothelium initially prevents further thrombosis. With time, however, the ischemic damage to the endothelial cells results in thrombosis of the distal arterial tree. With prompt removal of the offending embolus, flow can be restored before irreversible damage occurs. Additionally, acute ischemia can rarely be the presenting symptom of a myocardial infarction with mural

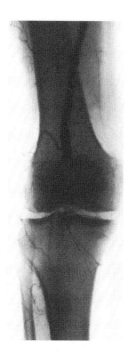

FIGURE 1 Acute embolic occlusion of the right popliteal artery demonstrating a meniscus.

thrombus. The clot thus formed during the infarction embolizes to the end organ where acute ischemia is induced.

The next common clinical scenario for acute ischemia is that of acute arterial thrombosis. In this setting, preexistent arterial disease, either occlusive or aneurysmal, leads to slowing of flow and thrombosis. Usually, chronic disease allows adequate time for collateral formation in the extremity. In unusual cases, plaque rupture or loss of collaterals may lead to acute ischemia. In these patients, there is often a significant previous vascular history of claudication or rest pain. This clue to the existence of prior disease implies the need for more extensive reconstruction in most cases. For the majority of patients with acute thrombosis, removal of thrombus will need to be supplemented with endovascular intervention or open bypass. Only by treating the underlying disease can a permanent solution be provided.

There are a number of other clinical situations where acute ischemia can occur. These are usually scenarios where the sudden obstruction of blood flow occurs secondary to a disruption in the vessel itself, such as a dissection. This can occur secondary to hypertensive vessel dissection or traumatic injury to the vessel wall itself. The result is a sudden decrement in blood flow often associated with a short-segment vessel thrombosis secondary to the injury to the vessel itself. Generally, a history of direct trauma or pain in the area of thrombus precedes the onset of ischemia itself.

Finally, intrinsic thrombosis due to local or generalized hypercoagulability can rarely occur in patients with severe dysfunction of their clotting systems. While this may result in a more generalized event rather than a localized one, disruptions in the coagulation system can present as either a thrombotic or an embolic event occurring because of more distant clot formation. While these are technically either local thromboses or embolic events, the underlying etiology is the hypercoagulable state rather than other anatomic pathologies (26).

DEMOGRAPHICS

The patient population at risk for acute ischemia depends on the etiology as discussed above. For example, emboli arising from the heart increase with age, resulting in an increasingly elderly population at risk for embolic events. On the other hand, thrombosis of atherosclerotic lesions tends to occur in patients with aggressive premature atherosclerosis, a younger population than that traditionally seen with ischemic cardiac disease. Plaque prone to ulceration, rupture, and thrombosis tends to be more active, generally an earlier stage than the calcific chronic plaque seen in the elderly. Therefore, thrombosis tends to occur in younger patients than those with embolization. Unfortunately, the overlap in age is broad, preventing easy categorization as to etiology. Gender prevalence can also be related to the underlying etiology of the acute ischemia. Typically, embolic events have a relatively equal sex distribution, while occlusions associated with thrombosis are male predominant, as are most atheroscleroses.

DIAGNOSIS

The diagnosis of acute ischemia is a clinical one, relying on history and physical findings to define the disorder. First and foremost are the historical elements related to onset. As discussed above, with embolic occlusion, the onset is instantaneous, with the patient usually aware of the exact moment of onset. Typically, the onset of paresthesias, the first "P," is rapidly followed by pain in the ischemic distribution. There may be pallor and invariably pulselessness will be associated with the event. Finally, paralysis develops to complete the diagnostic pentad. With these, the diagnosis is assured and only the etiology remains to be defined. Unfortunately, acute ischemia does not always present with an obvious diagnosis.

PRESENTATION

By definition, patients with acute ischemia present within two weeks of the onset of their ischemia. In most cases, the presentation is even more acute, often within minutes of the initiation of ischemia. The patient will usually present in significant discomfort, often with dramatic symptoms. These symptoms are usually severe enough to require urgent or emergent care.

Embolic Arterial Occlusion

Embolic occlusions, as discussed above, typically occur from a cardiac source (22–25). Therefore, while the clinical presentation is one of acute limb ischemia, the secondary symptoms revolve around the symptoms of underlying cardiac disease. Usually the patient presents with cardiac arrhythmias, most commonly atrial fibrillation or flutter. Nonetheless, atrial or ventricular ectopy can present with remote embolization as well. If a myocardial infarction has caused a mural thrombus, which has embolized, ventricular ectopy will be common because of the amount of ischemic myocardium. Over 80% of patients with cardiac origin emboli will present with a cardiac rhythm other than normal sinus.

Obviously, chest pain or evidence of congestive heart failure may be present in these patients as well. Therefore, if an acute embolus is suspected, a careful cardiac history will be essential as will a careful cardiac examination. Evidence of rales by auscultation of the lungs may be a sign of cardiac dysfunction; in more severe cases, an abdominal fluid wave or a pulsatile liver may hint at severe right heart failure. Although the embolus is acute, the underlying cardiac pathology is less so, often with cardiac signs or symptoms of a more chronic nature than the acute extremity event.

Acute Arterial Thrombosis

The presentation of patients with acute thrombotic occlusion centers on two divergent histories: first, one with chronic symptoms prior to the acute event; and second, one with an acute event without antecedent symptoms. While the former is much more common than the latter, both can be seen and both must be understood to not miss an episode of acute thrombosis. Both of these presentations are difficult to manage, but for different reasons. While both may benefit from thrombolytics, the acute presentation requires thrombolysis in many cases to open outflow for possible reconstruction.

In the most common scenario, preexistent arterial disease leads to acute thrombosis with propagation of thrombus for a variable distance into the distal arterial tree (Fig. 2). Typically, the patient has symptoms of claudication prior to the event or may have a similar history in the contralateral extremity. While pulse examination will obviously be abnormal on the involved side, often the opposite extremity has an abnormal pulse examination as well. An invariable component of the acute presentation is the lack of adequate collateral circulation. If the occlusion occurs in a controlled fashion, then collateral formation may be sufficient to avoid an acute presentation. When collaterals are limited in some fashion, acute symptoms develop, which are unlikely to be ignored. Similarly, a hypercoagulable state may lead to sudden occlusion without collateral compensation. In these settings, symptoms of acute ischemia may vary from severe claudication to rest pain to compromised sensation and motion. The determining factors are the extent of the thrombosis and the degree of collateral compensation.

In the second scenario, the thrombosis of the distal circulation is the overwhelming issue, limiting any reconstruction of distal flow. This is most commonly seen in popliteal aneurysm thrombosis, as the outflow is often compromised by distal embolization and there are often no target vessels distally for reconstruction. In this scenario, infusion thrombolysis is often essential to success, to provide an outflow bed for possible reconstruction. These patients are at high risk for extremity amputation even with thrombolytic infusion.

TREATMENT

First and foremost, the treatment of acute ischemia is the rapid and complete restoration of nutrient blood flow. The mechanism by which this is accomplished is variable, but the goal is the same, whether performed by endovascular or open techniques. The intent is to remove all obstructing clot, treat any underlying pathology, and reperfuse the extremity successfully. With significant ischemia, fasciotomy to allow the extremity to swell is both prudent and often necessary.

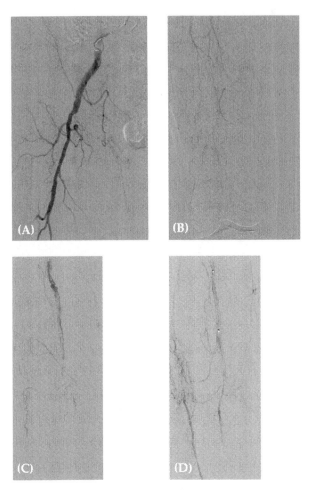

FIGURE 2 Acute arterial thrombosis. (**A**) Right common femoral arteriogram, showing chronic superficial femoral artery occlusion. (**B**) Absence of blood vessels in the above knee popliteal artery. (**C**) Thrombus in popliteal artery after selective catheterization. (**D**) Limited runoff from popliteal artery, presumably leading to thrombosis.

With the recognition of acute ischemia, early anticoagulation is important to preserve the meager blood flow remaining in the extremity (23,27,28). By limiting the growth of extremity thrombus, preservation of collateral flow may limit short-term damage as well as ease the difficulty of reperfusion. After a short overall assessment confirms the diagnosis and rules out any potential sources of hemorrhage, full systemic anticoagulation should be administered using intravenous unfractionated weight-based heparin. Intravenous unfractionated heparin is preferred because of its rapid onset of action and its potential reversibility with protamine. Once anticoagulated, the treatment can be rapidly planned and executed to restore oxygenation to the extremity.

INITIAL APPROACH

All treatments for acute arterial ischemia should ideally begin with adequate intra-arterial imaging. While there may be many mitigating factors that prevent angiography from being performed, the modern treatment of acute ischemia begins (and often ends) with percutaneous access for diagnosis and for treatment. Therefore, if the patient is a candidate for arteriography and the facilities and staff are readily available, percutaneous access for diagnosis is warranted and appropriate. If obtaining angiographic images will delay treatment, then it may be appropriate to forego imaging to allow more urgent treatment.

The angiographic approach to a patient with acute ischemia is often remote access away from the site of acute ischemia. With modern imaging, access to the area of ischemia is usually easily performed and the remote access avoids interference with any operative procedure that may ultimately be needed. Once the catheter is in position, arteriography is performed. The presence of collaterals from normal proximal vessels suggests long-standing disease, which may have developed in response to chronic atherosclerotic occlusion, and the offending thrombus is often distal to the chronic disease. Therefore, great care must be taken to ensure that delayed images are obtained to demonstrate any distal vessels that may be present. With acute embolic occlusion, the classic finding will be a proximal meniscus from the occluding embolus within the vessel, with no collateral formation and very poor visualization of the distal arterial tree. In this setting, delayed images will show no named arteries in many cases.

If no distal vessels can be visualized with delivery of angiographic contrast into the normal proximal artery, then a decision to enter the distal vessel must be made depending on the expertise and the equipment available. The occurrence of acute thrombosis of preexistent atherosclerotic disease may require subintimal angioplasty to cross the occluded segment to define any distal targets available for treatment. Typically, as the chronic occlusion is crossed, a thrombus-filled vessel will be encountered where adjunctive injection of thrombolytics may be of benefit. This acutely occluded vessel is the target for intraoperative thrombolysis to define what options may exist. At each level, dye is injected (with delayed imaging) to better define what vessels are available distally for intervention. As an alternative, open exploration of distal vessels may be undertaken but is fraught with challenges.

In any given patient, the acute ischemia requires demonstration of several key features (Table 2). The features seen will make the diagnosis of the cause of

TABLE 2 Thrombolytic Agents and Their Features

Agents for thrombolysis	
Agent	Features
Streptokinase	Antigenic, indirect plasminogen activator, variable efficacy
Urokinase	Direct plasminogen activator, limited availability
Tissue plasminogen activator	Recombinant human protein
Retaplase	Modified version of tPA, primarily used for cardiac
Tenecteplase	Engineered version of tPA, longer half-life, resistance to plasminogen activator inhibitors
Plasmin	Recently FDA approved

Abbreviation: tPA, tissue plasminogen activator.

the ischemia in most cases and may provide a head start on treatment. From this initial angiographic evaluation, all treatments will follow.

THROMBOLYSIS

While the natural thrombolytic mechanisms responsible for maintaining blood flow are overwhelmed by the acute ischemic event, increasing the lysis of thrombus by the use of exogenous pharmacologic agents can improve or correct the ischemia. The most important treatment for acute ischemia is the rapid and early administration of heparin. The function of this treatment is severalfold. First, heparin prevents new clot formation in the obstructed outflow bed. This may delay or limit the damage done by the occlusion and provide a margin of safety in reperfusion. Second, the clotting process is a balance between the formation of clot (thrombosis) and the breakdown of clot (thrombolysis). By stopping new clot formation, the patient develops a relatively thrombolytic state, allowing improvement in the patient's perfusion. While revascularization is still needed, heparin will stop the coagulation process to temporarily avoid further deterioration.

Perhaps the simplest concept to restore flow is to dissolve the offending clot using thrombolysis. While many agents (Table 3) have been used for thrombolysis, the most commonly used agent today is tissue plasminogen activator (tPA). tPA has a half-life of three to five minutes, breaking down fibrin into degradation products. One of these breakdown products is the D-dimer, only produced from clot breakdown by thrombolysis. While this breakdown product is widely used as a screening test for deep venous thrombosis, it can be found any time that clot is broken down under any circumstance. With exogenous administration of a thrombolytic agent, the breakdown of the fibrin strands by plasmin is the overall goal. By increasing the production of plasmin from plasminogen by administration of these pharmacologic agents, the lysis of clot can be increased dramatically.

In its simplest form, thrombolysis is enhanced by infusion of agents into or near the clot, which accelerate its breakdown (29–35). The method of infusion may be systemic or regional depending on the goals of the therapy. In the setting of arterial ischemia, intra-arterial infusion is often preferred in an effort to speed up the process of clot dissolution. This intra-arterial treatment is often combined with mechanical adjuncts in an effort to speed up the process further (see below). The use of mechanical adjunct allows the thrombolytic process to be sped up, decreasing the dose of thrombolytic agent and therefore decreasing the bleeding risk associated with thrombolysis. While traditional infusion thrombolysis using urokinase often continued for two to three days, the newer protocols are shorter,

TABLE 3 Angiographic Features in Acute Ischemia

Angiographic features in acute ischemia	
Location	Anatomic concerns
Proximal inflow	Presence of atherosclerosis, collaterals, meniscus
Collaterals	Vessels supplied, extent
Distal vessels	Evidence of thrombus, collaterals

often being completed in a single treatment episode. This dramatically decreases risk, resources, and cost for treatment of patients with thrombolysis.

The challenge in arterial thrombolysis is resolving not only the fresh thrombus associated with the acute event, but also the chronic component that was associated with the initiation of the ischemia. In the event of an embolus, the inciting thrombus has often originated from a chronic source in the proximal circulation, usually the heart. This thrombus may have been present in the circulation for a long time and therefore may be resistant to thrombolysis. In the case of in situ arterial thrombosis, the underlying stenosis may have associated chronic thrombus of variable age. Finally, with acute popliteal aneurysm thrombosis, the laminar thrombus within the aneurysm often embolizes and may be reticent to thrombolysis, similar to cardiac origin thrombus.

Catheter-directed thrombolysis is a focused effort to resolve arterial ischemia more quickly. By placement of a catheter into the occluded artery, directed thrombolytic delivery can significantly improve thrombolysis compared with systemic administration with decreased complications. In the earliest protocols, the infusion was through end-hole catheters imbedded into the area of thrombosis. Referred to as the McNamara protocol (32) after the first proponent of this technique, this technique requires frequent catheter repositioning to continue to infuse into the clot for maximal lysis. This can be resource intense, with multiple angiographic procedures to keep active thrombolysis. Nonetheless, rapid intra-arterial lysis of clot can be achieved using this approach.

With the development of multi-side-hole catheters, an alternative to the McNamara protocol became possible. While it was known that guidewire traversal was possible in many of the patients with thrombosis, infusion could not proceed faster than the clot lysis could be produced. The next major infusion protocol, the Bookstein protocol (36–40), utilized wire traversal and the side-hole catheter for two purposes. First, the side-hole catheter was used to "pulse spray" thrombolytic into the clot throughout its length. This intraclot injection of agent dramatically sped up the process of clot lysis. Second, infusion thrombolysis was performed through the same side-hole catheter, potentially infusing the entire length of clot present. Using side-hole catheters, the process of thrombolytic infusion can be significantly shortened.

MECHANICAL ADJUNCTS FOR THROMBOLYSIS

While the use of thrombolytic agents may be sufficient without mechanical adjuncts, often mechanical devices are combined with thrombolysis to speed up the process of clot removal. The mechanical devices may speed up the actual process of thrombolysis or they may simply remove small pieces of clot to debulk the clot that thrombolysis is used for. Generally, the mechanical adjunct is designed to speed the pharmacologic process by either mechanism.

Perhaps the most widely used mechanical adjunct for thrombolysis is the AngioJet thrombectomy catheter (Possis Corporation, Minneapolis, Minnesota, U.S.) (41–48). The AngioJet catheter is a percutaneous catheter that removes clot by fragmentation and suction, allowing both acute and chronic clot to be removed (Fig. 3). While older clot is more difficult to fragment and remove than fresh thrombus, using thrombolytics with the AngioJet catheter allows improved clot removal.

As an additional adjunct, the AngioJet catheter has been used to deliver thrombolytic agent using the "power pulse" technique (47,49). To use this

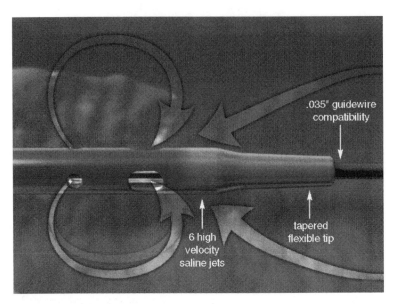

FIGURE 3 AngioJet catheter. Alternating infusion of saline with suction creates a venturi effect, which fragments clot and allows its removal.

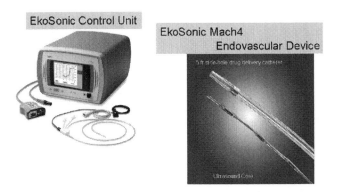

FIGURE 4 EKOS System. Control unit (*left*) and ultrasonic core and side-hole catheter (*right*) allow drug delivery with ultrasonic agitation of clot.

technique, the outflow suction port of the AngioJet catheter is shut off and concentrated thrombolytic agent is attached to the inflow pump. With this configuration, thrombolytic agent is driven into the offending clot under pressure to speed the lysis of the thrombus by improving delivery. After dwelling, the thrombus is then removed using the same catheter.

A more recent addition to the treatment of arterial clot has been the Ekosonic endovascular system (EKOS Corporation, Bothell, Washington, U.S.) (50,51) (Fig. 4). For many years, ultrasound has been known to speed thrombolysis. While the exact mechanism for this acceleration is unknown, it appears that the ultrasound "opens" the interstices of the clot, allowing the thrombolytic agent better access to the bound plasminogen within the clot (52–54). Thus, the thrombolytic agent works much quicker, allowing for shorter infusion times than would currently be possible. While the results with this device are preliminary, it appears that thrombolysis can be accelerated significantly using this technology.

OPEN MANAGEMENT

The open treatment of acute ischemia has changed over the years, but the underlying concept remains the same: physical removal of the offending clot. As discussed above, initial angiography is often invaluable to assist with diagnosis and treatment planning. While this adjunct may not always be possible, it should be a standard part of the approach to acute extremity ischemia whenever possible.

If angiography has not been done, then the approach reverts to the standard open treatment traditionally performed. Typically, an arteriotomy is performed just above the level of ischemia or above the level where the pulse is lost. Embolic occlusions tend to occur at the bifurcation of arteries, since the decrease in arterial caliber ultimately prevents further distal migration of the offending embolus. With thrombotic occlusion, the atherosclerotic process typically leads to occlusion back to a major vessel branch bifurcation. Therefore, arteriotomy will usually be performed above vessel bifurcations in either situation.

With the invention of the embolectomy catheter in 1963, removal of clots remote to the site of access became possible (55–58). Typically, a transverse arteriotomy is made after controlling the vessels proximally and distally. With the inflow occluded, the embolectomy catheter is passed down the occluded vessel blindly, taking care to "feel" the ease of passage and noting the extent to which the catheter will pass. Resistance to passage may represent the presence of chronic disease or imply that the catheter may be lodged in a smaller side branch. Ultimately, the catheter is passed to the maximum length and then inflated slowly as the catheter is withdrawn. Many authors advocate the use of air in the embolectomy catheter balloon, particularly in smaller, tapered vessels such as the profunda femoris artery or one of the trifurcations vessels. The key to the use of the embolectomy catheter is the avoidance of excessive force on the arterial wall to avoid arterial rupture or complete denudation of the endothelial surface (59–62). In spite of the best techniques, up to 80% of the endothelial surface is denuded by a single passage of the embolectomy catheter (60).

As the clot is removed, it is grasped with forceps and tractioned longitudinally to avoid fracture and to allow removal of the most clot possible with each catheter passage. The embolectomy catheter is passed until two clean sequential passes of the catheter occur. At this point, repeat arteriography is routine to document the presence of residual thrombus. Clinical studies have documented that over 80% of patients will have residual thrombus after this sequence (63,64).

With the acquisition of endovascular skills, the possibility of improving open thrombectomy became realized. First, selective distal catheterization allows the intraoperative infusion of thrombolytic agents to maximize outflow after thrombectomy. In the event of popliteal trifurcation thrombosis, injection of aliquots of thrombolytic agent into each distal vessel can help clear the distal vasculature and allow restoration of maximal flow. Similarly, selective distal catheterization after open femoral thrombectomy can allow trifurcation vessel thrombectomy from a remote approach by passing over-the-wire embolectomy catheters into the distal circulation. In this manner, open popliteal exploration can be avoided, limiting operative trauma yet improving clot removal. Endovascular adjuncts to open thrombectomy improve clearance of thrombus and limit surgical trauma.

If the embolectomy catheter will not pass to its full length, then the likelihood of chronic atherosclerosis becomes significantly higher. In this setting, repeat angiography is needed to find some distal target for operative exploration. In the absence of a distal target, blind exploration has been advocated by some authors, but the results in the long term are generally poor. If the vessel distally is patent but there is limited runoff, then distal thrombolysis may be appropriate. Obviously, infusion thrombolysis becomes significantly more complicated once a surgical incision has been made secondary to the increased risk of surgical site bleeding.

If an embolic occlusion is found, then revascularization is relatively simple and the main issue is adequate clot removal. In advanced ischemia, distal arterial thrombosis of the native artery is a bad prognostic sign, since this implies endothelial damage of sufficient severity to limit vessel patency after reperfusion. With diffuse distal thrombosis, aggressive heparin therapy after maximal clot removal is the only hope for improving patency. Endothelial damage should heal relatively rapidly, but the initial 48 hours are critical to the success of treatment.

In atherosclerotic acute ischemia, reconstruction of the vasculature is necessary to restore flow. While this may be difficult technically, the major issue in most cases is the underlying operative risk of the patient for a prolonged surgical procedure. The acutely ischemic patient is often medically compromised, dramatically increasing risk. Therefore, careful preoperative evaluation and good surgical judgment are essential for a successful outcome. The bypass technique is similar to that seen with chronic revascularization and requires a reasonable target vessel for successful bypass surgery.

As with acute ischemia of any cause, the restoration of flow brings with it the possibility of reperfusion injury and extremity swelling. The swelling often requires adjunctive fasciotomy to allow the limb to swell beyond the confines of the fascia. The technique of fasciotomy in this setting is no different than that seen commonly with acute trauma. In general, any concern about the extent of extremity swelling is only going to increase in the postoperative period, and therefore, early fasciotomy at the first operation is often warranted.

CLINICAL RESULTS FOR OPEN TREATMENT VS. THROMBOLYSIS

While most studies of thrombolysis were performed during the urokinase era, the results obtained remain a foundation on which current thrombolytic therapy is based. While not all of the studies can be applied to acute ischemia and its management, many of the studies include at least some patients with acute ischemia. Nonetheless, in spite of several prospective randomized trials, thrombolysis remains a niche therapy, often relegated to high-risk patients or those with occluded bypass grafts. While the discussion below will focus on acute ischemia, current management of chronic ischemia is usually by open surgery or endovascular techniques, as thrombolysis has not been shown to be beneficial in these patients.

The Rochester Trial
The Rochester trial (65) was undertaken to evaluate the use of thrombolytic therapy in patients with severe acute ischemia. At the time, it was well recognized that open surgical treatment in these patients carried a high amputation and death rate. Therefore, this study was undertaken to define the role of thrombolysis and whether better outcomes could be achieved. Over the course of three years, 114 patients with ischemia due to embolus or thrombosis of less than seven days duration were randomized to intra-arterial urokinase or immediate open surgery.

While no difference was seen in major amputation at 12 months (about 18% in both groups), there was a dramatic decrease in mortality in the urokinase-treated group at 12 months (16% vs. 42%). Further analysis showed that almost all of the operative mortality difference was secondary to a higher rate of cardiopulmonary complications in surgical patients. Surgical patients appeared to be poorly prepared for operative intervention, resulting in a higher rate of cardiopulmonary complications. In patients with cardiopulmonary complications in the urokinase group, the mortality was essentially the same as that seen in the operative group with cardiopulmonary complications. Therefore, the difference appears to be the higher rate of cardiopulmonary complications seen with patients treated with emergent or urgent operation.

About two-thirds of patients in the urokinase group required open surgery. The difference was that the urokinase patients were converted to elective treatment by the thrombolysis, allowing routine management of the patients when full support was available. Additionally, there was no difference seen in the cost of treatment or the duration of hospitalization in the two groups.

The STILE Trial
In the Surgery Versus Thrombolysis for Ischemia of the Lower Extremity (STILE) trial, tPA and urokinase were compared with open surgery in the treatment of patients with symptoms of ischemia of less than six-month duration (66). While this was designed for a broad range or durations, subgroup analysis of 112 patients (out of 375 randomized) with 14 days of ischemia or less was presented as part of this analysis. In this group, while there was no difference in the composite clinical outcome, surgical patients with acute ischemia demonstrated a trend toward increased major amputations (17.9% vs. 5.7% for thrombolysis, $p = 0.061$). In both the surgical group and the thrombolysis group, a high rate of ongoing/recurrent ischemia was seen in the group with acute ischemia (43.7% overall vs. 20.8% in the chronic patients treated with surgery). Mortality was not seen to be increased in the acute ischemia treated with surgery, in contrast to the Rochester trial.

Interestingly, there was no difference seen between tPA and urokinase in this trial in spite of a dose of tPA that would be considered excessive in today's treatment algorithms (5–10 mg/hr vs. 1–2 mg/hr currently). Native arterial occlusions of any cause were noted to respond poorly to thrombolytic therapy.

The TOPAS Trial
The Thrombolysis or Peripheral Artery Surgery (TOPAS) trial consisted of two separate studies: a dose-ranging study of urokinase in 244 patients (67) and a comparison of surgery versus thrombolysis for patients with 14 days of ischemia or less (68). This trial was not only randomized but was also multicenter, with

113 centers around the world participating. A total of 544 patients were randomized to surgery or thrombolysis. In contrast to the Rochester trial, one-year amputation-free survival was similar in the surgery and thrombolysis groups (70% vs. 65%, p = 0.23). One significant difference between the two groups was a significantly higher bleeding rate in the thrombolysis group; when mandatory heparin was deleted from the protocol, bleeding rates decreased considerably. Finally, considerably fewer surgical procedures were performed in the thrombolysis group compared with the surgery group despite similar one-year outcomes. Thus, either open surgery or primary thrombolysis was equivalent after this well-run trial.

SUMMARY
Acute ischemia represents a life- and limb-threatening event. While ischemic extremity may be the symptom that leads a patient to seek treatment, the underlying pathophysiology can often be even more significant than the acute ischemia. Treatments continue to evolve, but, increasingly, hybrid endovascular and open treatments are the norm. Additionally, thrombolysis is often combined with mechanical adjuncts or surgery to provide more rapid return of perfusion to the extremity. These combination treatments are not yet fully developed, but incremental improvements have been realized. The future of acute ischemia management will inevitably include some of these elements to maximize limb salvage while minimizing morbidity and mortality. Newer techniques and devices will only improve our results further.

REFERENCES
1. Rutherford RB, Baker JD, Ernst C, et al. Recommended standards for reports dealing with lower extremity ischemia: revised version. J Vasc Surg 1997; 26(3):517–538.
2. Badhwar A, Forbes TL, Lovell MB, et al. Chronic lower extremity ischemia: a human model of ischemic tolerance. Can J Surg 2004; 47(5):352–358.
3. Kuntscher MV, Schirmbeck EU, Menke H, et al. Ischemic preconditioning by brief extremity ischemia before flap ischemia in a rat model. Plast Reconstr Surg 2002; 109(7):2398–2404.
4. Holoman M, Záhorec R, Kusý J, et al. Biochemical monitoring in patients during revascularization surgery. Vasa 1995; 24(1):23–28.
5. Ikizler M, Ovali C, Dernek S, et al. Protective effects of resveratrol in ischemia-reperfusion injury of skeletal muscle: a clinically relevant animal model for lower extremity ischemia. Chin J Physiol 2006; 49(4):204–209.
6. Kharbanda RK, Mortensen UM, White PA, et al. Transient limb ischemia induces remote ischemic preconditioning in vivo. Circulation 2002; 106(23):2881–2883.
7. Magnoni F, Pedrini L, Palumbo N, et al. Ischemia: reperfusion syndrome of the lower limbs. Int Angiol 1996; 15(4):350–353.
8. Petrasek PF, Homer-Vanniasinkam S, Walker PM. Determinants of ischemic injury to skeletal muscle. J Vasc Surg 1994; 19(4):623–631.
9. Sako H, Hadama T, Miyamoto S, et al. Limb ischemia and reperfusion during abdominal aortic aneurysm surgery. Surg Today 2004; 34(10):832–836.
10. Yassin MM, Harkin DW, Barros D'Sa AA, et al. Lower limb ischemia-reperfusion injury triggers a systemic inflammatory response and multiple organ dysfunction. World J Surg 2002; 26(1):115–121.
11. Bulkley GB. Free radical-mediated reperfusion injury: a selective review. Br J Cancer Suppl 1987; 8:66–73.
12. Bulkley GB. The role of oxygen free radicals in human disease processes. Surgery 1983; 94(3):407–411.

13. Im MJ, Hoopes JE, Yoshimura Y, et al. Xanthine: acceptor oxidoreductase activities in ischemic rat skin flaps. J Surg Res 1989; 46(3):230–234.

14. Perler BA, Tohmeh AG, Bulkley GB. Inhibition of the compartment syndrome by the ablation of free radical-mediated reperfusion injury. Surgery 1990; 108(1):40–47.

15. Ratych RE, Chuknyiska RS, Bulkley GB. The primary localization of free radical generation after anoxia/reoxygenation in isolated endothelial cells. Surgery 1987; 102(2):122–131.

16. Schiller HJ, Reilly PM, Bulkley GB. Tissue perfusion in critical illnesses. Antioxidant therapy. Crit Care Med 1993; 21(2 suppl):S92–S102.

17. Im MJ, Shen WH, Pak CJ, et al. Effect of allopurinol on the survival of hyperemic island skin flaps. Plast Reconstr Surg 1984; 73(2):276–278.

18. Koyama I, Bulkley GB, Williams GM, et al. The role of oxygen free radicals in mediating the reperfusion injury of cold-preserved ischemic kidneys. Transplantation 1985; 40(6):590–595.

19. Parks DA, Bulkley GB, Granger DN, et al. Ischemic injury in the cat small intestine: role of superoxide radicals. Gastroenterology 1982; 82(1):9–15.

20. Buchbinder D, Karmody AM, Leather RP, et al. Hypertonic mannitol: its use in the prevention of revascularization syndrome after acute arterial ischemia. Arch Surg 1981; 116(4):414–421.

21. Magovern GJ Jr., Bolling SF, Casale AS, et al. The mechanism of mannitol in reducing ischemic injury: hyperosmolarity or hydroxyl scavenger?Circulation 1984; 70(3 pt 2): I91–I95.

22. Jivegard L, Bergqvist D, Holm J, et al. Preoperative assessment of the risk for cardiac death following thrombo-embolectomy for acute lower limb ischaemia. Eur J Vasc Surg 1992; 6(1):83–88.

23. Blaisdell FW, Steele M, Allen RE. Management of acute lower extremity arterial ischemia due to embolism and thrombosis. Surgery 1978; 84(6):822–834.

24. Cambria RP, Abbott WM. Acute arterial thrombosis of the lower extremity. Its natural history contrasted with arterial embolism. Arch Surg 1984; 119(7):784–787.

25. Allermand H, Westergaard-Nielsen J, Nielsen OS. Lower limb embolectomy in old age. J Cardiovasc Surg (Torino) 1986; 27(4):440–442.

26. Pedrinelli R, Dell'Omo G, Barchielli A, et al. Fibrinogen and mortality in chronic critical limb ischaemia. J Intern Med 1999; 245(1):75–81.

27. Hanlon CR, Paletta FX, Copper T, et al. Acute arterial occlusion in the lower extremity. Clinical and experimental studies of muscular ischemia. J Cardiovasc Surg (Torino) 1965; 6:11–14.

28. Dale WA. Differential management of acute ischemia of the lower extremity. J Cardiovasc Surg (Torino) 1973; Spec No:8–12.

29. Sicard GA, Schier JJ, Totty WG, et al. Thrombolytic therapy for acute arterial occlusion. J Vasc Surg 1985; 2(1):65–78.

30. Comerota AJ, White JV, Grosh JD. Intraoperative intra-arterial thrombolytic therapy for salvage of limbs in patients with distal arterial thrombosis. Surg Gynecol Obstet 1989; 169(4):283–289.

31. Dawson KJ, Reddy K, Platts AD, et al. Results of a recently instituted programme of thrombolytic therapy in acute lower limb ischaemia. Br J Surg 1991; 78(4):409–411.

32. McNamara TO, Bomberger RA, Merchant RF. Intra-arterial urokinase as the initial therapy for acutely ischemic lower limbs. Circulation 1991; 83(2 suppl):I106–I119.

33. Allen DR, Smallwood J, Johnson CD. Intra-arterial thrombolysis should be the initial treatment of the acutely ischaemic lower limb. Ann R Coll Surg Engl 1992; 74(2): 106–110; discussion 111.

34. Giddings AE, Walker WJ. Intra-arterial thrombolysis should be the initial treatment of the acutely ischaemic lower limb. Ann R Coll Surg Engl 1992; 74(4):301.

35. Lang EV, Stevick CA. Transcatheter therapy of severe acute lower extremity ischemia. J Vasc Interv Radiol 1993; 4(4):481–488.

36. Bookstein JJ, Fellmeth B, Roberts A, et al. Pulsed-spray pharmacomechanical thrombolysis: preliminary clinical results. AJR Am J Roentgenol 1989; 152(5):1097–1100.

37. Valji K, Bookstein JJ. Pulsed-spray thrombolysis accelerates clot dissolution. Diagn Imaging (San Franc) 1991; 13(12):58–63.
38. Valji K, Roberts AC, Davis GB, et al. Pulsed-spray thrombolysis of arterial and bypass graft occlusions. AJR Am J Roentgenol 1991; 156(3):617–621.
39. Bookstein JJ, Valji K. Pulse-spray pharmacomechanical thrombolysis. Cardiovasc Intervent Radiol 1992; 15(4):228–233.
40. Bookstein JJ, Bookstein FL. Augmented experimental pulse-spray thrombolysis with tissue plasminogen activator, enabling dose reduction by one or more orders of magnitude. J Vasc Interv Radiol 2000; 11(3):299–303.
41. Kasirajan K, Gray B, Beavers FP, et al. Rheolytic thrombectomy in the management of acute and subacute limb-threatening ischemia. J Vasc Interv Radiol 2001; 12(4):413–421.
42. Ansel GM, George BS, Botti CF, et al. Rheolytic thrombectomy in the management of limb ischemia: 30-day results from a multicenter registry. J Endovasc Ther 2002; 9(4): 395–402.
43. Singh M, Tiede DJ, Mathew V, et al. Rheolytic thrombectomy with AngioJet in thrombus-containing lesions. Catheter Cardiovasc Interv 2002; 56(1):1–7.
44. Siablis D, Liatsikos EN, Goumenos D, et al. Percutaneous rheolytic thrombectomy for treatment of acute renal-artery thrombosis. J Endourol 2005; 19(1):68–71.
45. Barbato JE, Wholey MH. Use of AngioJet mechanical thrombectomy for acute peripheral ischemia associated with stent fracture. Catheter Cardiovasc Interv 2007; 70(6):795–798.
46. Lin PH, Mussa FF, Hedayati N, et al. Comparison of AngioJet rheolytic pharmaco-mechanical thrombectomy versus AngioJet rheolytic thrombectomy in a porcine peripheral arterial model. World J Surg 2007; 31(4):715–722.
47. Shammas NW, Dippel EJ, Shammas G, et al. Dethrombosis of the lower extremity arteries using the power-pulse spray technique in patients with recent onset thrombotic occlusions: results of the dethrombosis registry. J Endovasc Ther 2008; 15(5): 570–579.
48. Kasirajan K, Haskal ZJ, Ouriel K. The use of mechanical thrombectomy devices in the management of acute peripheral arterial occlusive disease. J Vasc Interv Radiol 2001; 12(4):405–411.
49. Allie DE, Hebert CJ, Lirtzman MD, et al. Novel simultaneous combination chemical thrombolysis/rheolytic thrombectomy therapy for acute critical limb ischemia: the power-pulse spray technique. Catheter Cardiovasc Interv 2004; 63(4):512–522.
50. Mahon BR, Nesbit GM, Barnwell SL, et al. North American clinical experience with the EKOS MicroLysUS infusion catheter for the treatment of embolic stroke. AJNR Am J Neuroradiol 2003; 24(3):534–538.
51. Wissgott C, Richter A, Kamusella P, et al. Treatment of critical limb ischemia using ultrasound-enhanced thrombolysis (PARES Trial): final results. J Endovasc Ther 2007; 14(4):438–443.
52. Prokop AF, Soltani A, Roy RA. Cavitational mechanisms in ultrasound-accelerated fibrinolysis. Ultrasound Med Biol 2007; 33(6):924–933.
53. Soltani A, Soliday C. Effect of ultrasound on enzymatic activity of selected plasminogen activators. Thromb Res 2007; 119(2):223–228.
54. Lutsep HL. Mechanical endovascular recanalization therapies. Curr Opin Neurol 2008; 21(1):70–75.
55. Cranley JJ, Krause RJ, Strasser ES, et al. Peripheral arterial embolism: changing concepts. Surgery 1964; 55:57–63.
56. Fogarty TJ, Cranley JJ. Catheter technic for arterial embolectomy. Ann Surg 1965; 161:325–330.
57. Fogarty TJ. Catheter technic for arterial embolectomy. J Cardiovasc Surg (Torino) 1967; 8(1):22–28.
58. Fogarty TJ. The balloon catheter in vascular surgery. Rev Surg 1967; 24(1):9–19.
59. Barone GW, Conerly JM, Farley PC, et al. Endothelial injury and vascular dysfunction associated with the Fogarty balloon catheter. J Vasc Surg 1989; 9(3):422–425.

60. Barner HB, Fischer VW, Beaudet L. Effects of dilation with a balloon catheter on the endothelium of the internal thoracic artery. J Thorac Cardiovasc Surg 1992; 103(2): 375–380.
61. Doornekamp FN, Borst C, Haudenschild CC, et al. Fogarty and percutaneous transluminal coronary angioplasty balloon injury induce comparable damage to the arterial wall but lead to different healing responses. J Vasc Surg 1996; 24(5):843–850.
62. Doornekamp FN, Borst C, Post MJ. Endothelial cell recoverage and intimal hyperplasia after endothelium removal with or without smooth muscle cell necrosis in the rabbit carotid artery. J Vasc Res 1996; 33(2):146–155.
63. Norem RF II, Short DH, Kerstein MD. Role of intraoperative fibrinolytic therapy in acute arterial occlusion. Surg Gynecol Obstet 1988; 167(2):87–91.
64. Garcia R, Saroyan RM, Senkowsky J, et al. Intraoperative intra-arterial urokinase infusion as an adjunct to Fogarty catheter embolectomy in acute arterial occlusion. Surg Gynecol Obstet 1990; 171(3):201–205.
65. Ouriel K, Shortell CK, DeWeese JA, et al. A comparison of thrombolytic therapy with operative revascularization in the initial treatment of acute peripheral arterial ischemia. J Vasc Surg 1994; 19(6):1021–1030.
66. Results of a prospective randomized trial evaluating surgery versus thrombolysis for ischemia of the lower extremity. The STILE trial. Ann Surg 1994; 220(3):251–266; discussion 266–268.
67. Ouriel K, Veith FJ, Sasahara AA. Thrombolysis or peripheral arterial surgery: phase I results. TOPAS Investigators. J Vasc Surg 1996; 23(1):64–73; discussion 74–75.
68. Ouriel K, Veith FJ, Sasahara AA. A comparison of recombinant urokinase with vascular surgery as initial treatment for acute arterial occlusion of the legs. Thrombolysis or Peripheral Arterial Surgery (TOPAS) Investigators. N Engl J Med 1998; 338(16):1105–1111.

Major Lower Extremity Amputation

Traci A. Kimball and Mark R. Nehler
University of Colorado Denver, Anschutz Medical Campus, Section of Vascular Surgery, Department of Surgery, Aurora, Colorado, U.S.A.

INTRODUCTION

According to *Dorland's Illustrated Medical Dictionary*, 28th edition, amputation is derived from the Latin word *amputare*, to cut away, from *amb* (about) and *putare* (to prune), although this word has been reserved to indicate punishment for criminals. In the surgical context, the word can be found in many forms in 16th century French texts and from early English writers. Synonyms such as "extirpation" (16th century French texts tended to use extirper), "disarticulation," and "dismemberment" (from the Old French desmembrer) were more commonly used before the 17th century to describe limb loss or removal. However, the English derivation, "amputation" was first used in surgical references in the early 17th century, and by the century end, this term was used ubiquitously as the accepted medical translation (1).

Historical Point

The history of human amputation is best described using frames of reference defined by eras or time periods. Initially amputations occurred as the result of trauma or *nonsurgical* removal for many thousands of years. It was not until around the 15th century that intentional surgical removal began, primarily military casualties suffering from extensive trauma and gangrene. This distinction was marked by the choice of the patient and the aim of saving a life and achieving a healed stump, despite the difficulties with infection and the lack of effective control of pain and blood loss.

Advancements in surgical techniques combined with improved hemorrhage control in the 19th century and ether anesthesia in the 1840s as well as Listerian infection control nearly 20 years later made amputations much more humane and mainstream (Fig. 1). A review of 19th century amputations from the surgical logs of the Royal Berkshire Hospital in Reading nicely summarized the amputation experience of this facility dating over 40 years (3). Of the 276 amputations carried out between 1839 and 1879, over half were due to trauma with a minority due to "diseases of the affected limb." In today's operative suites, we have come a long way from battlefield facilities with our technological improvements and advanced rehabilitation options allowing for the increased use of state-of-the-art prosthetic limbs and the attainment of higher levels of rehabilitation.

This chapter summarizes the epidemiology and natural history of amputations and amputees and data on functional outcomes and multidisciplinary rehabilitation. Indications and level of amputation, specifically pre- and perioperative issues, complications, and the principles of postoperative care of the amputee will be addressed. Amputation techniques will conclude the review. As the majority of literature on amputations comes from outside of the United States, many of our references are from Europe.

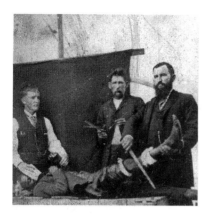

FIGURE 1 A black-and-white photograph depicting preparation for an amputation. The photographic image, probably made between 1855 and 1860, shows Dr. Crawford Long of Athens, Georgia, demonstrating the use of ether anesthesia in surgery. The scene was staged to portray Dr. Long's original discovery and use of anesthesia in 1842, four years before it was demonstrated at Massachusetts General Hospital by William T. Morton. Dr. Long's claim was eventually verified. *Source*: From Ref. 2.

EPIDEMIOLOGY AND NATURAL HISTORY

Most of modern day major limb amputations are performed for critical limb ischemia (CLI) (4–7). The reported incidence of major amputation varies considerably from 84 to 500 per million patients per year (4–8). Despite advances in revascularization in the last decade (9), amputation rates remain high and continue to increase presumably because of the aging population (10). An Italian study of 1560 CLI patients found that age affected all outcomes studied, including amputation rate. The group found that each year of age over 70 increased the risk of having a major limb amputation by about 2% (11).

When controlling for age, the presence of peripheral arterial disease (PAD) and diabetes remain major risk factors for lower extremity amputation (12). Diabetics represent 70% of the CLI population undergoing major amputation (13,14), many presenting with significant pedal necrosis (14,15), compared with nondiabetics (Table 1). Patients with diabetes have a 10-fold greater risk for amputation than those without diabetes (16). This is likely multifactorial, but strongly indicative of the lack of education and negative perception of amputation

TABLE 1 Details Regarding Presenting Foot Lesions in 132 Limbs with Foot Necrosis Undergoing Major Lower Extremity Amputation

Location	n (%) ulceration n = 25	n (%) dry gangrene n = 56	n (%) sepsis n = 51	Total (%) n = 132
Forefoot				
Digit single	4 (16)	4 (7)	3 (6)	11 (8)
Digit multiple	6 (24)	11 (20)	2 (4)	19 (14)
MTH single	2 (8)	3 (5)	5 (10)	10 (8)
MTH multiple	0 (0)	6 (11)	8 (16)	14 (11)
Malleolar	1 (4)	3 (5)	2 (4)	6 (5)
Midfoot	4 (16)	5 (9)	16 (31)	25 (19)
Heel	6 (24)	13 (23)	10 (20)	29 (22)
Global[a]	2 (8)	11 (20)	5 (10)	18 (13)

Categorization based on gross appearance of the foot necrosis on preoperative physical examination alone.
[a]Either complete breakdown of prior amputations, extremities that had large gangrenous defects or extremities that presented nonviable at either the foot or calf level.
Abbreviation: MTH, metatarsal head.
Source: From Refs. 15 and 78.

in this patient population (17). Diabetics will delay care, leaving amputation as the only treatment option at presentation. Therefore educational efforts and prevention are critical (18) in this at-risk subgroup with aggressive screening programs, vigilant foot care, and prompt patient referrals and treatment.

The ratio of above-knee amputations (AKAs) to below-knee amputations (BKAs) performed worldwide is roughly 1 (16,19). Many of the AKAs performed are done so on the basis of lack of rehabilitation potential, rather than the inability for them to eventually heal a BKA. Significant ongoing morbidity occurs in both the remaining BKA stump and the contralateral limb following major lower extremity amputation. Overall, 60% of BKAs heal by primary intention, 15% heal after secondary procedures, and at two years, 15% of patients with an initially successful BKA will convert to an above-knee amputee, and another 15% will suffer a major contralateral amputation (19).

Survival in the amputee for CLI is poor. The perioperative mortality rate for a BKA approximates 8% and double that for AKA (19). Patient survival is significantly worse at one and five years for those receiving AKAs (50.6% and 22.5%) than BKAs (74.5% and 37.6%) (20), emphasizing the palliative nature of these procedures. Compared with the 2% perioperative mortality rate published in the recent Veterans Affairs multicenter small aneurysm trial (21), major amputations are statistically more dangerous—obviously not because of the complexity of the procedures but rather because of the patient population requiring them. Available data suggest the presence of significant medical comorbidities including poor nutrition, anemia, and a deconditioned state secondary to immobility/pain (15) make these patients challenging to care for.

Functional Outcomes

Amputation is the operation vascular surgeons perform having the greatest emotional and functional impact on their patients; therefore, reasonable postoperative goals should be set for all amputees. Modest numbers of patients will ambulate independently and/or wear prostheses, but the majority will return to their home. In a review of 172 amputations in 154 patients from our institution, 29% of patients were able to walk outside their homes with a prosthesis, 42% used a prosthetic limb, and 92% of patients were able to return to community living (15). Globally, the incidence of vascular amputees that ambulate and wear prostheses postoperatively varies but is limited to those receiving BKAs. Ultimately ambulatory amputees decline over time because of a variety of issues (22–24). Many elderly vascular patients are unable to complete an arduous rehabilitation program and ambulate to any extent with the use of a prosthesis (25). Current data suggest this is likely due to their age and preoperative disabilities—one of the most important being loss of proprioception (25,26).

Multidisciplinary Care

A number of different providers will care for the amputee, each with different levels of training, expertise, and goals. These include medical and surgical teams, nurses, physiatrists, occupational therapists, pain specialists, prosthetists, and social workers. The coordinated efforts of such a multidisciplinary group of providers, that is, an integrated pathway, is essential if early discharge, reduced readmission, and increased homebound rates are to be achieved (27). A dedicated, multidisciplinary team approach clearly improves the ultimate outcome of the amputee, especially in diabetics as found by Gibbons et al. The published algorithms are evidence based, resulting in improved limb salvage or amputation stump healing (28).

INDICATIONS FOR AMPUTATION

Indications for amputation found in clinical series vary greatly (15,29,30), but are categorized by patient presentation due to either acute ischemic, CLI, or complications of diabetic neuropathy with normal pedal circulation. Of these, CLI remains the major etiology for amputation (15,30), manifesting a significant role of the vascular surgeon in this area. Abou-Zamzam et al. attempted to categorize the indications for major amputation to explain why amputations continue to be performed despite aggressive revascularization programs (30). In their series of 131 consecutive major lower extremity amputations, several patient scenarios influenced the decision to amputate; delayed presentation of acute limb ischemia, CLI with exhausted anatomic/conduit options or extensive pedal gangrene/sepsis, as well as patient comorbidities/nonambulatory status affecting their outcomes. A summary of their findings can be found in Table 2; the most common etiology was exhausted options for CLI revascularization.

A major preventable factor in limb loss is delayed referral secondary to lack of diagnosis, health care access, or ineffective treatment (minor amputation in the setting of insufficient circulation). Abou-Zamzam et al. found that a mean wait of 8.6 weeks did not have a statistically significant impact on the type of treatment (primary amputation vs. revascularization); it was a small series, and more than half underwent primary amputation (31). Other studies have similar findings. Nehler et al. found that the mean time to vascular surgery consultation for pedal tissue loss was 73 days and for rest pain was 27 days (15), possibly explaining the high primary amputation rate encountered. Furthermore, Bailey et al. showed that only one of four CLI patients were perceived as needing "urgent" vascular consultation, with a mean duration of symptoms prior to vascular evaluation of eight weeks (32). It is reasonably safe to conclude that a percentage of major lower extremity amputations are potentially preventable, again underscoring the need of patient and physician awareness and education.

Given this reality for the CLI population, many patients will currently present late with limited options. When is a primary amputation most appropriate, especially given the poor survival in CLI? The elderly want to spend their remaining days in their home environment with their families rather than undergo multiple procedures and prolonged hospitalizations—with the real

TABLE 2 Indications for Major Amputation

Indication for major amputation	Number of cases (%), $n = 131$
Critical limb ischemia with failed revascularization	51 (39)
Extensive pedal gangrene	20 (15)
Unreconstructable arterial anatomy	15 (11)
Overwhelming pedal sepsis	12 (9)
Excessive surgical risk	12 (9)
Nonviable, acutely ischemic foot	11 (8)
Nonambulatory status	10 (8)

Source: From Refs. 30 and 78.

possibility of eventual limb loss regardless. An approach we have used is to look at the problem from three sides: the technical issues of the revascularization, the pedal wounds/ultimate function, and patient comorbidities. Patients with marginal prospects in more than one category are generally not considered reasonable limb salvage candidates. For example, alternate vein conduit for a tibial bypass would be reasonable for a patient with manageable toe gangrene and modest comorbidity, but would not be reasonable for a patient on home oxygen or with a large heel defect. Subgroups with severe comorbidities like those with end-stage renal disease, who may survive the procedure because of modern anesthesia, but are unlikely to survive the follow-up required to heal incisions/wounds and undergo rehabilitation, would also not be offered extensive limb salvage (33).

AMPUTATION LEVEL DETERMINATION

The goals of major lower extremity amputation for CLI are (*i*) removal of ischemic or infected tissue with wound healing, (*ii*) appropriate stump length for rehabilitation/function, and (*iii*) minimize postoperative morbidity. Ideally, both patient and surgeon would like to maximize each of these goals, but in reality compromise of one over the other is needed. As previously mentioned, many patient and system factors will direct the overall recovery and outcome of life and limb. For example, a patient with a healed amputation (AKA or BKA) that can independently transfer and take a few limited steps but remains in the community is acceptable and is the end result for the majority of elderly amputees. Conversely, multiple operations and significant near-term morbidity could be acceptable in a young trauma patient if the end result is ambulation. Therefore, because of the limited life expectancy of the CLI population, the surgeon must shift from limb-focused to patient-focused goals.

The length of the preserved limb has important implications on rehabilitation. A stump that includes the knee joint will allow a prosthesis providing the below-knee amputee with a means to ambulate with lower energy expenditures compared with above-knee amputees (34). Unfortunately, as mentioned previously, the prevalence of patients who use a prosthesis and of those who ambulate postoperatively steadily declines over time (15,22–24,35,36).

While anyone would agree that the longer the residual stump, the better the chances are for superior patient function, unfortunately in the CLI patient population, any incision below-the-knee joint is often problematic, with healing times measured in months rather than weeks (15). In general, BKAs take longer to heal and suffer greater morbidity than AKAs (15,19). There is an increasing interest in through-knee amputations in CLI for this very reason—an opportunity to provide a better compromise between healing level and ultimate function.

Despite the failure of an amputation to heal being multifactorial, a tremendous amount of research has focused on defining a single surrogate marker [toe pressure, pulse volume recordings, transcutaneous oxygen tension ($TcPO_2$)] that has the best accuracy of predicting stump healing. Although these measures are concrete and depending on the surgeon's vascular lab, easy to measure, no single test will ever predict stump healing 100%. Several papers using various modalities to predict healing have variable revision rates, especially with minor amputations (15,30,34,36,37). Amputation revisions are additional morbidity and a mortality rate around 5% (34).

The optimal circulatory parameter for selecting the appropriate amputation level remains uncertain. Most studied include physical findings alone (pulses, extent of foot ischemia/infection, skin temperature) (34,38,39,41) or are paired with clinical judgment (40,41), noninvasive hemodynamic tests (absolute segmental and toe pressures) (34,41–43), angiographic scoring systems (38,44,45), and physiologic tests (^{99m}Tc-sestamibi skin perfusion, transcutaneous oxygen measurements, and multispatial spectroscopy of regional microcirculation, e.g., hyperspectral imaging) (46–49). The specifics regarding the utility of these measurements are beyond the scope of this chapter, but as a general point, many of these techniques used alone are neither reliable nor practical or both in clinical practice; and furthermore, the more advanced optical imaging options are purely experimental to date. A pulse just above the level of amputation (popliteal pulse above a BKA) is helpful, but the absence of a pulse does not preclude healing. Clinical judgment paired with other objective parameters, like $TcPO_2$ more than 40 mmHg, can yield an accurate assessment of a viable level in several large clinical series (15,40,41,47,48).

THE PREOPERATIVE EVALUATION

The CLI population requiring amputation is as ill as any in modern medicine bringing with them a multitude of comorbidities. An episode of aspiration pneumonitis, subendocardial infarct, or exacerbation of congestive failure perioperatively can easily prove fatal and is responsible for the high mortality rates discussed previously.

Depending on the etiology for amputation, the preoperative evaluation may be more or less expeditious. Acute limb ischemia may focus on removal of nonviable tissue and obtaining consent from the patient or family as a primary issue with stabilization focused on the immediate need for operation/anticoagulation. In the setting of CLI, patients are considered high surgical risk with some time to potentially modify the same. The evaluation and assessment of cardiac disease is important—active signs and symptoms of decompensated heart failure, unstable angina, or morbid ventricular arrythmias [serial preventricular contractions (PVCs) or complete heart block] must be recognized and treated as these clinical factors have been linked to poor outcomes (50). Absent these findings, aggressive risk stratification with invasive tests and interventions, that is, percutaneous transluminal coronary angioplasty (PTCA) or coronary artery bypass grafting (CABG) are not typically done, but some authors have advocated routine β-blockade (51,52).

PERIOPERATIVE COMPLICATIONS

As previously stated, the perioperative mortality rates for major lower extremity amputations are high (15,16,20), challenging that an amputation exposes a patient to lower physiologic stress/risk than that of revascularization—when comparing mortality rates, cardiovascular complications, and sepsis, including pneumonia, are the leading causes for early mortality (15,53,54). Stroke is often common in the perioperative period, but rarely causes mortality (54).

Several authors have published improved mortality rates of less than 5% following major lower extremity amputation (53,55), attributing their success to the liberal use of invasive cardiac monitoring and pharmacologic agents directed at improving cardiac function. This reduction in overall mortality following amputation is predominately attributed to the reduction of cardio-vascular complications and subsequent cardiac death, thought due to multiple factors including improved anesthesia care and the use of perioperative car-dioprotective drugs such as antiplatelet agents and β-blockade (56–59).

Sepsis can originate from a number of sources in this patient population around the time of surgery (60). Typical sites of origin include the lungs (pneumonia), the urinary tract, indwelling central venous catheters, decubiti, infections, or existing prosthetic from failed bypass or dialysis access, or stump healing failure. It is imperative that a diagnostic evaluation ensues with sub-sequent goal-directed therapy, specifically culture-specific antibiotics, targeted glycemic control and also adequate hemodynamic support (61).

The incidence of deep venous thrombosis in this population is substantial (1 in 10) mandating some level of anticoagulation (55). The judicious use of heparin in these patients is useful in preventing thrombembolism and likely also has some cardiac effects, but also increases the incidence of wound hematomas and potential stump breakdown.

The presence of delayed or failed primary stump healing is typically reported as the most frequently encountered local complication. In additional to this, part of the difficulty in wound healing is related to falls and stump trauma. The rates of primary BKA stump failure range from 20% to 30% of patients (19,30,35,62). Of these, 10% to 15% of the patients will require revisions to a higher level (19,20).

One of the most important morbidities in the amputee is postoperative pain. This can be categorized as acute or chronic in nature found in either the residual stump or the phantom limb, although acute phantom limb pain (PLP) is hard to define. Acute postoperative residual limb pain invariably occurs to some degree in all amputees. The typical patient is easily managed with intrathecal or parenteral narcotics perioperatively, and then oral pain medications in the out-patient setting with resolution measured in days. Prolonged, severe postopera-tive pain in the residual stump following amputation should raise concerns about ongoing ischemia, hematoma, or infection. Severe residual pain at the stump site following healing and during prosthetic use is suspicious for neuroma formation and can be managed by temporary and permanent injections.

Chronic PLP occurs in 50% to 80% of limb amputees after the stump has healed (63,64) Both central and peripheral pain mechanisms appear to be involved, including ectopic activity originating from afferent fibers in a neu-roma, compounded by cortical reorganization and spinal cord sensitization (65). Both primary and secondary prevention strategies have been describe and studied. Some data suggest that the duration and intensity of preamputation limb pain play a role in late onset (>6 months) amputation residual limb and PLP (66–68), emphasizing problems with delayed amputation. Primary pre-vention with the use of preoperative epidural blockade for 72 hours prior to amputation resulted in a significant reduction in the incidence of PLP at six months (69). However when tested under a prospective, randomized, blinded study design starting 18 hours prior to amputation, Nikolajsen et al. found no difference in the incidence of PLP at 3, 6, and 12 months following amputation (65). Since preamputation pain is a risk factor for late onset amputation pain, extension of these follow-up times may yet yield improvement. While this arena needs more study, in the acute setting, epidural anesthesia is very effective. In addition, an even a stronger association has been found between PLP and passive coping strategies, especially catastrophizing (i.e., the exaggerated orientation toward the pain stimulus, and it is associated with a heightened pain experience, reported pain intensity, and disability) before amputation (70). This knowledge may assist in the development of novel preemptive techniques focusing on tempering the patient's psyche before undergoing this life-changing event with the overall goal of reducing the incidence of PLP.

Secondary prevention strategies using virtual reality or the use of mirrors have been tried. These modalities arose out of the theory that PLP may be induced by a conflict between visual feedback and proprioception of the amputated limb (71). Three recent studies describe these techniques and provided variable results in the improvement of subject PLP (72–74). Both strategies (immersive virtual reality and mirrors) did increase subjects' abilities to move their phantom limbs but ironically led to an increased incidence of phantom limb phenomenon, including PLP (64,71). Whether or not these techniques have any use broadly in clinical practice is yet to be determined.

OPERATIVE PRINCIPLES
General Considerations

Regardless of the clinical presentation and level of amputation chosen by the consulting surgeon, there are a number of general principles that need to be observed to optimize the outcome of surgery. Most importantly, tissue handling should be as atraumatic as possible. The surgeon should handle tissues without the use of instruments such as forceps, which can further compromise marginal tissue and impair ultimate wound healing. Second, all necrotic and nonviable tissues require excision, and should infection exist, as is often the case in the diabetic patient, these areas too need to be incised and drained. With this scenario however, formation of a definitive amputation stump should be delayed until active infection has subsided. In, addition, the surgical plan should include dividing muscles with the minimum number of firm clean cuts to eliminate the macerating effect of multiple incisions. With few exceptions, bone should be transected rather than disarticulated and have its periosteum removed. Bone edges should be rounded, and prominences bevelled to optimize subsequent prosthetic fitting. The use of a power saw to divide bone avoids the splintering encountered with bone cutters and reduces the risk of collateral tissue damage that can result from the use of a handsaw. This is particularly crucial in transtibial amputations. When bone is resected, the operative field should be irrigated with saline to wash out any dust or bone fragments. Finally, flaps should be kept thick to avoid unnecessary dissection between soft tissue planes (75).

Nerves should be transected under traction to facilitate retraction into the adjacent soft tissue. Occasionally absorbable suture ligation of larger nerves is required to control bleeding from nutrient vessels, but any suture will promote neuroma formation. In general, it is preferable to control bleeding by meticulous suture ligation of bleeding points using fine absorbable sutures. This method is preferred over a mass ligation technique, and if adequate hemostasis cannot be achieved, a closed-system suction drain should be employed in the wound depths, placing one vacuum drain over the bone end and one in a more superficial plane. These drains are not sutured in place to facilitate ease of removal. The excessive use of cautery should be discouraged, as thermal damage to adjacent soft tissue can impair wound healing (75–77). Skin edges should be apposed without tension using a nonabsorbable monofilament suture or skin staples. Adhesive paper strips are a satisfactory alternative or adjunctive means of skin closure and help minimize tension.

Polymicrobial antibiotic prophylaxis is mandatory to reduce perioperative infection risk. A combination of a penicillin and metronidazole covers the most likely pathogens, although where active infection is present, antibiotics appropriate to the most recent bacteriologic cultures should also be administered in combination with clostridial prophylaxis to avoid subsequent gas gangrene (78).

Tourniquets

Historically, the use of tourniquets in amputation surgery has not been advocated, primarily because of the prevalence of PAD and circulatory compromise of the surgical site (78). Recently two studies challenged this dogma, supported by successful knee arthroplasty performed using tourniquets in the elderly (79,80). Choksy et al. published a negative study (79), showing no improvement in revision rates and healing times in the tourniquet group, while Wolthuis et al. found the opposite; the use of a pneumatic tourniquet reduced revision rates by over 50%, and with a subsequent cost savings (80). Not surprising both studies found that pneumatic tourniquet use lowered absolute blood loss and patient transfusion requirements. It is our practice to use tourniquets for BKAs as long as the patient's arterial calcification does not prevent their effectiveness.

Control of Sepsis

Amputation in the presence of infection is a major cause of morbidity and mortality. Removal of all irreversibly ischemic tissue, adequate drainage of abscesses, and allowance for the wound to close by secondary intention is the accepted practice. The use of adjunctive intravenous antibiotics is critical.

A guillotine two-stage amputation, a high primary amputation or cryoamputation are the viable options and choosing the appropriate technique to perform depends on the patient scenario. If there is any ambiguity regarding the level at which the limb is irreversibly threatened or the infection is extremely invasive, a guillotine amputation followed by formal amputation several days later has been shown to have lower complication rates than definitive primary amputation (81). It is our practice to err on the side of conservatism in this regard and perform many two-stage BKAs. The diabetic patient presenting with extreme forefoot sepsis and severe ketoacidosis who is too unstable to undergo guillotine amputation can be offered physiologic cryoamputation until the medical comorbidities are stabilized and the patient can safely undergo definitive amputation proximal to the level of cooling (82,83).

Postoperative Care

Postoperatively the amputation site must be protected from trauma, and direct weight bearing should be avoided until the site has healed completely, although the use of appropriate pressure-distributing devices may enable early mobilization. Various methods are described in the literature with the goal of protecting the residual BKA stump to achieve improved healing rates and shorten the time delay before the application of a prosthetic. Much of the initial pioneering work behind this "immediate fitting principle"(84) occurred in the mid- to late 1960s (85). Application of soft, elastic dressings, semirigid to rigid plaster casts, or, more recently, silicon or gel-liners are offered as the main options; however, a consensus regarding their efficacy is lacking. A recent systematic review attempted to elucidate which of these methods would offer patients a benefit in terms of wound healing, edema reduction, and functional outcome (86). This meta-analysis showed a trend in favor of rigid and semirigid dressings for achieving acceptable healing rates and reducing stump volume. The authors could not render an evidence-based opinion to the effect on functional outcomes. Shortly after this publication materialized, a small randomized controlled study of 50 consecutive below-knee amputees surfaced comparing groups receiving immediate postoperative removable rigid dressing (RRD) (fiberglass casting) versus standard soft dressing (SSD) (87). The intention-to-treat analysis showed a strong trend toward faster wound healing in the RRDs group, although the difference of two weeks did not reach true statistical significance ($p = 0.07$), likely because of small numbers. However, RRDs appear to protect patients from stump revisions due to falls. Four patients fitted with RRDs fell with zero incidence of injury compared with half of the patients fitted with SSDs who fell; all required surgical revision and two-thirds ultimately required AKA. These data are in line with other published series regarding the protective effects of RRDs against injury and stump revision surgery (88,89). It is our practice to use RRDs in all BKAs—although the timing is usually postoperative day 2 to 3.

TECHNICAL STRATEGIES
The techniques described herein will be limited to major amputations only, including BKA variations (e.g., skew, sagittal, long posterior flaps, etc.), through-knee amputation, and AKA.

Transtibial (Below-Knee) Amputation
The commonly described BKAs utilize (*i*) a long posterior myocutaneous flap on the basis of the gastrocnemius muscle, (*ii*) equal length anterior and posterior myocutaneous flaps (fish-mouth technique), (*iii*) equal length medial and lateral myocutaneous flaps via sagittal incisions, (*iv*) equal length anteromedial and posterolateral fasciocutaneous flaps, known as the skew flap technique, and (*v*) a medially based fasciocutaneous flap (Fig. 2). It is useful to understand the various flap types as patients with prior failed bypasses may be best served with one of the less used flap configurations because of prior incisions.

Both the long posterior flap and the skew flap are in common use, with neither having shown any distinct advantage over the other in terms of healing or revision rates (90,91). The skew flap technique can accommodate tissue loss extending more proximally, provided the gastrocnemius remains viable. It also takes the suture line further away from potential pressure points, avoids "dog-ears," and prevents the typical bulbous shape of the long posterior flap. Both techniques have been described in great detail by Robinson (76), so only the salient points are described here.

Long Posterior Flap
Technique
As for any BKA, the patient is positioned supine with a soft pad such as a rolled towel behind the lower thigh and the knee joint opposite the break in the table. Once the diseased part of the limb has been removed, the end of the table can be dropped if desired, allowing the surgeon to sit facing the stump and thus to work comfortably and effectively to achieve flap hemostasis and closure.

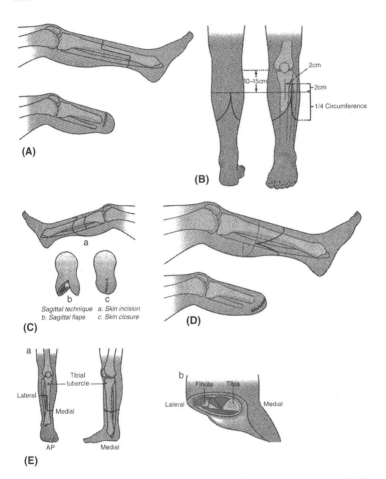

FIGURE 2 Transtibial amputations: skin flaps. (**A**) Long posterior flap. (**B**) Skew flap incisions. (**C**) Sagittal flaps. (**D**) Equal anterior and posterior flaps. (**E**) Medially based flap. *Source*: From Ref. 78.

The proximal skin incision is marked at a point one handsbreadth below the tibial tuberosity. The incision should encompass between one half and two-thirds of the calf circumference at this level. Too wide a flap has dog-ear deformities, making it hard to shape and fit for a prosthesis. Too narrow a flap may have inadequate blood supply distally. A posterior flap somewhat greater than one-third of the calf circumference is a useful compromise, thus the flap extends from the medial and lateral ends of the proximal transverse incision, along the axis of the limb for a distance equal to at least half the length of the transverse incision—the posterior transverse incision completes the flap (Fig. 2A). It is prudent to fashion the posterior flap slightly longer than will ultimately be required to ensure good skin apposition after trimming to length.

Generally we use the knife through subcutaneous tissue and deep fascia, care being taken to avoid separation of skin from underlying fascia, and major bleeding points are ligated. At the level selected for transaction of the tibia, the muscles of the anterior compartment are divided transversely with cautery with

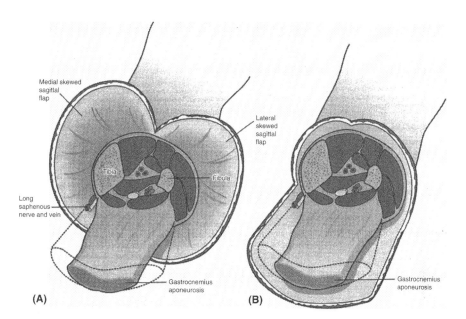

FIGURE 3 (**A**) Skew flap technique. Note the oblique skin flaps and the underlying myofascial flap based on gastrocnemius. This flap is placed obliquely over the bone ends, trimmed, and sutured to the anterior periosteum and deep fascia (see Fig. 4). (**B**) Long posterior flap. Although the myofascial flap is almost identical to the skew flap, it remains attached to the overlying skin of the posterior flap and is then placed anteriorly and sutured to the anterior fascia and periosteum parallel with the skin incisions. *Source*: From Ref. 78.

suture ligation of the anterior tibial vessels, transection of the peroneal nerve under tension, and incision of the interosseous membrane. The lateral and posterior aspect of the tibia is cleaned of its attachments at the level of section, and then the tibia is divided with a power saw at the level of the anterior incision. The fibula is cleaned of proximal attachments for 2 cm, and then divided at a level 1 to 2 cm proximal to the tibia transaction with a Gigli saw. Next the flap is finished by removing most or all of the deep compartment. The myocutaneous flap is based on gastrocnemius plus/minus soleus both tapered distally to reduce the bulk of the stump as in the skew flap technique (Fig. 3). In large patients there is little need to preserve any of soleus. The authors prefer to first develop the plane between gastrocnemius and soleus by gentle finger dissection at the level of tibial transection, where there is rarely significant fusion of the two muscles. The transverse division of the deep compartment muscles is then continued through the soleus until it meets with this plane, and thereafter the plane is developed distally to the point at which gastrocnemius is divided transversely at the distal extent of the flap. Hemostasis is then achieved with suture ligatures, and the tibial nerve is transacted sharply under tension. The aponeurotic end of gastrocnemius is then sutured to the anterior tibial periosteum with interrupted absorbable sutures and the sutures are inverted to bury the knots. The muscle length may be reduced to ensure a snug fit over the bone end, without tissue tension or undue redundancy. Thereafter the skin is trimmed to enable apposition with interrupted nylon sutures and/or adhesive paper strips and any dog-ears at the lateral wound edges excised.

Skew Flap

Technique

The patient is positioned as described for the long posterior flap. The posterior superficial muscle flap utilized in this amputation is exactly the same as outlined for the long posterior flap. The only difference is in the creation of anteromedial and posterolateral fasciocutaneous flaps, which are separated from the deeper tissues and based on the cutaneous blood supply of the lower limb. Accurate flap design is critical. Flaps are marked at the level previously described, one handsbreadth below the tibial tuberosity. A piece of tape or thread is used to measure the circumference of the calf at the level of tibial section. Halving this tape distance is the length of the base for each flap. The anterior junction of the flaps is a point 2.5 cm from the tibial crest, over the anterior muscle compartment, and the half tape is then passed around the calf at this point to identify the posterior junction of the flaps. The tape is then quartered, and the midpoint of the base of each flap marked. The quartered tape is then used in the style of a compass to identify the apex of each flap and mark out equal semicircular flaps as shown (Fig. 2B). At the anterior junction of the two flaps, a 2-cm proximal incision is marked to facilitate access to the line of bone section.

The incisions are then made extending through skin and subcutaneous tissue with the knife. Veins are divided between absorbable ligatures, and nerves divided under tension. Thereafter the fasciocutaneous flaps can be reflected proximally to enable the remainder of the amputation to continue as described above for the long posterior flap. The key to success is the correct shaping of the gastrocnemius tendon and fascia. It does not correspond to the skin flap but is cut approximately 5 m longer and more directly posterior than the skin flap. Caution is therefore required not to carry the skin incisions of the posterior parts of the skin flaps any deeper than the subcutaneous fat. On completion, the gastrocnemius can be slightly narrowed and trimmed before being brought obliquely forward and sutured to the anterior tibial periosteum. The myofascial flap coverage of the bone ends confers much of the benefit of this operation (Fig. 4). Skin can be approximated with either suture or adhesive paper strips or preferably both. If hemostasis is less than perfect, two vacuum drains are positioned, one over the end of the tibia and the other more superficially. They are not sutured to the skin so that they can be drawn out at 24 to 48 hours without disturbing the dressing.

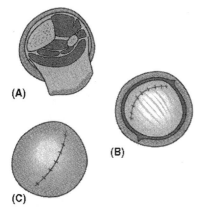

FIGURE 4 Completing the skew flap stump. (**A**) The posterior myofascial flap of gastrocnemius and deep fascia. (**B**) The flap is rotated obliquely forward over the tibia and sutured to deep fascia. (**C**) The skin flaps are then opposed, and the suture line does not overlie the bone end or the myofascial suture line. *Source*: From Ref. 78.

Sagittal Flap
Technique

This technique is an alternative to the skew flap in the patient whose limb infection, ischemia, prior scars, or necrosis encroaches on a proposed long posterior flap. It involves the creation of anterolateral and posteromedial musculocutaneous flaps based on the underlying muscle groups (Fig. 2C), and therefore does not require a viable distal gastrocnemius muscle, making it particularly useful after a short guillotine open operation. The procedure involves a myoplasty over the tibia with the anterior compartment muscles and the medial gastrocnemius. Readers are referred to Persson (92) for a full description of the technique.

Equal Anterior and Posterior Flaps
Technique

This technique involves the creation of equal posterior and anterior myocutaneous flaps to reduce the requirement for adequate posterior tissue, and was in common use until the introduction of the long posterior flap (Fig. 2D). The main disadvantage with this technique stems from the tenuous nature of the skin and subcutaneous tissue overlying the anterior tibia. As a result the technique has little to offer to recommend it to the surgeon who is comfortable with either skew or sagittal flaps.

Medially Based Flap
Technique

The medially based flap that is offset some 30° to 70° medial to the conventional posterior flap (Fig. 2E), and has been described for use in patients who are not suitable for the standard long posterior flap on the basis of thermographic studies (93). A fasciocutaneous flap is fashioned from the medial skin, which has a better blood flow, and the tibia is covered using a gastrocnemius flap trimmed to give good cover of the tibia. The technique may prevent unnecessary AKA in a minority of patients, but patient selection requires the use of thermographic techniques that are not widely available.

Through-Knee Amputation
Technique

The procedure can be undertaken using equal medial and lateral fasciocutaneous flaps (Fig. 5). These flaps must be cut generously since the main cause of failure of this operation is tension of the skin over the condyles. The patellar tendon is detached from its tibial insertion and sutured to the divided cruciate ligaments, along with the hamstring tendons, bringing the skin suture line to lie between the femoral condyles (Fig. 5C). This procedure does require a suction drain to be placed in the joint cavity at surgery, as prolonged leakage of synovial fluid can be a problem.

The Gritti-Stokes operation has been recommended by some authors (94,95). In this procedure, the femoral joint surface and condyles are excised and the patella advanced and fused to the distal femur to enable direct weight bearing and prosthetic fitting. A long anterior flap is used to cover the stump, but the end result does not offer any clear advantage over the simpler

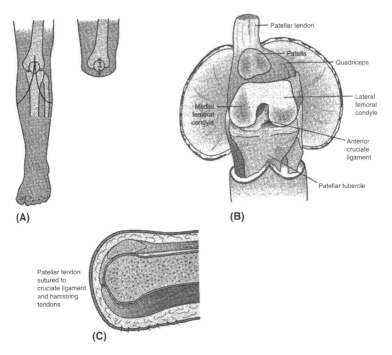

FIGURE 5 Through-knee amputation. (**A**) Equal sagittal skin flaps for a through-knee amputation. (**B**) The limb prior to disarticulation of the knee joint by division of the cruciate ligaments. (**C**) The completed stump with the patellar tendon sutured to the cruciate ligament and hamstring tendons. *Source*: From Ref. 78.

through-knee disarticulation. There has been a resurgence of through-knee amputation interest using these techniques. Both these procedures are described in detail by Robinson (76).

Transfemoral (Above-Knee) Amputation
Technique
The level of transfemoral amputation is in part determined by the tissue available for flap construction, but as long a length of femoral shaft as possible should be preserved, transecting the femur approximately 12 cm from the knee joint. A myoplastic stump construction is advised to maximize proprioception, optimize stump shape, and to reduce late hip flexion deformities. The commonest incision involves creation of equal anterior and posterior flaps, each equal to half the circumference of the thigh at the point of proposed femoral transection. The flaps should meet at the level of femoral transection and extend distally to a level approximately two fingerbreadths above the patella (Fig. 6). After marking flaps in this fashion, skin and subcutaneous tissue are divided in a single incision, with the knife blade angled proximally. The incision is then extended down to bone, dividing muscles with cautery in an oblique manner as the skin and subcutaneous tissues, such that the point of femoral transection is reached. Periosteum should then be elevated from the bone at this point, and the bone drilled at three positions, to give six holes for suturing, just proximal to the point of femoral

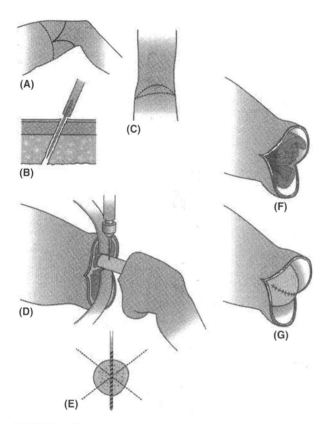

FIGURE 6 Transfemoral amputation. (**A**) Anterior and posterior skin flaps. (**B**) Beveling the subcutaneous fat. (**C**) Extra convexity is cut on the posterior flap to minimize puckering of tissues when the wound edges are opposed. (**D**) The femur is drilled before its division. (**E**) Sites of drill holes in femur just proximal to the level of amputation. (**F**) Lateral and medial muscle bundles sutured to the bone with nonabsorbable sutures. (**G**) Anterior and posterior muscles and deep fascia sutured across the bone end. *Source*: From Ref. 78.

transection (Fig. 6). The lateral (vastus lateralis) and medial (adductor) muscle groups are divided at the proposed level of bone section while the anterior (quadriceps) and the posterior (hamstrings) are divided two to three finger-breadths beyond the proposed level of bone section. The femur is then divided, preferably with a power saw, the bone end is rounded off with a rasp and the myoplasty achieved by suturing the lateral and medial muscle groups to the bone end with fine nonabsorbable sutures. Thereafter the quadriceps and hamstrings are sutured to each other over the end of the stump, using an absorbable suture placed in the fascia rather than the muscle tissue, providing a second layer of cover over the bone end. In this procedure the center part of posterior flap tends to retract as a result of muscle retraction, and this can be prevented by cutting an extra convexity to the posterior flap as shown in the figure. Alternative skin flaps can be used on the basis of a circumferential skin incision centered 2 to 3 cm distal to the point of femoral transection. The skin should then be closed with sutures and/or paper strips and a light bandage applied.

SUMMARY

The aim of this chapter was to provide readers with a broad overview of major lower extremity amputation. The authors presented the epidemiology and natural history of the amputee along with expected functional outcomes. The perioperative evaluation of a patient needing an amputation including indications for amputation and level determination along with perioperative considerations were provided to give readers the tools to workup and treat these patients. Finally operative principles and the technical aspects of major lower amputation were outlined to provide a surgical atlas for the clinician performing these procedures.

REFERENCES

1. Wikipedia. Amputation. Available at: http://en.wikipedia.org/wiki/Amputation.
2. The University of Texas Health Science Center. San Antonio Libraries Digital Repository. Available at: http://www.learningobjects.library.uthscsa.edu/u?/HOM,2613.
3. Galland RB. Nineteenth century amputations at the Royal Berkshire Hospital, Reading. Ann R Coll Surg Engl 2003; 85(6):393–395.
4. Eskelinen E, Lepantalo M, Hietala EM, et al. Lower limb amputations in Southern Finland in 2000 and trends up to 2001. Eur J Vasc Endovasc Surg 2004; 27(2):193–200.
5. Melillo E, Nuti M, Bongiorni L, et al. [Major and minor amputation rates and lower critical limb ischemia: the epidemiological data of western Tuscany.] Ital Heart J Suppl 2004; 5(10):794–805.
6. Carmona GA, Hoffmeyer P, Herrmann FR, et al. Major lower limb amputations in the elderly observed over ten years: the role of diabetes and peripheral arterial disease. Diabetes Metab 2005; 31(5):449–454.
7. Wohlgemuth WA, Freitag MH, Wolfle KD, et al. [Incidence of major amputations, bypass procedures and percutaneous transluminal angioplasties (PTA) in the treatment of peripheral arterial occlusive disease in a German referral center 1996–2003.] Rofo 2006; 178(9):906–910.
8. Norgen L, Hiatt WR, Dormandy JA, et al.; for TASC II Working Group. Inter-Society Consensus for the Management of Peripheral Arterial Disease (TASC II). J Vasc Surg 2007; 45(suppl S):S5–S67.
9. Hallett JW Jr., Byrne J, Gayari MM, et al. Impact of arterial surgery and balloon angioplasty on amputation: a population-based study of 1155 procedures between 1973 and 1992. J Vasc Surg 1997; 25:29–38.
10. Fletcher DD, Andrews KL, Hallett JW Jr., et al. Trends in rehabilitation after amputation for geriatric patients with vascular disease: implications for future health resource allocation. Arch Phys Med Rehabil 2002; 83:1389–1393.
11. Bertele V, Roncagiloni MC, Pangrazzi J, et al. Clinical outcome and its predictors in 1560 patients with critical limb ischemia. Eur J Vasc Endovasc Surg 1999; 18:401–410.
12. Group TG. Epidemiology of lower extremity amputation in centers in Europe, North America and East Asia. The global lower extremity amputation study group. Br J Surg 2000; 87:328–337.
13. Sheahan MG, Hamdan AD, Veraldi JR, et al. Lower extremity minor amputations: the roles of diabetes mellitus and timing of revascularization. J Vasc Surg 2005; 42 (3):476–480.
14. Adam DJ, Raptis S, Fitridge RA. Trends in the presentation and surgical management of the acute diabetic foot. Eur J Vasc Endovasc Surg 2006; 31(2):151–156.
15. Nehler MR, Coll JR, Hiatt WR, et al. Functional outcome in a contemporary series of major lower extremity amputations. J Vasc Surg 2003; 38:7–14.
16. Feinglass J, Pearce WH, Martin GJ, et al. Postoperative and late survival outcomes after major amputation: findings from the Department of Veterans Affairs National Surgical Quality Improvement Program. Surgery 2001; 130(1):21–29.
17. Resnick HE, Valsania P, Phillips CL. Diabetes mellitus and nontraumatic lower extremity amputation in black and white Americans: the National Health and

Nutrition Examination Survey Epidemiologic Follow-up Study, 1971–1992. Arch Intern Med 1999; 159:2470–2475.

18. Bruckner M, Mangan M, Godin S, et al. Project LEAP of New Jersey: lower extremity amputation prevention in persons with type 2 diabetes. Am J Manag Care 1999; 5:609–616.

19. Dormandy J, Heeck L, Vig S. Major amputations: clinical patterns and predictors. Semin Vasc Surg 1999; 12:154–161.

20. Aulivola B, Hile CN, Hamdan AD, et al. Major lower extremity amputation: outcome of a modern series. Arch Surg 2004; 139:395–399.

21. Lederle FA, Wilson SE, Johnson GR, et al. Immediate repair compared with surveillance of small abdominal aortic aneurysms. N Engl J Med 2002; 346:1437–1444.

22. Ecker ML, Jacobs BS. Lower extremity amputation in diabetic patients. Diabetes 1970; 19:189–195.

23. Hagberg E, Berlin OK, Renstrom P. Function after through-knee compared with below-knee and above-knee amputation. Prosthet Orthot Int 1992; 16:168–173.

24. Siriwardena GJ, Bertrand PV. Factors influencing rehabilitation of arteriosclerotic lower limb amputees. J Rehabil Res Dev 1991; 28:35–44.

25. Schoppen T, Boonstra A, Groothoff JW, et al. Physical, mental, and social predictors of functional outcome in unilateral lower-limb amputees. Arch Phys Med Rehabil 2003; 84:803–811.

26. Taylor SM, Kalbaugh CA, Blackhurst DW, et al. Preoperative clinical factors predict postoperative functional outcomes after major lower limb amputation: an analysis of 553 consecutive patients. J Vasc Surg 2005; 42(2):227–235.

27. Schaldach DE. Measuring quality and cost of care: evaluation of an amputation clinical pathway. J Vas Nurs 1997; 15:13–20.

28. Gibbons GW. Lower extremity bypass in patients with diabetic foot ulcers. Surg Clin North Am 2003; 83:659–669.

29. Malone JM. Lower extremity amputations. In: Moore WS, ed. Vascular Surgery: A Comprehensive Review. Philadelphia: WB Saunders, 2002:875–917.

30. Abou-Zamzam AM Jr., Teruya TH, Killeen JD, et al. Major lower extremity amputation in an academic vascular center. Ann Vasc Surg 2003; 17:86–90.

31. Abou-Zamzam AM Jr., Gomez NR, Molkara A, et al. A prospective analysis of critical limb ischemia: factors leading to major primary amputation versus revascularization. Ann Vasc Surg 2007; 21:458–463.

32. Bailey CM, Saha S, Magee TR, et al. A 1 year prospective study of management and outcome of patients presenting with critical lower limb ischaemia. Eur J Vasc Endovasc Surg 2003; 25:131–134.

33. Nehler MR, Hiatt WR, Taylor LM Jr. Is revascularization and limb salvage always the best treatment for critical limb ischemia? J Vasc Surg 2003; 37:704–708.

34. DeFrang RD, Taylor LM, Porter JM. Basic data related to amputations. Ann Vasc Surg 1991; 5:202–207.

35. McWhinnie DL, Gordon AC, Collin J, et al. Rehabilitation outcome 5 years after 100 lower-limb amputations. Br J Surg 1994; 81:1596–1599.

36. Toursarkissian B, Shireman PK, Harrision A, et al. Major lower-extremity amputation: contemporary experience in a single Veterans Affairs institution. Am Surg 2002; 68:606–610.

37. Anthony T, Roberts J, Modrall JG, et al. Transmetatarsal amputation: assessment of current selection criteria. Am J Surg 2006; 192:e8–e11.

38. Dwars BJ, van den Broek TA, Rauwerda JA, et al. Criteria for reliable selection of the lowest level of amputation in peripheral vascular disease. J Vasc Surg 1992; 15:536–542.

39. Spence VA, Walker WF, Troup IM, et al. Amputation of the ischemic limb: selection of the optimum site by thermography. Angiology 1981; 32:155–169.

40. Harris JP, Page S, Englund R, et al. Is the outlook for the vascular amputee improved by striving to preserve the knee? J Cardiovasc Surg (Torino) 1988; 29:741–745.

41. Wagner WH, Keagy BA, Kotb MM, et al. Nonivasive determination of healing of major lower extremity amputation: the continued role of clinical judgement. J Vasc Surg 1988; 8:703–710.

42. Nguyen TH, Gordon IL, Whalen D, et al. Transmetatarsal amputation: predictors of healing. Am Surg 2006; 72(10):973–977.
43. Vitti MJ, Robinson DV, Hauer-Jensen M, et al. Wound healing in forefoot amputations: the predictive value of toe pressure. Ann Vasc Surg 1994; 8:99–106.
44. Gu YQ. Determination of amputation level in ischaemic lower limbs. ANZ J Surg 2004; 74(1–2):31–33.
45. Toursarkissian B, Hagino RT, Khan K, et al. Healing of transmetatarsal amputation in the diabetic patient: is angiography predictive?Ann Vasc Surg 2005; 19(6):769–773.
46. Sarikaya A, Top H, Aygit AC, et al. Predictive value of (99m)Tc-sestamibi scintigraphy for healing of extremity amputation. Eur J Nucl Med Mol Imaging 2006; 33 (12):1500–1507.
47. Poredos P, Rakovec S, Guzic-Salobir B. Determination of amputation level in ischaemic limbs using tcPO2 measurement. Vasa 2005; 34(2):108–112.
48. Keyzer-Dekker CM, Moerman E, Leijdekkers VJ, et al. Can transcutaneous oxygen tension measurement determine re-amputation levels?J Wound Care 2006; 15(1): 27–30.
49. Khaodhiar L, Dinh T, Schomacker KT, et al. The use of medical hyperspectral technology to evaluate microcirculatory changes in diabetic foot ulcers and to predict clinical outcomes. Diabetes Care 2007; 30(4):903–910.
50. McFalls E, Ward H, Moritz T, et al. Clinical factors associated with long-term mortality following vascular surgery: outcomes from the Coronary Artery Revascularizaion Prophylaxis (CARP) Trial. J Vasc Surg 2007; 46:694–700.
51. Krupski WC, Nehler MR, Whitehill TA, et al. Negative impact of cardiac evaluation before vascular surgery. Vasc Med 2000; 5:3–9.
52. McFalls E, Ward H, Moritz T, et al. Coronary-artery revascularization before elective major vascular surgery. N Engl J Med 2004; 351:2795–2804.
53. Bunt TJ, Manship LL, Bynoe RP, et al. Lower extremity amputation for peripheral vascular disease. A low-risk operation. Am Surg 1984; 50:581–584.
54. Inderbitzi R, Buettiker M, Enzler M. The long-term mobility and mortality of patients with peripheral arterial disease following bilateral amputation. Eur J Vasc Endovasc Surg 2003; 26(1):59–64.
55. Yeager RA, Moneta GL, Edwards JM, et al. Deep vein thrombosis associated with lower extremity amputation. J Vasc Surg 1995; 22:612–615.
56. Hiatt WR. Preventing atherothrombotic events in peripheral arterial disease: the use of antiplatelet therapy. J Intern Med 2002; 251:193–206.
57. Auerbach AD, Goldman L. beta-Blockers and reduction of cardiac events in noncardiac surgery: scientific review. JAMA 2002; 287:1435–1444.
58. Feringa HH, Bax JJ, Schouten O, et al. Protecting the heart with cardiac medication in patients with left ventricular dysfunction undergoing major noncardiac vascular surgery. Semin Cardiothorac Vasc Anesth 2006; 10(1):25–31.
59. Fleisher LA, Beckman JA, Brown KA, et al. ACC/AHA 2007 guidelines on perioperative cardiovascular evaluation and care for noncardiac surgery: a report of the American College of Cardiology/American Heart Association Task Force on Practice Guidelines (Writing Committee to Revise the 2002 Guidelines on Perioperative Cardiovascular Evaluation for Noncardiac Surgery): developed in collaboration with the American Society of Echocardiography, American Society of Nuclear Cardiology, Heart Rhythm Society, Society of Cardiovascular Anesthesiologists, Society for Cardiovascular Angiography and Interventions, Society for Vascular Medicine and Biology, and Society for Vascular Surgery. Circulation 2007; 116(17):e418–e499.
60. Rush DS, Huston CC, Bivins BA, et al. Operative and late mortality rates of above-knee and below-knee amputations. Am Surg 1981; 47:36–39.
61. Dellinger RP, Levy MM, Carlet JM, et al. Surviving sepsis campaign: international guidelines for management of severe sepsis and septic shock: 2008. Crit Care Med 2008; 36:296–327.
62. Keagy BA, Schwartz JA, Kotb M, et al. Lower extremity amputation: the control series. J Vasc Surg 1986; 4:321–326.

63. Dijkstra PU, Geertzen JHB, Stewart R, et al. Phantom pain and risk factors: a multivariate analysis. J Pain Symptom Manage 2002; 24:578–585.
64. Richardson CD, Glenn S, Nurmikko T, et al. Incidence of phantom limb pain 6 months after major lower limb amputation in patients with peripheral vascular disease. Clin J Pain 2006; 22:353–358.
65. Nikolajsen L, Ilkjaer S, Christensen JH, et al. Randomised trial of epidural bupivacaine and morphine in prevention of stump and phantom pain in lower-limb amputation. Lancet 1997; 13:477–485.
66. Hanley MA, Jensen MP, Smith DG, et al. Preamputation pain and acute pain predict chronic pain after lower extremity amputation. J Pain 2007; 8(2):102–109.
67. Schott GD. Delayed onset and resolution of pain: some observations and implications. Brain 2001; 124:1067–1107.
68. Katz J, Melzack R. Pain memories in phantom limbs: review and clinical observations. Pain 1990; 43:319–336.
69. Bach S, Noreng MF, Tjelden NU. Phantom limb pain in amputees during the first 12 months following limb amputation after preoperative lumbar epidural blockade. Pain 1988; 33:297–301.
70. Richardson C, Glenn S, Horgan M, et al. A prospective study of factors associated with the presence of phantom limb pain six months after major lower limb amputation in patients with peripheral vascular disease. J Pain 2007; 8(10):793–801.
71. Ramachandran VS, Hirstein W. The perception of phantom limbs. Brain 1998; 121:1603–1630.
72. Brodie EE, Whyte A, Niven CA. Analgesia through the looking-glass? A randomized controlled trial investigating the effect of viewing a "virtual" limb upon phantom limb pain, sensation and movement. Eur J Pain 2007; 11(4):428–436.
73. Murray CD, Pettifer S, Howard T, et al. The treatment of phantom limb pain using immersive virtual reality: three case studies. Disabil Rehabil 2007; 29(18):1465–1469.
74. Chan BL, Witt R, Charrow AP, et al. Mirror therapy for phantom limb pain. N Engl J Med 2007; 357(21):2206–2207.
75. Smith DG. Amputation: preoperative assessment and lower extremity surgical techniques. Foot Ankle Clin 2001; 6:271–296.
76. Robinson KP. Amputations in vascular patients. In: Bell PRF, Jamieson CW, Ruckley CV, eds. Surgical Management of Vascular Disease. London: WB Saunders, 1992:609–635.
77. Atnip RG. Introduction and general principles. J Op Tech Gen Surg 2005; 7:62–66.
78. Woodburn KR, Ruckley V. Lower extremity amputation: technique and perioperative care. In: Rutherford RB, ed. Vascular Surgery. 6th ed. Philadelphia: Elsevier-Saunders, 2003:2460–2473.
79. Choksy SA, Lee CP, Smith C, et al. A randomised controlled trial of the use of a tourniquet to reduce blood loss during transtibial amputation for peripheral arterial disease. Eur J Vasc Endovasc Surg 2006; 31(6):646–650.
80. Wolthuis AM, Whitehead E, Ridler BM, et al. Use of a pneumatic tourniquet improves outcome following trans-tibial amputation. Eur J Vasc Endovasc Surg 2006; 31(6):642–645.
81. Fisher DF Jr., Clagett GP, Fry RE, et al. One-stage versus two-stage amputation for wet gangrene of the lower extremity: a randomized study. J Vasc Surg 1988; 8:428–433.
82. Hunsaker RH, Schwartz JA, Keagy BA, et al. Dry ice cryoamputation: a twelve-year experience. J Vasc Surg 1985; 8:812–816.
83. Winburn GB, Wood MC, Hawkins ML, et al. Current role of cryoamputation. Am J Surg 1991; 162:647–650.
84. Tooms RE. General principles of amputation. In: Canale ST, ed. Campbell's Operative Orthopaedics. St. Louis: Mosby, 1998:521–528.
85. Berlemont M, Weber R, Wilot JP. Ten years of experience with the immediate application of prosthetic devices to amputees of the lower extremities on the operating table. Prosthet Int 1969; 3:8–17.
86. Nawijn SE, van der LH, Emmelot CH, et al. Stump management after trans-tibial amputation: a systematic review. Prosthet Orthot Int 2005; 29(1):13–26.

87. Deutsch A, English RD, Vermeer TC, et al. Removable rigid dressings versus soft dressings: a randomized, controlled study with dysvascular, trans-tibial amputees. Prosthet Orthot Int 2005; 29(2):193–200.
88. Woodburn KR, Sockalingham S, Gilmore H, et al. A randomized trial of rigid stump dressing following trans-tibial amputation for peripheral arterial insufficiency. Prosthet Orthot Int 2004; 28:22–27.
89. Hughes S, Solomon N, Wilson S. Use of a removable rigid dressing for trans-tibial amputees rehabilitation: a Greenwich Hospital experience. Aust J Physiother 1998; 44:135–137.
90. Ruckley CV, Stonebridge PA, Prescott RJ. Skewflap versus long posterior flap in below-knee amputations: multicenter trial. J Vasc Surg 1991; 13:423–427.
91. Allcook PA, Jain AS. Revisiting transtibial amputation with the long posterior flap. Br J Surg 2001; 88:683–686.
92. Persson BM. Sagittal incision for below-knee amputation in ischaemic gangrene. J Bone Joint Surg 1974; 56B:110.
93. Jain AS, Steward CPU, Turner MS. Transtibial amputation using a medially-based flap. J R Coll Surg Edinb 1995; 40:263–265.
94. Yusuf SW, Baker DM, Wenham PW, et al. Role of Gritti-Stokes amputation in peripheral vascular disease. Ann R Coll Surg Engl 1997; 79:102–104.
95. Faber DC, Fielding P. Gritti-Stokes (through-knee) amputation. Should it be reintroduced?South Med J 2001; 94(10):997–1001.

14 Long-Term Management and Surveillance in the Treatment of Critical Limb Ischemia

Charlie C. Cheng and Michael B. Silva, Jr.
Department of Surgery, The University of Texas Medical Branch, Galveston, Texas, U.S.A.

INTRODUCTION

When managing a patient with critical limb ischemia (CLI), the goal of any treatment is to relieve pain, preserve functional tissue, and maintain mobility of the individual. Vascular surgeons in general agree on the criteria used to assess the success or failure of open surgical treatments. Is the bypass graft patent? Is the limb still attached? Has our patient's health been adversely affected in some unexpected way by the procedure we performed? Are the answers to these questions the same at six months, one year, and five years?

There is less agreement on the criteria that should be used to assess endovascular procedures, and no consensus on what specific endovascular modality should be used in which patient, or even if some endovascular devices should be used at all. These questions are persistent echoes of those raised a decade or more ago when the reluctance to widely adopt endovascular techniques grew from the arguments that durability, efficacy, and safety concerns would prove to be worse for endovascular procedures. But, a lot has changed in 10 years.

We now know definitively that patients prefer minimally invasive procedures to those with incisions. This is such a natural and forceful bias that the durability of an endovascular procedure may not need to be equivalent to that of a bypass as long as the other issues—pain resolution and wound healing—are resolved. If the problems recur, patients are less reluctant to accept an additional "touch-up" endovascular procedure than general anesthesia and open bypass. We have realized when comparing Endo versus Open that if safety is better and efficacy the same, durability can be less and Endo will still carry the day.

But what are the data for efficacy, durability, and safety for endovascular procedures? It seems a straightforward question but to answer with confidence, we have had to address a number of issues.

Historically, there has been an argument that data accumulated comparing competing therapies would reflect the bias of those who performed one kind of procedures but not the alternative. Interventionalists, for instance, were skeptical when surgeons reported that they could perform open procedures with good results and minimal morbidity ("Carotid Endarterectomy with a 1–2% stroke rate? Not in my hospital . . . "), and open surgeons were equally skeptical when endovascular therapies were reported as having 98% technical success rates and excellent one-year success rates based on no need for target vessel reintervention—a concept foreign to most surgical studies. Now, studies comparing competing therapies are being reported by groups with individuals who can perform both therapies, so the bias argument is less credible. We have seen as well that patients with CLI and nonhealing wounds can have endovascular procedures that work long enough to allow healing, and the patient becomes asymptomatic. As long as the patient remains asymptomatic a year later and has not needed any additional intervention, isn't that enough to label the procedure a success?

There has also been a problem interpreting studies performed during the period of rapid evolutionary advancement of endovascular devices. Some studies have taken long enough to complete that the devices used toward the end are better than those used early in the trial. The message from these types of trials can be difficult to discern. Now, for many devices and techniques there has been so much refinement that we can be confident that we are in a period where true, and one hopes good, results are obtainable.

Just as devices mature and get better, so do interventionalists. This can be seen in studies where complications in the earlier phases are higher, and then improve as the trial continues. We explain these results by speaking of the learning curve of procedure or device—a graphic depiction of decreasing complication rates or improving efficacy rates as the experience of the individual performing the procedure with a device improves with time. A learning curve phenomenon results from one of two possibilities—either the device is technically nuanced or challenging to use or the practitioner is improving on his or her endovascular skills. The past decade has seen a dramatic expansion and democratization of endovascular skills as training programs were developed for practicing surgeons, and fellowships began to require substantive catheter skills as part of their curricula. The interventionalists' technical experience is now becoming less of an issue. Currently, if a study reports data demonstrating a significant learning curve, it is more likely a reflection of the complexity of the device than the inexperience of the practitioner.

We are then in an ideal time to assess the relative efficacy, durability, and safety of "Endo versus Open" in the treatment of CLI. There are many more new members on the Endo team to evaluate compared with the tried and true champions of team Open—prosthetic and autogenous bypass. For the most part, trials to date assessing various endovascular techniques have relied on comparison with historical rates of success for traditional bypass grafting. We will begin with a review of the most common endovascular procedures being used in the management of CLI, with emphasis on early and midterm results and the methods of surveillance and long-term management used in these trials. We will review the accepted methods for open surgical surveillance and follow-up and the data leading to that acceptance. Many of these topics will be covered in greater detail in other chapters. Finally, we will discuss our preferred use of duplex ultrasound (DU) in the long-term management of our patients treated for CLI and review the protocols we use at the University of Texas Medical Branch, Texas Vascular Center.

SUBINTIMAL ANGIOPLASTY

In 1987, Bolia et al. (1) first described the technique of subintimal angioplasty for the treatment of occluded femoropopliteal arteries. Their early results were first reported in 1989. The authors later extended this technique to the treatment of tibial arteries with good initial success (86%). In this technique, the subintimal plane is purposely dissected, beginning at the proximal segment of the arterial occlusion. Using this plane, the lesion is transversed, and the true arterial lumen is reentered distal to the occlusion. A new flow channel is thus established within a subintimal plane, circumventing the occluded true lumen entirely. Intuitively, subintimal angioplasty alone would not be predicted to have the same durability and primary patency results as either open surgical procedures or endovascular procedures using adjuvant techniques. Nonetheless, proponents quote acceptable limb salvage rates, and this technique has a loyal following.

From his own early experience, Bolia (2) reported his results for 28 limbs in 27 patients with infrapopliteal lesions; 61% of limbs had ulcerations and 25% had gangrene. The technical success rate was 82%. At one year, the primary patency was 53% and the limb salvage rate 85%. Duplex ultrasonography and selective arteriography were used to assess patency.

In a larger series recently, Lazaris et al. (3) reported their experience of 112 limbs with infrainguinal lesions in 99 patients; 55% of lesions extended from femoral to popliteal, 29% from popliteal to crural, while 15% extended from femoral to crural arteries. The technical success was 89%. Kaplan-Meier life-table analysis was used to analyze clinical success and limb salvage. The clinical success at 12, 24, and 36 months was 74%, 72%, and 65% in nondiabetics, and 69%, 63%, and 54% in diabetics, respectively. The limb salvage rate at 36 months was 88% overall (90% in nondiabetics and 82% in diabetics).

Met et al. (4) echoed similar results in a systematic review of the literature with analysis of 23 cohort studies. There were a total of 1549 patients. The technical success rates varied between 80% and 90%. At one year, the primary patency rate was around 50% and limb salvage varied from 80% to 90%. Again DU was used as the first-line determinant of primary patency.

One of the first long-term outcomes of subintimal angioplasty was reported by Scott et al. (5,6); 104 patients with 159 occlusions in the iliac ($n = 10$), superficial femoral artery (SFA) ($n = 185$), popliteal ($n = 48$), and tibial ($n = 16$) were treated. The primary patency was 55%, 43%, and 35% at 12, 24, and 36 months, respectively. Multivariate analysis revealed CLI to be the only predictor of reduced primary patency. Limb salvage rate was 54% and 43% at 12 and 36 months, respectively. These are not good primary patency and limb salvage rates.

Most recently, the same authors published the results of the largest review on subintimal angioplasty in 472 patients with 506 limbs; 63% of patients presented with CLI, the remaining with disabling claudication; 47% of limbs had isolated SFA occlusions, 40% had femoropopliteal occlusions, and 13% had occlusions beginning in SFA and extending into tibial arteries. Most of the lesions treated were either TransAtlantic Inter-Society Consensus (TASC) C or D. Stenotic lesions were not included. Technical success was 87%, with 73% of failure due to inability to reenter the true lumen. Bare-metal stent was used in 20.3% of successful cases. The median follow-up was 12.4 months (range 0–48 months). The mean increase in ankle-brachial index (ABI) was 0.27, from 0.50 ± 0.16 to 0.77 ± 0.23. The primary patency was 45%, 30%, and 25% at 12, 24, and 36 months, respectively. These are not good numbers. There was reduction in the patency rate with progressive distal segment of occlusion. At 36 months, the primary patency was 31% for isolated SFA occlusion, 20% for femoropopliteal occlusions, and 16% for femorotibial occlusions. Again, these are not very impressive results. As one would expect, patency was increased in limbs treated for claudication, while reduced patency was significantly associated with femorotibial occlusions and CLI. At three years, primary potency was 30% for claudication and 21% for CLI. Surprisingly, in their experience, stent use was not associated with improved patency. Limb salvage for CLI was a respectable 88% at 12 months, 81% at 24 months, and 75% at 36 months. This was significantly reduced for femorotibial occlusions compared with isolated SFA occlusions. Claudication was improved in 96.8% of limbs and sustained in 67% at 36 months. Overall, the results of subintimal angioplasty as a stand-alone procedure for CLI have been underwhelming in our view, and adjuvant endovascular procedures have been developed to improve primary and late-term efficacy. The majority of studies to date have used a combination of ultrasound and angiography to follow these patients.

BALLOON ANGIOPLASTY

Andreas Grüntzig performed the first balloon angioplasty of the SFA over three decades ago in 1974. In 1975, he dilated an iliac artery. Since then, endovascular technology and operator experience have advanced significantly. The technique involves crossing the arterial lesion transluminally with a guidewire. A balloon is advanced over the wire and inflated at the location of the lesion. The treatment is considered successful if the residual stenosis is less than 30% or there is no pressure gradient across the area treated.

The STAR registry reporting a multicenter experience with angioplasty was published by Clark et al. (7). The authors evaluated angioplasty of femoropopliteal lesions in 205 patients with 219 limbs. Patients were followed prospectively with clinical outcomes as well as objective testing using angiogram and/or DU. The primary patencies at 12, 24, and 36 months for all limbs were 87%, 80%, and 69%. At 48 and 60 months, it was 55%. A negative predictor of long-term patency was found to be poor tibial runoff—specifically single tibial vessel runoff with 50% to 99% stenosis or occlusion. Diabetes or renal failure was also associated with lower patency. Long-term patency was higher with American Heart Association (AHA) category 1 lesions.

Atherosclerosis is a systemic disease that affects all vascular beds. Patients with chronic lower limb ischemia often have multisegmental occlusive disease involving the iliac arteries, femoral arteries, and tibial circulation. Regardless of the therapeutic modality chosen, poor tibial runoff is associated with lower primary patency if only proximal lesions are treated. With increased operator experience and the advent of smaller guidewires and low-profile balloons, tandem lesions and more distal lesions are frequently treated in a single setting.

Dorros et al. (8,9) published the feasibility of angioplasty in tibioperoneal vessels in a nonrandomized series of 312 patients with 417 vessels and 657 lesions. Overall technical success was 92% (98% in stenotic and 77% in occlusive lesions). Thirteen cases required stenting for intimal flap or dissection refractory to prolonged inflation. Success was higher in patients with claudication. More specifically, claudication was relieved in 98% of patients with stenoses and in 86% presenting with occlusions. Resolution of CLI was noted in 98% when stenotic lesions were treated and in 77% of patients with occlusions.

In a subsequent report, the same authors evaluated their five-year experience for these same patients, but focused on those with CLI. There were 284 limbs in 235 patients with 529 lesions in the tibioperoneal vessels; 167 (59%) limbs required concomitant dilatation of the inflow lesions to access the distal vessels.

Follow-up was obtained in 215 (97%) of successfully treated patients. Eight percent of the limbs required bypass surgery and 9% required amputation, giving an overall limb salvage rate of 91% at five years. As expected, Fontaine class III patients had significantly less bypass surgeries and amputations compared with class IV patients.

Giles et al. (10) reported similar results in a contemporary series of infrapopliteal lesions causing CLI. In their series of 163 patients with 176 limbs, 76% of patients presented with tissue loss and 15% had rest pain. All lesions were evenly distributed in the four TASC classes. The technical success was 93%, with 58% requiring concomitant dilatation of the femoropopliteal lesions and 8% requiring adjunctive stenting, most commonly for residual stenosis. Similar to above, the success was higher for less severe lesions (100% for TASC A–C, 75% for TASC D, $p < 0.0001$). Dorros et al. (8,9), however, did not describe their lesions using the TASC classification. Follow-up was performed at two weeks, then every three months for one year, and every six months thereafter. Measurement of patency used DU and angiogram when indicated, and followed Society for Vascular Surgery (SVS) reporting standard criteria for patency. At one year, freedom from restenosis, reintervention, or amputation for TASC A to D was 50%, 39%, 53%, and 14%, respectively. This was significantly lower for TASC D lesions, and was predicted by both univariate and multivariate analysis to have a lower rate. Primary patency at one year for TASC A to D was 53%, 58%, 67%, and 37%. Again, TASC D was a predictor of lower rate by multivariate analysis. Limb salvage at one year was 84%, with TASC D lesion as a predictor for loss of limb.

Kudo et al. (11) published a 10-year experience of angioplasty for CLI. There were 138 limbs in 111 patients, and the most distal lesions treated were 33% in iliac, 30% in femoropopliteal, and 37% in below knee group; 91% of the lesions were TASC C and D. Reporting standard followed SVS criteria. Follow-up intervals and the studies used were similar to the report by Giles et al. (10) above. Using Kaplan-Meier analysis, the primary patency and limb salvage rates for femoropopliteal and below knee groups at three year were 59.4% and 92.7%, and 23.5% and 77.3%, respectively. Significant independent risk factors for outcomes included multiple segment, more distal, and TASC D lesions.

Mwipatayi et al. (12) reported a contemporary meta-analysis comparing balloon angioplasty with stenting for the treatment of femoropopliteal lesions. The authors performed a systemic review of the literature that was published between September 2000 and January 2007. The search included studies that reported long-term results of at least one year. They found that seven RCT studies comparing angioplasty with stenting and were used for this meta-analysis. This gave a total of 934 patients, with 452 patients who were treated with balloon angioplasty and stenting in the remaining. The one-year primary patency rate for the angioplasty group ranged from 45% to 84.2%, and for two-year rate, it ranged from 25% to 77.2%. A four-year primary patency of 44% was reported in one study. In a similar meta-analysis performed earlier from 1993 to 2000, there were 923 patients treated with balloon angioplasty and 473 patients with stents. The combined three-year patency rates after angioplasty were 61% for stenosis and claudication, 48% for occlusions and claudication, 43% for stenoses and critical ischemia, and 30% for occlusions and critical ischemia.

CUTTING BALLOON ANGIOPLASTY

The cutting balloon was originally designed for use in coronary arteries with high-pressure, balloon resistant de novo, or in-stent lesions. Its use in the peripheral arteries has been increasing. The balloon features three or four atherotomes or microsurgical blades mounted longitudinally on the surface of a noncompliant balloon. The blades score the lesion and dilate the vessels with less force than conventional balloon angioplasty.

Ansel et al. (13) reported their outcomes on the treatment of symptomatic limb ischemia in the popliteal and infrapopliteal arteries. Technical success rate in 73 patients with 93 vessels was 100%; 20% required adjunctive stenting due to severe intimal dissection or inadequate hemodynamic results. The one-year limb salvage rate was 89.5%.

Canaud et al. (14) reported a prospective, nonrandomized study evaluating the outcomes of infrainguinal lesions. There were 128 patients with 203 lesions consisting of 66 femoropopliteal and 69 infrapopliteal arterial segments. Using the TASC classification, 41.5% were A and 45.2% were B. The technical success rate was 96.3%. The one- and two- year results for patients with CLI were primary patency 64.4% and 51.9%, respectively; limb salvage 84.2% and 76.9%. In the same time periods, patients with claudication had primary patency rate of 82.1%. More distal lesions and TASC classification were significant independent risk factors for outcome ($p < 0.05$). Follow-up used clinical examination, routine DU, and selective arteriography.

Cotroneo et al. (15) reported a comparison of cutting balloon angioplasty with conventional angioplasty in 84 consecutive patients with a total of 142 focal (<3 cm) calcified femoropoliteal lesions treated; 40 patients were treated with conventional angioplasty, while 44 patients underwent cutting balloon angioplasty. The patients were followed clinically and with DU at intervals of two years. Technical success rate was 100%, with 6% of percutaneous transluminal angioplasty (PTA) lesions requiring adjunctive stenting and none in the cutting balloon angioplasty. The primary patency rate for PTA was 91.0% at 6 months, 83.1% at 12 months, and 66.6% at 2 years. For cutting balloon, it was 93.2%, 90.4% ($p < 0.001$), and 79.7% ($p < 0.001$), respectively. The authors concluded that cutting balloon achieved better patency at midterm compared to conventional PTA.

Recently, Amighi et al. (16) reported a prospectively randomized controlled trial comparing conventional balloon with cutting balloon angioplasty in the treatment of de novo, short (<5 cm) SFA lesions. Forty-three patients were randomly assigned, with 22 in PTA and 21 in cutting balloon angioplasty (CBA). They were followed clinically and with ultrasound. At six months, the restenosis rate according to ultrasound with a greater than 50% reduction in arterial diameter was 32% for PTA versus 62% in CBA. Clinically, 73% of PTA while 38% of cutting balloon angioplasty (CBA) patients remained asymptomatic. However, there was no significant difference in ABI between the two groups. The authors concluded that CBA was not superior to PTA and showed increased restenosis rate at six months.

Angiosculpt

This new endovascular device is similar in concept to the cutting balloon and is intended for treatment of complex infrapopliteal lesions. It has three spiral struts made of highly flexible nitinol that encircle a semi-compliant conventional balloon catheter. This allows for focal concentration of the dilating force along the edges of the scoring element with improved luminal expansion compared with conventional balloon angioplasty. This device is also designed to minimize slippage and resultant vessel wall injury outside the intended treatment zone.

Recently, results from five centers in Europe have been encouraging. Scheinert et al. (17) reported 42 patients with 56 infrapopliteal lesions. The study classified lesions according to the amount of calcification and also evaluated device slippage during deployment; 38 patients (90.5%) had limb-threatening ischemia with Rutherford category more than 4, and 13 patients were originally planned for amputation. The device was successfully deployed in 98.2% of lesions, with 10.7% requiring adjunctive stenting. The overall slippage rate was 0.09 ± 0.20. The authors noted decreased dissection rate compared with the historical experience with conventional balloons. All 13 patients with planned amputation achieved limb salvage. However, there was no long-term follow-up in this study.

A new study is currently ongoing evaluating the use of this cutting balloon in femoropopliteal lesions. It is expected to be finished in late 2009.

CRYOPLASTY

A balloon modality that is gaining acceptance for infrapopliteal intervention is the balloon cryoplasty, The PolarCath Peripheral Dilatation System. It provides both mechanical dilatation and cryotherapy through the use of nitrous oxide. The gas is used to fill the angioplasty balloon and to cool its surface to –10°C. As the balloon is inflated, it exerts both mechanical and biological effects. The cooling promotes apoptosis, which reduces excess thickening from intimal hyperplasia of smooth muscle cells after angioplasty, and should result in reduced restenosis.

Early studies were published by Laird et al. (18,19) in a prospective multicenter trial involving patients with femoropopliteal disease and treated with stand-alone cryoplasty. There were 102 patients from 16 centers. The technical success rate was 85.3%. At nine months, clinical patency with freedom from revascularization was 82.2%. Primary patency determined by DU was 70.1%. In their subsequent report of long-term results, follow-up was achieved in 70 patients with a mean of 31 months (range 11 to 41 months). The clinical patency rate calculated by the Kaplan-Meier method was 83.2% after the original follow-up period of 300 days. This was maintained at 75.0% after more than three years (1253 days). No objective measurement or diagnostic study was performed.

Results for treatment of infrapopliteal lesions were studies in the prospective multicenter trial from the below-the-knee chill study. The study enrolled 108 patients with 111 limbs conducted in 16 centers. The technical success rate was 97.3%. At 180 days, the rate of freedom from major amputation was 93.4%. The amputation rate was higher in diabetics.

Recently, Samson et al. (20) reviewed their long-term results for the treatment of SFA and popliteal lesions; 92 lesions in 64 consecutive patients were treated and followed up for a median of 16 months. Most of the lesions were TASC A. The technical success rate was 88%, being limited by calcified lesions. Hemodynamic improvement was noted in ABI, with increase from mean of 0.73 to 0.89. At one-month follow-up, DU of all successfully treated lesions showed no hemodynamic compromise using velocity profiles. At 12- and

24-month follow-up, freedom from restenosis was 47% and 38%. The authors concluded that with the added cost of this technology, there was no improved efficacy compared with conventional angioplasty. In a recent review of literature of published cryoplasty studies, Wildgruber and Berger (21) obtained a similar conclusion.

ATHERECTOMY

Atherectomy is the physical removal of atherosclerotic plaque material from the blood vessel. Technologic advances in the past several years have led to the development of atherectomy devices that allow for treatment of CLI using endovascular therapy. The theoretic benefit is that it removes the obstructing plaque rather than displacing it as angioplasty and stenting. This has become a growing therapeutic modality in the treatment of limb ischemia with multilevel and small-vessel disease. There are two main categories for atherectomy devices. Excisional atherectomy catheters remove and collect the atheroma while ablative devices fragment the atheroma into small particles.

The dominant directional atherectomy device currently in use is the SilverHawk Plaque Excision System. The FDA approved it in 2003 for the treatment of peripheral arterial disease. The device debulks by self-apposing on the atheroma using a hinge system. A carbide cutter rotates at speeds up to 8000 rpm, and shaves the atherosclerotic plaque material from the luminal surface of the arterial wall. This material is collected in a storage chamber. A drive unit with a thumb switch allows for a single-operator use. The device can be used alone or with adjunctive modalities such as balloon angioplasty or stenting.

Yancy et al. (22) reviewed their results on consecutive 17 limbs in 16 CLI patients with TASC C femoropopliteal diseases. All patients also had at least another level of lesion, 5 with primarily inflow and 12 with primarily tibial/ pedal diseases. Technical success rate was high (88%) and resulted in resolution of symptoms in 12 patients with partial healing in two others. Three patients required early amputation within one month; all had severe inframalleolar disease at presentation. ABIs improved from 0.39 ± 0.08 before surgery to 0.75 ± 0.08 in the early postoperative period ($p = 0.02$). The one-year stenosis-free patency was 22%, with an overall limb salvage rate of 70% and 62% for those with tissue loss. The late ABI had returned toward baseline at an average of six months after surgery, with a mean of 0.48 ± 0.07. Again follow-up was more symptom-based than image-based.

Keeling et al. (23) published their outcome of 70 procedures on 66 limbs in 60 patients during a period of 17 months. All patients were assigned SVS ischemia scores and TASC lesion criteria. DU follow-up was performed at 1, 3, 6, and 12 months. Atherectomized arterial segments included common femoral, superficial femoral, popliteal, and tibial arteries. The technical success rate was high (87.1%), but 20% required adjunctive balloon angioplasty and 4% adjunctive stenting. The preoperative ABI was 0.53 ± 0.03 and mean toe pressure was 41.3 ± 5.7 mmHg, and increased by a mean of 0.27 ± 0.04 and 21.6 ± 7 mmHg, respectively, after procedure. The primary patency was 61.7% for the entire cohort and was significantly improved for SVS grades 2 to 3 and TASC lesions A and B; 17.1% of the lesions developed recurrent disease detected at a mean of 2.8 ± 0.7 months. The limb-salvage rate was 86.2% at 12 months.

Zeller et al. (24,25) published their early and long-term results after atherectomy of femoropopliteal lesions. Lesions were grouped into primary stenoses, native vessel restenoses, and in-stent restenoses. In their early publication, there were 52 patients with 71 lesions; 58% required adjuvant balloon angioplasty and 6% required stenting. At six months, the restenosis rate was not significantly different in primary lesions (27%) compared with other groups (41% for restenoses and 36% for in-stent restenoses). Greater than 80% of the patients were symptom free or had no lifestyle-limiting claudication. In their long-term follow-up, there were 84 patients with 131 lesions. Again, the lesions were grouped similarily: primary lesions, native vessel restenoses, and in-stent restenoses. Primary patency was 84%, 54%, and 54% at 12 months and 73%, 42%, and 49%, respectively. Target lesion revascularization rate was 16%, 44%, and 47% at 12 months and 22%, 56%, and 49% at 18 months. ABI was significantly improved after 12 and 18 months in all groups. Their only independent predictor for restenosis was treatment of restenotic lesions.

Most recently, Sarac et al. (26) published data on 167 vessels treated in 73 patients. Vessels treated included 64% in the femoral above-knee popliteal segment, 12% in the below-knee popliteal-tibial segment, and 25% in both; 87 vessels were occluded, while 80 were stenotic; 63 vessels required adjunctive treatments. The mean preoperative ABI was $0.57 + 0.19$ and increased to $0.81 + 0.21$ ($p < 0.001$). There was symptomatic relief in most of the patients: 81% in claudicants, 76% with rest pain, and 78% with tissue loss. The one-year patency and limb salvage were 43% and 75%, with no difference in the location of vessel treated by TASC classification. Also, treatment of multiple vessels did not influence patency or limb salvage. Recurrence of symptoms preceded and paralleled that of recurrent disease. Adjunctive therapy did not improve results. Clinical symptoms and noninvasive imaging studies were used for documenting patency.

Currently, there is no randomized controlled trial for excisional atherectomy with the SilverHawk device in the treatment of CLI. The largest registry is the TALON (Treating Peripherals with SilverHawk: Outcomes Collections) registry and includes 19 U.S. centers. The technical success was 97.6% with adjunctive therapy required in 21.7% of patients. The 6- and 12-month rates of survival free of target lesion reintervention (TLR) were 90% and 80%, respectively. Lesion length more than 50 mm was associated with a 2.9-fold increased risk for TLR, while lesion length more than 100 mm was 3.3-fold increase.

Surveillance was performed at baseline and every three months thereafter. Clinical symptoms and selective nonimaging studies were performed.

LASER ATHERECTOMY

This modality falls into the category of ablative atherectomy devices. The device is a cold-tipped laser that delivers bursts of ultraviolet/xenon energy in short pulse durations. This allows for exact energy control, decreasing perforation, and thermal injury to the treated vessels. The ultraviolet light ablates 5 μm of tissue on contact without a rise in surrounding tissue temperature. Its key feature is the ability to debulk tissue without damaging surrounding tissue, minimizing restenosis.

Early studies were published by Scheinert et al. (27), and they compared laser-assisted percutaneous transluminal angioplasty versus PTA alone for long, total SFA occlusions. The technical success was similar in both groups (85% in the laser group and 91% in the PTA group). The one-year patency rate was also similar, 49% for both groups.

Zhou et al. (28) retrospectively reviewed their results in 15 patients with 19 lesions. Arterial segments treated included femoral, popliteal, and tibial arteries. Technical success rate was 84% with a perforation of a tibial vessel without consequence. The average initial follow-up occurred at six months with patency rate of 71% for femoral, 65% for popliteal, and 25% for tibial lesions. Limb salvage at six month was 93%.

Stoner et al. (29) published their midterm result with 47 lesions in 40 patients. Lesions were grouped into femoropopliteal and infrapopliteal segments and classified using the TASC classification. The technical success rate was 88%, with 75% requiring adjunctive angioplasty and 13% requiring stenting; 75% had hemodynamic improvement; increase in ABI of at least 0.1 or 5 mm in pulse volume recording tracing. During the mean follow-up of 461 ± 49 days, primary patency was achieved in 23 of 40 cases. Kaplan-Meier life-table analysis showed primary patency and limb salvage probabilities at 12 months were 43.8% ± 0.1% and 55.0% ± 0.2%, respectively.

The largest trial was the LACI (Laser Angioplasty for Critical Limb Ischemia) phase II study that involved 14 sites in the United States and Germany. There were 145 patients with 155 limbs and 423 lesions: 41% SFA, 15% popliteal, 41% infrapopliteal, and 70% combination of stenoses. Technical success was achieved in 86% of limbs, with most lesions in TASC C and D. Limb salvage at six months was 93%.

Similar results were achieved by a five-center registry in Belgium. Bosiers et al. (30) presented outcomes of 48 patients with 51 limbs in Rutherford category 4, 5, or 6 who were poor candidates for bypass surgery. The limb salvage at six months was 90.5%.

STENTING

Sabeti et al. (31,32) reported their experience with stainless steel and nitinol self-expanding stents for treatment of femoropopliteal diseases in a retrospectively reviewed, nonrandomized study; 175 consecutive patients presented with claudication (in 150 patients) and CLI (25 patients). Stents were placed electively following balloon angioplasty failure due to residual stenosis or flow-limiting dissection. This resulted in 123 patients receiving stainless steel stents and 52 nitinol stents. The choice of stents was at the discretion of the interventionist. The length of the lesions treated ranged from 5 to 6 cm. DU with angiographic confirmation was used for follow-up. The cumulative patency rates at 6, 12, and 24 months were 85%, 75%, and 69%, respectively, for nitinol stenting versus 78%, 54%, and 34%, respectively for stainless steel stenting. The authors noted significantly improved primary patency rates for nitinol stents.

The same authors also reported their early experience with long lesions at least 10 cm in the femoropopliteal segment. Only nitinol stents were used and placed after primary failure of balloon angioplasty as above. The median length of the stented segments was 16 cm. The median follow-up was eight months, with in-stent restenosis noted in 40% of patients. The overall cumulative freedom from restenosis at 6 and 12 months was 79% and 54%. This was not affected by stent length or the number of stents used. However, patency was decreased in diabetics.

The authors later randomly assigned 104 patients with stenotic or occlusive SFA lesions to undergo primary stenting (51 patients) or angioplasty (53 patients) with optional stenting (32% receiving stents). The mean length of the lesions was 13.2 cm for the stent group and 12.7 cm for the angioplasty group. At six months, the rate of restenosis was 24% in the stent group and 43% in the angioplasty group. At 12 months, the rate was 37% and 63%, respectively. These results were sustained at two years. In a subsequent report of the same patient group, the authors noted a restenosis rate of 45.7% for the stent group versus 69.2% for the angioplasty group. During this period, reintervention was also lower in the primary stenting group (37% vs. 53.8%).

Vogel et al. (33) also reported their results of primary stenting. There were 41 patients with femoropopliteal disease; 37 patients had TASC B lesions and four had TASC D lesions. The mean lesion length was 6.69 cm. Primary patency rates using Kaplan-Meier analysis at six months, one year, and two year were 95%, 84%, and 84%, respectively. The limb salvage rate during similar period was 92%, 89%, and 89%, respectively. The lesions treated in this study were shorter than those reported by Sabeti et al. above.

Midterm results were published by Mewissen (34). There were 122 patients with femoropopliteal lesions in 137 limbs; 125 limbs presented with TASC B and C lesions. The mean length of the lesion was 12.2 cm and the technical success was 98%. The primary patency rates at 6, 12, 18, and 24 months were 92%, 76%, 66%, and 60%, respectively.

Ferreira et al. (35) noted similar favorable results in a long-term report with long femoropopliteal lesions. In this report of 59 patients with 74 lesions, there were 16% lesions in TASC C and 61% in TASC D. The mean lesion length was 19 cm and the mean follow-up was 2.4 years. The primary patency rates estimated by Kaplan-Meier at 1, 2, 3, 4, and 4.8 years were 90%, 78%, 74%, 69%, and 69%, respectively. In another contemporary data, Baril et al. (36) also noted the sustained results of nitinol stent. The study retrospectively reviewed 125 patients with 108 TASC B and 32 C lesions. The mean follow-up period was 12.7 months. Forty-one limbs experienced restenosis or occlusion at eight months. Freedom from restenosis/occlusion at 12 months for the entire cohort was 58.9% and 47.9% at 24 months. There was no difference between TASC B and C lesions.

With advances in technology, angioplasty and stenting of infrapopliteal lesions is gaining acceptance. Kickuth et al. (37) recently reported their initial experience with a low-profile self-expanding nitinol stent. The authors treated 35 patients, with 19 having lifestyle limiting claudication and 16 with CLI. Selective stenting was performed after failed balloon angioplasty due to residual stenosis, elastic recoil, or flow-limiting dissections. Stent placement was performed in 22 patients with distal popliteal artery lesions and 13 in tibioperoneal artery lesions. Technical success was achieved in all patients. Follow-up studies were performed with DU and angiogram. The six-month primary patency rate was 82%. The authors noted the feasibility of treating infrapopliteal lesions with the new nitinol stent.

A contemporary meta-analysis was reported by Mwipatayi et al. (38) comparing balloon angioplasty with stenting for the treatment of femoropopliteal lesions. A systemic review of the literature was performed on reports published between September 2000 and January 2007. The search included studies that reported long-term results of at least one year. They found seven RCT studies comparing angioplasty with stenting and were used for this meta-analysis. This gave a total of 934 patients, with 482 patients who were treated with stenting and balloon angioplasty in the remaining. For the stent group, the one-year primary patency rates varied from 63% to 90% and two-year primary patency ranged from 46% to 87%. The use of stents did not improve the patency rate at one year.

Ihnat et al. (39) recently evaluated the effect of lesion severity with patency after stenting of femoropopliteal segment. There were 95 patients treated with 109 limbs; 71 patients (65%) were treated for claudication and 38 (35%) for CLI. The average lesion length was 15.7 cm. The type of the lesions according to the TASC classifications was 39% A, 14% B, 29% C, and 18% D. The average runoff score was 4.6. The overall 36-month primary patency rate was 52%. Limb salvage was 75% in patients with CLI. Decreased patency rates were noted in TASC D lesions and limbs with poor initial runoff score.

STENT GRAFT

One of the most widely used stent grafts in the treatment of chronic lower extremity ischemia is the Viabahn (WL Gore, Flagstaff, Arizona). It is contructed with expanded polytetrafluoroethylene (ePTFE) liner attached to an external nitinol stent. The inner surface is now bonded with heparin. This stent graft is extremity flexible, allowing it to conform closely to the anatomy of the SFA.

Railo et al. (40) first reported preliminary results in 15 patients with femoropopliteal lesions. The clinical presentation varied from claudication to acute leg ischemia, as well as one ruptured popliteal artery aneurysm. Primary patency rates at 1, 12, and 24 months were 100%, 93%, and 84%, respectively. There was no limb loss during the follow-up period.

Jahnke et al. (41) reported their midterm experience in 52 patients with medium- or long-segment occlusions and stenoses of the femoropopliteal artery. The technical success was 100%; with mean length of the covered segments was 10.9 cm $\pm$ 5.13. There was initial hemodynamic improvement with ABI increasing from 0.54 ± 0.12 to 0.89 ± 0.14. The mean follow-up duration was 23.8 months. Patients were followed with DU, and the primary patency rate at 12 and 24 months were 78.4% and 74.1%, respectively. The length of implanted stent graft did not affect the primary patency rates.

In a six-year experience, Fischer et al. (42) evaluated their outcome for 57 patients treated for stenoses (13%) or occlusions (87%) of the SFA. The average length of treated lesions was 10.7 cm; 10% suffered early thrombosis of the graft within 30 days. The mean follow-up was 55 months (8–78). The primary patency rates for 30 days, 1, 3, and 5 years were 90%, 6%, 57%, and 45%, respectively. In an earlier long-term publication, Bleyn et al. (43) treated 67 patients a mean lesion length of 14.3 cm. Their five-year primary patency rate was 47%.

The most recent results came from Shaikh et al. (44). They reported a series of 81 patients with 98 SFAs using 167 stent grafts; 80% of the interventions were for TASC C and D lesions. The one-year primary patency was 96%. In their second group, 43 patients were randomized to either stent graft or SilverHawk atherectomy interventions. Twenty-three patients were treated with Viabahn in 29 SFAs, while atherectomy had 20 patients with 23 SFAs. The technical success rate was 100% in both groups. There were significantly more complications in the atherectomy group (5 patients or 21%) than Viabahn (0 patients). The one-year primary patency rate was 90% for Viabahn and 57% for SilverHawk atherectomy.

Comparisons of the Viabahn with different treatment modalities have been reported by others as well. Saxon et al. (45) compared stent graft with percutaneous transluminal angioplasty alone in a multicenter, prospectively randomized study. The stent graft group had 97 patients and the PTA had 100. The stent-graft group had a significantly higher technical success rate (95% vs. 66%, $p < 0.0001$). Follow-up at one year using DU showed that the primary patency rate was 65% for stent graft and 40% for PTA alone. This improvement was noted for lesions at least 3 cm long.

Kedora et al. (46) compared Viabahn with above-knee surgical bypass with synthetic graft material in a prospective randomized study. Eighty-six patients with 100 limbs were randomized to 50 limbs each for the stent-graft and bypass. The mean length of artery stented was 25.6 cm. ABIs and DU were used for follow-up at 3, 6, 9, and 12 months. The primary patency at 3, 6, 9, and 12 months were 84%, 82%, 75.6%, and 73.5% for stent grafts, respectively. For bypass, it was 90%, 81.8%, 79.7%, and 74.2%, respectively. The authors noted similar reintervention and secondary patency rates as well.

DU SURVEILLANCE

DU has become the primary modality for following open and endovascular procedures. The majority of studies described above have utilized DU as their method of imaging follow-up. While very early studies and coronary trials have used routine postprocedure contrast angiography (at 6 months and 1 year), the ready availability, lower risk ratio, and proven sensitivity and specificity of DU have made it difficult to argue that trials designed today should require contrast angiographic follow-up. Routine surveillance with DU and selective angiography once a problem has been identified have become the standard.

The benefit of graft surveillance using DU in lower extremity bypass has been established. Reports from Idu et al. (47) and Buth et al. (48) both showed that all vein grafts progressed to occlusion when stenosis greater than 70% diameter reduction was detected by ultrasound surveillance. Buth et al. (48) further established the duplex criteria needed to identify high risk lesions; peak systolic velocity (PSV) at the site of the lesion exceeding 300 to 350 cm/sec or a velocity ratio exceeding 3.5 or 4. The ratio is calculated using the PSV at the site of the lesion divided by the PSV of a normal graft segment proximal to the lesion.

Using these duplex criteria, Mills et al. (49) studied the natural history of autogenous infrainguinal vein grafts with intermediate and critical stenosis. A PSV more than 300 cm/sec or ratio of more than 4 was used to detect critical stenosis. In grafts with the unrevised critical stenosis, nearly 80% progressed to occlusion, all within four months of ultrasound detection. For grafts with intermediate stenosis, the occlusion rate was not different from grafts without stenosis, and serial surveillance was safe and effective.

Calligaro et al. (50,51) established the utility of surveillance in prosthetic graft; 85 prosthetic bypasses in 59 patients were studied in a graft surveillance protocol. There were 35 femoropopliteal, 16 femorotibial, 15 iliofemoral, 13 axillofemoral, and 6 femorofemoral bypasses. The benefit of DU was compared with other noninvasive studies such as changes in symptoms or pulses and ABI. Follow-up was performed one week and every three months after the initial bypass or after graft revision for a mean of 11 months. DU was able to predict 81% of graft failures versus 24% using non-ultrasound findings. In the presence of a normal study, the likelihood of a graft failure was 7% using duplex criteria versus 21% with non-ultrasound studies. The DU was more sensitive in predicting prosthetic graft failure.

In a subsequent report, the same authors focused on 89 infrainguinal prosthetic grafts in 66 patients. The same surveillance protocol using DU and noninvasive studies was used. Results were compared between femoropopliteal and femorotibial bypasses. The authors supported the routine use of DU for graft surveillance of femorotibial but not femoropopliteal, prosthetic grafts.

In a contemporary report (2007), Carter et al. (52) studied the natural history of stenosis within the lower extremity bypass graft with duplex surveillance. There were 212 infrainguinal lower limb grafts in 197 patients and DU studies were performed at 0, 1, 3, 6, 12, and 18 months after surgery; 56.2% of grafts remained patent during this period. It was noted that prosthetic grafts and femorocrural bypasses tended to occlude without any prior documented stenosis; 40.5% of salvage procedures were performed at the six-month time point. In contrast, vein grafts were more likely to develop progressive stenosis prior to occlusion. The authors concluded that surveillance is a valid method for detecting high-risk lesions in vein graft but failed in prosthetic and femorocrural grafts. This is in contrast to the findings by Calligaro et al. above, where they found utility in prosthetic femorotibial grafts.

In a contemporary retrospective analysis, Tinder et al. (53) found other factors that enhanced the efficacy of DU surveillance. There were 353 infrainguinal vein bypasses performed in 329 patients. Factors that were predictive of stenosis detected during surveillance included were non-single segment saphenous vein conduit, warfarin drug therapy, and redo bypass grafting. Factors not predictive of graft revision were procedure indication, postoperative ABI level, statin drug therapy, and vein conduit orientation. Another predictive factor was abnormal initial duplex velocities [PSV (peak systolic velocity) of 180–300 cm/sec or ratio of 2–3.5]. Forty percent of these grafts had earlier revision and lower three-year assisted primary patency rate. In a report by Passman et al. (54), normal initial duplex velocities were not predictive of long-term patency; 31% of grafts had abnormal duplex results first detected more than six months after operation.

Lesion characteristics detected during ultrasound surveillance may also be used to determine the type of reintervention needed. Gonsalves et al. (55) found factors to be based on temporal and duplex data. PTA is recommended for short (<2 cm) stenoses in good caliber veins (3.5 mm or more) found more than three months after the bypass procedure. Direct surgical repair or replacement is recommended for early (<3 months) and/or long segment stenoses in small caliber veins.

Hagino et al. (56) also found other lesion characteristics to be of useful predictive value. Grafts treated for early lesions continued to have high failure rate regardless of modality used compared to late lesions. Lesions located at the anastamoses were better treated by surgical revision, although patency was not different from those treated with endovascular means. Endovascular therapy was recommended for focal, late-appearing lesions involving the mid-graft.

While the use of DU in endovascular follow-up is intuitive and consistent with the utility observed in management of surgical bypass, there are few large studies looking at its ability to predict failure and impact on long-term results. Tielbeek et al. (57) used DU surveillance, clinical exam, and ABI on femoropopliteal lesions successfully treated with endovascular interventions. Impending failure was diagnosed with a PSV ratio more than 2.5. Failure was diagnosed as occlusion or recurrent stenosis requiring intervention for severe symptoms. Treatment failure was predicted by DU with a sensitivity of 86% and a specificity of 75%, which is good, but interestingly ABI decrease was even more predictive with a sensitivity of 93% and specificity of 90%, respectively.

In another study by Spijkerboer et al. (58), 34 femoropopliteal segments were treated with PTA. The PSV ratio was determined with DU before PTA, one day and one year after PTA. Segments with residual stenosis detected on one day after PTA, all occluded within the year. In those segments with good initial ultrasound results after PTA, there was deterioration in 30%. This suggests the need for more frequent routine DU follow-up.

SUMMARY

During the last decade, advances and refinements in technology have brought a plethora of new tools to the disposal of the vascular specialist treating CLI. The new devices described in this chapter and elsewhere in this text, coupled with aggressive training initiatives targeted at disseminating skills to fellows and mature surgeons alike have led to an extraordinary paradigm shift. Endovascular techniques are routinely used as the initial treatment for virtually all levels of arterial occlusive disease and all severities of vascular symptoms including CLI. Although the many new modalities have given us the luxury of choice, there is little consensus as to the primacy of one technique over the others. Indeed, randomized trials comparing new devices and techniques head to head are lacking.

While we lack consensus on the best endovascular modality to use in most patients, we are certain of the need for routine follow-up and close involvement in all patients treated for CLI. The ultimate success of any intervention we perform, either endovascular or open surgical bypass, can be improved by a continued relationship with the patient and regular examination. We utilize smoking cessation counseling and adjuvant techniques such as medications and nicotine replacement to help our patients with this important aspect of their treatment. We also use indefinite administration of oral antiplatelet agents (81 mg ASA daily and 75 mg clopidagril daily) and aggressive lipid modification in all patients who have any intervention for CLI.

Duplex arterial ultrasound has gained wide acceptance as the modality of choice for surgical bypass graft surveillance, and it is also our first choice for following patients treated with endovascular therapy. Our practice guidelines include a baseline DU scan before intervention, another following the intervention to document improvement (the timing of this scan varies from 1 day to 2 weeks following the intervention), and then additional scans at three months and six months post procedure to assess continued efficacy. We then perform DU at six-month intervals thereafter. Evaluation of continued subjective clinical improvement and performance of ABIs are essential and simple adjunctive measures that should be performed at each visit.

CLI is often a hallmark of the beginning of the end game in the battle for survival in patients with diffuse atherosclerotic disease. The sobering reality is that the words in the title of this chapter referring to "long-term management and surveillance" are optimistic and misleading. With a known five-year survival of about 50% this population is extremely disadvantaged. Our best chance for helping this group of patients lies in providing the least invasive endovascular intervention that will provide pain relief, tissue healing, and limb salvage. We must provide close follow-up with appropriate counseling, intensive medical management with repeat interventions performed as clinical conditions warrant. These measures offer the best strategy for successful intervention and continued management of CLI. But, the final determinant of success for any strategy we propose is our patients' perception of an enhancement in the quality of their remaining years of life.

REFERENCES

1. Bolia A, Brennan J, Bell PR. Recanalization of femoro-popliteal occlusions: improving success rate by subintimal recanalization. Clin Radiol 1989; 40:325.
2. Bolia A, Sayers RD, Thompson MM, et al. Subintimal and intraluminal recanalization of occluded crural arteries by percutaneous balloon angioplasty. Eur J Vasc Surg 1994; 8:214–219.
3. Lazaris AM, Tsiamis AC, Fishwick G, et al. Clinical outcome of primary infrainguinal subintimal angioplasty in diabetic patients with critical lower limb ischemia. J Endovasc Ther 2004; 4:447–453.
4. Met R, Van Lienden KP, Koelemay W, et al. Subintimal angioplasty for peripheral arterial occlusive disease: a systematic review. Cardiovasc Intervent Radio 2008; 31:687–697.
5. Scott EC, Biuckians A, Light RE, et al. Subintimal angioplasty for the treatment of claudication and critical limb ischemia: 3-year results. J Vasc Surg 2007; 46:959–964.
6. Scott EC, Biuckians A, Light RE, et al. Subintimal angioplasty: our experience in the treatment of 506 infrainguinal arterial occlusions. J Vasc Surg 2008; 48:878–884.
7. Clark TW, Groffsky JL, Soulen MC. Predictors of long-term patency after femoropopliteal angioplasty: results from the STAR registry. J Vasc Interv Radiol 2001; 12:923–933.
8. Dorros G, Jaff MR, Murphy, KJ, et al. The acute outcome of tibioperoneal vessel angioplasty in 417 cases with claudication and critical limb ischemia. Cathet Cardiovasc Diagn 1998; 45:251–256.
9. Dorros G, Jaff MR, Dorros AM, et al. Tibioperoneal (outflow lesion) angioplasty can be used as primary treatment in 235 patients with critical limb ischemia. Five-year follow-up. Circulation 2001; 104:2057–2062.
10. Giles KA, Pomposelli FB, Hamdan AD, et al. Infrapopliteal angioplasty for critical limb ischemia: relation of TransAtlantic InterSociety Consensus class to outcome in 176 limbs. J Vasc Surg 2008; 48:128–136.
11. Kudo T, Chandra FA, Ahn SS. The effectiveness of percutaneous transluminal angioplasty for the treatment of critical limb ischemia: a 10-year experience. J Vasc Surg 2005; 41:423–435.
12. Mwipatayi BP, Hockings A, Hofmann M, et al. Balloon angioplasty compared with stenting for treatment of femoropopliteal occlusive disease: a meta-analysis. J Vasc Surg 2008; 47:461–469.
13. Ansel GM, Sample NS, Botti III CF Jr, et al. Cutting balloon angioplasty of the popliteal and infrapopliteal vessels for symptomatic limb ischemia. Catheter Cardiovasc Interv 2004; 61:1–4.
14. Canaud L, Alric P, Berthet JP, et al. Infrainguinal cutting balloon angioplasty in de novo arterial lesions. J Vasc Surg 2008; 48(5):1182–1188.
15. Cotroneo AR, Pascali D, Iezzi R. Cutting balloon versus conventional balloon angioplasty in short femoropopliteal arterial stenoses. J Endovasc Ther 2008; 15:283–291.

16. Amighi J, Schillinger M, Dick P, et al. De Novo superficial femoropopliteal artery lesions: peripheral cutting balloon angioplasty and restenosis rates-randomized controlled trial. Radiology 2008; 247:267–272.
17. Scheinert D, Peeters P, Bosiers M, et al. Results of the Multicenter First-in-Man Study of a Novel Scoring Balloon Catheter for the Treatment of Infra-Popliteal Peripheral Arterial Disease. Catheter Cardiovasc Interv 2007; 70:1034–1039.
18. Laird JR, Jaff MR, Biamino G, et al. Cryoplasty for the treatment of femoropopliteal arterial disease: results of a prospective, multicenter registry. J Vasc Interv Radiol 2005; 16:106–1073.
19. Laird JR, Biamino G, McNamara T, et al. Cryoplasty for the treatment of femoropopliteal arterial disease: extended follow-up results. J Endovasc Ther 2006; 13:1152–1159.
20. Samson RH, Showalter DP, Lepore M, et al. Cryoplasty therapy of the superficial femoral and popliteal arteries: a reappraisal after 44 month's experience. J Vasc Surg 2008; 48:634–637.
21. Wildgruber MG, Berger HJ. Cryoplasty for the Prevention of Arterial Restenosis. Cardiovasc Intervent Radiol 2008; 31(6):1050–1058.
22. Yancy AE, Minion DJ, Rodriguez C, et al. Peripheral atherectomy in TransAtlantic InterSociety Consensus type C femoropopliteal lesions for limb salvage. J Vasc Surg 2006; 44:503–509.
23. Keeling BW, Shames ML, Stone PA, et al. Plaque excision with the SilverHawk catheter: early results in patients with claudication or critical limb ischemia. J Vasc Surg 2007; 45:25–31.
24. Zeller T, Rastan A, Schwarzwalder U, et al. Percutaneous peripheral atherectomy of femoropopliteal stenoses using a new-generation device: six-month results from a single-center experience. J Endovasc Ther 2004; 11:676–687.
25. Zeller T, Rastan A, Sixt S, et al. Long-term results after directional atherectomy of femoropopliteal lesions. J Am Coll Cardiol 2006; 48:1573–1578.
26. Sarac TP, Altinel O, Bannazadeh M, et al. Midterm outcome predictors for lower extremity atherectomy procedures. J Vasc Surg 2008; 48(4):885–890.
27. Scheinert D, Laird JR, Schroder M, et al. Excimer laser-assisted recanalization of long, chronic superficial femoral artery occlusions. J Endovasc Ther 2001; 8:156–166.
28. Zhou W, Bush R, Lin P, et al. Laser atherectomy for lower extremity revascularization: an adjunctive endovascular treatment. Vasc Endovascular Surg 2006; 40:268–274.
29. Stoner MC, deFreitas DJ, Phade SV, et al. Mid-term results with laser atherectomy in the treatment of infrainguinal occlusive disease. J Vasc Surg 2007; 46:289–295.
30. Bosiers M, Peeters P, Elst FV, et al. Excimer laser assisted angioplasty for critical limb ischemia: results of the LACI Belgium Study. Eur J Vasc Endovasc Surg 2005; 29(6): 613–619.
31. Sabeti S, Schillinger M, Amighi J, et al. Primary patency of femoropopliteal arteries treated with nitinol versus stainless steel self-expanding stents: propensity score-adjusted analysis. Radiology 2004; 232:516–521.
32. Sabeti S, Mlekusch W, Amighi J, et al. Primary patency of long-segment self-expanding nitinol stents in the femoropopliteal arteries. J Endovasc Ther 2005; 12: 6–12.
33. Vogel TR, Shindelman LE, Nackman GB, et al. Efficacious use of nitinol stents in the femoral and popliteal arteries. J Vasc Surg 2003; 38:1178–1184.
34. Mewissen MW. Self-expanding nitinol stents in the femoropopliteal segment: technique and mid-term results. Tech Vasc Interv Radiol 2004; 7:2–5.
35. Ferreira M, Lanziotti L, Monteiro M, et al. Superficial femoral artery recanalization with self-expanding nitinol stents: long-term follow-results. Eur J Vasc Endovasc Surg 2007; 34:702–708.
36. Baril DT, Marone LK, Kim J, et al. Outcomes of endovascular interventions for TASC II B and C femoropopliteal lesions. J Vasc Surg 2008; 48:627–633.

37. Kickuth R, Keo HH, Triller J, et al. Initial clinical experience with the 4-F self-expanding XPERT stent system for infrapopliteal treatment of patients with severe claudication and critical limb ischemia. J Vasc Interv Radiol 2007; 18:703–708.

38. Mwipatayi BP, Hockings A, Hofmann M, et al. Balloon angioplasty compared with stenting for treatment of femoropopliteal occlusive disease: a meta-analysis. J Vasc Surg 2008; 47:461–469.

39. Ihnat DM, Doung ST, Taylor ZC, et al. Contemporary outcomes after superficial femoral artery angioplasty and stenting: the influence of TASC classification and runoff score. J Vasc Surg 2008; 47:967–974.

40. Railo M, Roth WD, Edgren J. Preliminary results with endoluminal femoropopliteal thrupass. Ann Chir Gynaecol 2001; 90:15–18.

41. Jahnke T, Andresen R, Muller-Hulsbeck S. Hemobahn stent-grafts for treatmemt of femoropopliteal arterial obstructions: midterm results of a prospective trial. J Vasc Interv Radio 2003; 14:41–51.

42. Fischer M, Schwabe C, Schulte KL. Value of the hemobahn/viabahn endoprosthesis in the treatment of long chronic lesions of the superficial femoral artery: 6 years of experience. J Endovasc Ther 2006; 13:281–290.

43. Bleyn J, Schol F, Vanhandenhove I, et al. Endovascular reconstruction of the superficial femoral artery. Controversies and updates in Vascular & cardiac Surgery 2004; 14:87–91.

44. Shaikh F, Mami-hani MD, Solis J, et al. Percutaneous endovascular treatment of SFA disease using the Gore Viabahn endoprosthesis. Do the procedure success and 1-year follow-up data make this the treatment of choice? Endovasc Today 2007; (suppl):4–8.

45. Saxon RR, Dake MD, Volgelzang RL, et al. Randomized, multicenter study comparing expanded polytetrafluoroethylene-covered endoprosthesis placement with percutaneous transluminal angioplasty in the treatmemt of superficial femoral artery occlusive disease. J Vasc Interv Radiol 2008; 19:823–832.

46. Kedora J, Hohmann S, Garrett W, et al. Randomized comparison of percutaneous Viabahn stent grafts vs prosthetic femoral-popliteal bypass in the treatment of superficial femoral arterial occlusive disease. J Vasc Surg 2007; 45:10–16.

47. Idu MM, Blankenstein JD, de Gier P, et al. Impact of a color-flow duplex surveillance program on infrainguinal vein graft patency: a five-year experience. J Vasc Surg 1993; 17:42–53.

48. Buth J, Disselhoff B, Sommeling C, et al. Color-flow duplex criteria for grading stenosis in infrainguinal. J Vasc Surg 1991; 4:716–728.

49. Mills JL Sr, Wixon, CL, James DC, et al. The natural history of intermediate and critical vein graft stenosis: recommendations for continued surveillance or repair. J Vasc Surg 2001; 33(2):273–278.

50. Calligaro KD, Musser DJ, Chen AY, et al. Duplex ultrasonography to diagnose failing arterial prosthetic grafts. Surgery 1996; 120:455–459.

51. Calligaro KD, Doerr K, McAffee-Bennett S, et al. Should duplex ultrasonography be performed for surveillance of femoropopliteal and femorotibial arterial prosthetic bypasses?Ann Vasc Surg 2001; 15:520–524.

52. Carter A, Murphy MO, Halka AT, et al. The natural history of stenoses within lower limb arterial bypass grafts using a graft surveillance program. Ann Vasc Surg 2007; 21:695–703.

53. Tinder CN, Chavanpun JP, Bandyk DF, et al. Efficacy of duplex ultrasound surveillance after infrainguinal vein bypass may be enhanced by identification of characteristics predictive of graft stenosis development. J Vasc Surg 2008; 48:613–618.

54. Passman MA, Moneta GL, Nehler MR, et al. Do normal early color-flow duplex surveillance examination results of infrainguinal vein grafts preclude the need for late graft revision?J Vasc Surg 1995; 22:476–481.

55. Gonsalves C, Bandyk DF, Avion AJ, et al. Duplex features of vein graft stenosis and the success of percutaneous transluminal angioplasty. J Endovasc Surg 1999; 6:66–72.

56. Hagino RT, Sheehan MK, Jung I, et al. Target lesion characteristics in failing vein grafts predict the success of endovascular and open revision. J Vasc Surg 2007; 46:1167–1172.

57. Tielbeek AV, Rietjens E, Buth J, et al. The value of duplex surveillance after endovascular intervention for femoropopliteal obstructive disease. Eur J Vasc Endovasc Surg 1996; 12:145–150.
58. Spijkerboer AM, Nass PC, de Valois JC, et al. Evaluation of femoropopliteal arteries with duplex ultrasound after angioplasty. Can we predict results at one year? Eur J Vasc Endovasc Surg 1996; 12:418–423.

15 Economic Impact of CLI

Carlo Setacci and Gianmarco de Donato
Unit of Vascular and Endovascular Surgery, Policlinico Le Scotte,
University of Sienna, Sienna, Italy

INCIDENCE OF CRITICAL LIMB ISCHEMIA

Critical limb ischemia (CLI) is the end stage of lower extremity peripheral arterial disease (PAD), in which severe obstruction of blood flow results in ischemic rest pain, ulcers, and a significant risk of limb loss.

The total prevalence of PAD, which commonly results from a progressive narrowing of the arteries in the lower extremities, secondary to atherosclerosis, has been evaluated in several epidemiologic studies as being in the range of 5% to 30% in the adult population in industrialized countries (1–3). Consequently, we can estimate that about 50 to 100 per 100,000 patients suffer from CLI every year, leading to significant morbidity and mortality as well as consuming large portions of health care and social care resources.

The real prevalence of asymptomatic PAD can only be estimated by using noninvasive measurements in the general population. Data from the 1999 to 2000 National Health and Nutrition Examination Survey in the United States (3) revealed that PAD, defined as an ankle-brachial index of less than 0.90 in either leg, was 4.3% (95% CI 3.1–5.5%) in adults aged 40 years and older. This means approximately five million individuals in the United States (95% CI, 4 to 7 million) are expected to have PAD.

Among those aged 70 years or older, the prevalence was 14.5% (95% CI, 10.8–18.2%). Moreover, in age- and gender-adjusted logistic regression analyses, black race/ethnicity (OR 2.83; 95% CI, 1.48–5.42), current smoking (OR 4.46; 95% CI, 2.25–8.84), diabetes (OR 2.71; 95% CI, 1.03–7.12), hypertension (OR 1.75; 95% CI, 0.97–3.13), hypercholesterolemia (OR 1.68; 95% CI, 1.09–2.57), and low kidney function (OR 2.00; 95% CI, 1.08–3.70) were positively associated with PAD.

Using similar diagnostic criteria, other studies, such as the Framingham Offspring Study (4), the Atherosclerosis Risk in Communities Study (5), the Honolulu Heart Program, and the Cardiovascular Health Study (6), confirmed that the prevalence of PAD ranged from 3% to 4% among middle-aged adults and between 13% and 14% in the elderly.

The incidence and prevalence of PAD increases substantially with age in both males and females (7–12). The prevalence of PAD determined by non-invasive ankle-brachial blood pressure measurement is higher than that of the disease defined by symptoms of intermittent claudication. Even if intermittent claudication is the main symptom of PAD, it does not always predict the real incidence of the disease. Despite having severe PAD, some patients may not have claudication because other conditions limit their exercise, while other patients with claudication may have a nonvascular origin of the problem (e.g., spinal arthrosis). It can be concluded that for every patient with symptomatic

PAD there are another three to four subjects with PAD who do not meet the clinical criteria for intermittent claudication.

In addition these studies have clearly shown that PAD is associated with a significantly elevated risk of cardiovascular disease–related morbidity and mortality (6,13,14). PAD is also strongly associated with traditional cardiovascular disease risk factors, such as smoking, diabetes, hypertension, and hypercholesterolemia: 95% of persons with prevalent PAD having at least one of these risk factors. Together, the systemic atherosclerosis triad of PAD, coronary artery disease (CAD), and cerebrovascular disease (CVD) account for approximately half of the rates of morbidity and mortality in the adult population aged 50 years and older (15). PAD serves as an important marker for advanced systemic atherosclerosis yet, despite its prevalence and association with high rates of morbidity and mortality, it still remains underdiagnosed and undertreated.

Management of patients with PAD appears to be moving in the direction of more aggressive lifestyle modifications and medical therapy, to provide earlier identification and treatment similar to CAD, with the clear goal of decreasing cardiovascular risk. However, ageing populations, the increasing prevalence of diabetes and its lower limb–related complications, and the failure thus far to substantially reduce tobacco consumption mean that despite advances in medical therapies, the number of patients needing lower limb revascularization for severe limb ischemia will probably increase in the foreseeable future.

Economic evaluations of preventive therapies for CAD are relevant for patients with vascular disease since CAD and peripheral arterial occlusive disease commonly occur together and share risk factors, pathophysiology, and response to preventive therapy. Cost-effectiveness analysis has shown that modification of vascular risk factors such as tobacco use, hypertension, and hypercholesterolemia improve clinical outcomes at cost-effectiveness ratios of usually less than $20,000 per year of life saved, making medical management for the reduction of cardiovascular risk factors generally cost-effective (16).

ECONOMIC BURDEN OF CRITICAL LIMB ISCHEMIA

Two methods have been used to assess the economic impact of the various techniques and treatments. The first is a cost-benefit analysis, which converts all benefits into monetary value so that very disparate treatments can be compared, but is not widely used. The second is a cost-effectiveness analysis where the outcome is measured in clinically relevant scales, such as years of life gained. This measures the cost per unit of health improvement, and is more frequently applied.

The economic burden of CLI is typically considered to consist of three components: the direct costs, that is, the resources used to treat the disease; the indirect costs, that is, the loss of productivity of the patients or their carers; and thirdly, intangibles, that is, the reduction in quality of life through pain or suffering associated with the disease (Table 1).

The total direct costs for patients with PAD include the managed care organization costs and patient cost-share amounts. The health care resources include medication, outpatient/physician office visits, laboratory/diagnostic procedures, emergency department visits, and hospitalization.

A diagnosis of PAD not only imposes a severe burden on patients and their families, but it also significantly increases the use of health care resources and the associated costs. It has been reported that by the end of year one from

TABLE 1   Economic Burden of Critical Limb Ischemia

Direct costs	- The number and cost of general practitioner consultations and prescriptions
	- The number and cost of inpatient procedures
	- The amount and cost of long-term and community care services
	- The number and cost of hospital outpatient referrals
	- The number and cost of diagnostic procedures
	- The amount and cost of ambulance transport
Indirect costs	- Loss of productivity of the patients
	- Loss of productivity of their carers
Intangible costs	- The reductions in quality of life through pain or suffering associated with the disease

the diagnosis of CLI, this burden is comparable with a diagnosis of myocardial infarction.

Several studies have compared the cost-effectiveness of primary limb amputation and arterial reconstruction in patients with CLI, and different surgical revascularization strategies (percutaneous transluminal angioplasty ± stenting or bypass surgery). However, the recent publication of the TransAtlantic Inter-Society Consensus (TASC) document has highlighted the lack of good-quality data concerning the cost-effectiveness of intervention in lower limb arterial disease.

Davies et al. (17) compared the cost-effectiveness of primary limb amputation and arterial reconstruction and found that the latter option resulted in lower overall costs. This was due to the relatively low use of rehabilitation and community care services by patients in the arterial reconstruction treatment group. On the other hand, although the rationale for primary amputation assumes that patients will ambulate successfully with a prosthesis, many do not, and thus costs for institutionalization must be included in the equation.

Hunick et al. (18) compared the relative benefits and cost-effectiveness of revascularization for femoropopliteal disease via percutaneous translumenal angioplasty or bypass surgery, using a decision analysis model based on data from the literature for mortality, morbidity, potency, and cost. The conclusion was that, in patients with disabling claudication and femoropopliteal stenosis or occlusion and in patients with chronic critical ischemia with stenosis, angioplasty is the preferred initial interventional treatment. In contrast, bypass surgery was found to be the preferred initial treatment in patients with chronic critical ischemia and femoropopliteal occlusion.

In a nonrandomized study (19), the cost of endovascular treatment for CLI ($9161) was remarkably similar to that of open surgery ($10,585). In a prospective study (20), the hospital costs related to distal reconstruction for CLI showed that the median costs for revascularization were $7200, in contrast to $28,433 for secondary amputation, including rehabilitation and the cost of the prosthesis. These costs were similar to those reported by Singh et al. (21), who showed a cost of $11,277 for successful revascularization compared with $21,545 for failed revascularization.

The recently published Bypass versus Angioplasty in Severe Ischaemia of the Leg (BASIL) trial (22), which randomized patients with CLI into a bypass surgery-first strategy group versus a balloon angioplasty–first strategy group, showed the cost benefit of angioplasty at one year, with similar clinical outcomes. However, patients assigned to receive surgery spent significantly longer in hospital and needed significantly more care in the high-dependency unit and intensive therapy unit for the first 12 months than those assigned to the angioplasty group. A high occurrence of cardiovascular, infective, and wound complications, and a small but clinically significant reintervention rate for graft revision, thrombectomy, and evacuation of hematoma were recorded in the surgical group. The mean cost of inpatient hospital treatment during the first 12 months of follow-up in patients assigned to a surgery-first strategy was estimated as £23,322 (£20,096 hospital stay, £3225 procedure costs), which is about a third higher than the £17,419 (£15,381/£2039) for patients assigned to an angioplasty-first strategy.

In the long term, that is, after two years, surgery seemed to be associated with a significantly reduced risk of future amputation, death, or both; that is, if a patient was alive with his or her legs intact two years after randomization, he or she seemed to be more likely to remain alive and with legs intact in the future if he or she had been assigned to receive surgery first rather than angioplasty first. This finding could suggest the encouraging possibility that, despite the increased short-term morbidity and the higher costs, patients could benefit more in the long term from a surgery-first than an angioplasty-first strategy.

However, the BASIL trial did not attempt to quantify the use and associated costs of health and social services outside the hospitals, which probably represents a large additional financial burden for certain patients, especially for those who ultimately need amputation.

Other nonrandomized studies have recently published data on the cost of treating CLI by surgical revascularization, percutaneous transluminal angioplasty and stenting, and primary amputation (23–25). Whatever the treatment considered, the costs are multiplied by a factor 2 to 4 when the initially planned procedure fails, for example, angioplasty requiring immediate or delayed crossover grafting, a bypass requiring revision after thrombosis or secondary amputation, and when renal and pulmonary comorbidities or complications are present. Results are consistent across countries, although the individual costs of procedures vary. The order of magnitude for the cost of angioplasty is around $10,000 ($20,000 if the procedure fails initially or later), the cost for bypass grafting is around $20,000 ($40,000 if revision is required), and the cost for amputation is around $40,000 (Table 2). Adding rehabilitation will usually double the costs.

Diabetic patients represent another impending problem. Amputations of the leg, foot, or toe are much more likely to occur in individuals with diabetes: two-thirds of all lower extremity amputations in industrialized countries are directly linked to the disease. While the risk of amputation increases with age for all individuals, the rate of amputation is far greater for people with diabetes, and patients hospitalized with diabetes are 28 times more likely to undergo an amputation than patients without diabetes.

Moreover multiple hospitalizations are common among individuals with diabetes, and certain vulnerable populations are more likely to experience multiple hospital stays. The complications associated with diabetes result in significant costs to the health care system, particularly for public insurance programs, and are largely preventable.

The worldwide prevalence of diabetes now exceeds 200 million, and is predicted to rise to more than 300 million in the next 20 years. Up to 15% of patients with diabetes have a foot ulcer at some stage, and over one million

TABLE 2 Cost-Effectiveness Analysis

Authors (Ref.)	Surgery	Angioplasty	Amputation
Singh et al. (21)	$11,277	NA	$21,545 (secondary)
Panayiotopoulos et al. (20)	~$7,200	NA	~$21,200 (primary) ~$28,300 (secondary)
Hunick et al. (18)	Preferred in patients with CLI	Preferred in patients with disabling claudication	NA
Ballard et al. (19)	$10,585	$9,161	NA
Adam et al. (22)	£23,322 (£20,096—hospital stay; £3,225—procedure cost)	£17,419 (£15,381—hospital stay; £2,039—procedure cost)	NA
Cardenas et al. (23)	~$20,000 (~$40,000 if revision is required)	~$10,000 (~$20,000 if the procedure fails initially)	~$20,000 (primary) ~$40,000 (secondary)

amputations for diabetes-related complications occur every year. It is high time for health care planners and health care professionals to turn their attention to a condition that is a source of major morbidity and mortality, and that often afflicts those who are least able to cope. Although evidence is scarcely available, poor socioeconomic status has been empirically accepted as a risk factor for diabetic foot complications, even in the International Consensus on Guidelines of the Diabetic Foot by the International Working Group on the Diabetic Foot (26).

Flores Rivera (27) has focused on the influence of acculturation and socioeconomic status on the prevalence of diabetes and obesity. In his analysis he studied amputation risk factors, including demographic information, and systemic factors, and found that significant risk factors in logistic regression analysis were lacking diabetes education (OR 17.5), neuropathy (OR 13.1), and high blood cholesterol (OR 5.9).

Diabetic foot ulcers and amputations result in huge societal costs and high costs for individual patients. Topical wound treatments and inpatient care account for the largest fraction of costs over time until the patient is completely healed. The costs of materials, staff, and transportation, as well as the frequency of dressing changes, the rate of healing, and the final outcome are factors that can effect the total costs and cost-effectiveness of topical treatments. The majority of costs for infected diabetic foot ulcers that healed after an amputation occurs between amputation and complete healing and is mainly related to topical treatments. Total direct costs for healing infected ulcers not requiring amputation are approximately US$17,500, compared with lower extremity amputation, which typically ranges from $30,000 to $33,500 (28). Prevention of foot ulcers and amputation is therefore the best cost-saving strategy.

Rehabilitation programs could represent another important economic impact factor of CLI. Rehabilitation plans for patients with amputations can be conducted on an inpatient or outpatient basis. The amputation rehabilitation team must be composed of many skilled professionals, including an orthopedist/orthopedic surgeon, physiatrist, rehabilitation nurse, physical therapist, occupational therapist, social worker, psychologist/psychiatrist, recreational therapist, case manager, and vocational counselor.

The rehabilitation program must be designed to meet the needs of the individual patient, and the active involvement of the patient and his or her family is vital to the success of the program.

The goal of rehabilitation after an amputation is to help the patient return to the highest level of function and independence possible, while improving his or her overall quality of life—physically, emotionally, and socially.

Although no studies have ever focused on the total cost of such a rehabilitation program, the real socioeconomic impact of this organization is extremely high.

CONCLUSIONS

In summary, severe limb ischemia imposes a very high human cost as well as a major economic burden on health and social care resources, not only in developed countries, but also increasingly in developing countries. Patients who undergo revascularization for severe limb ischemia, either by surgery or angioplasty, seem to represent the tip of an iceberg, the true dimensions of which are not yet completely defined.

Economic evaluation is important for all treatments, and cost-effectiveness should be part of any planned randomized controlled trial. This is applicable to populations rather than the individual patient. Nevertheless, clinicians should recognize that economic considerations are becoming increasingly important in the treatment of the individual. The cost-effectiveness of any procedure probably reinforces the prejudice of vascular surgeons working within strictly defined health care budgets.

The main aim of treatment for chronic CLI is the avoidance of amputation. However, primary amputation is more cost-effective than secondary amputation. In fact the median cost of managing a patient following amputation is almost twice that of successful limb salvage, thus justifying an aggressive revascularization policy. However, justification of such a policy on economic grounds requires that salvage failure episodes must be minimized as they increase costs considerably.

REFERENCES

1. Criqui MH, Fronek A, Barrett-Connor E, et al. The prevalence of peripheral arterial disease in a defined population. Circulation 1985; 71:510–551.
2. Hiatt WR, Hoag S, Hamman RF. Effect of diagnostic criteria on the prevalence of peripheral arterial disease. The San Luis Valley Diabetes Study. Circulation 1995; 91:1472–1479.
3. Selvin E, Erlinger TP. Prevalence of and risk factors for peripheral arterial disease in the United States: results from the National Health and Nutrition Examination Survey, 1999–2000. Circulation 2004; 110:738–743.
4. Murabito JM, Evans JC, Nieto K, et al. Prevalence and clinical correlates of peripheral arterial disease in the Framingham Offspring Study. Am Heart J 2002; 143:961–965.
5. Zheng ZJ, Sharrett AR, Chambless LE, et al. Associations of ankle-brachial index with clinical coronary heart disease, stroke and preclinical carotid and popliteal atherosclerosis: the Atherosclerosis Risk in Communities (ARIC) Study. Atherosclerosis 1997; 131:115–125.
6. Newman AB, Shemanski L, Manolio TA, et al. Ankle-arm index as a predictor of cardiovascular disease and mortality in the Cardiovascular Health Study: the Cardiovascular Health Study Group. Arterioscler Thromb Vasc Biol 1999; 19:538–545.

7. Kannel WB, McGee DL. Update on some epidemiologic features of intermittent claudication: the Framingham Study. J Am Geriatr Soc 1985; 33:13–18.
8. Smith GD, Shipley MJ, Rose G. Intermittent claudication, heart disease risk factors, and mortality: the Whitehall Study. Circulation 1990; 82:1925–1931.
9. Bainton D, Sweetnam P, Baker I, et al. Survival and association with risk factors in the Speedwell prospective heart disease study. Br Heart J 1994; 72:128–132.
10. Meijer WT, Hoes AW, Rutgers D, et al. Peripheral arterial disease in the elderly: the Rotterdam study. Arterioscler Thromb Vasc Biol 1998; 18:185–192.
11. Curb JD, Masaki K, Rodriquez BL, et al. Peripheral arterial disease and cardiovascular risk factors in the elderly: the Honolulu Heart Program. Arterioscler Thromb Vasc Biol 1996; 16:1495–1500.
12. Newman AB, Siscovick DS, Manolio TA, et al. Ankle-arm index as a marker of atherosclerosis in the Cardiovascular Health Study. Circulation 1993; 88:837–845.
13. Murabito JM, Evans JC, Larson MG, et al. The ankle-brachial index in the elderly and risk of stroke, coronary disease, and death: the Framingham Study. Arch Intern Med 2003; 163:1939–1942.
14. Criqui MH, Langer RD, Fronek A, et al. Mortality over a period of 10 years in patients with peripheral arterial disease. N Engl J Med 1992; 326:381–386.
15. Murray CJ, Lopez AD. Alternative projections of mortality and disability by cause 1990-2020: Global Burden of Disease Study. Lancet 1997; 349:1498–1504.
16. West JA. Cost-effective strategies for the management of vascular disease. Vasc Med 1997; 2:25–29.
17. Davies LM, Noone M, Drummond MF, et al. Technology assessment in the development of guidelines for vascularising the ischaemic leg. CHE/HYEC Discussion Paper 89, York, University of York, 1991.
18. Hunick MG, Wong JB, Donaldson MC, et al. Revascularization for femoropopliteal disease. A decision and cost-effectiveness analysis. J Am Med Assoc 1995; 274(2):165.
19. Ballard JL, Bergan JJ, Singh P, et al. Aortoiliac stent deployment versus surgical reconstruction: analysis of outcome and cost. J Vasc Surg 1998; 28:94–101.
20. Panayiotopoulos YP, Tyrrell MR, Owen SE, et al. Outcome and cost analysis after femorocrural and femoropedal grafting for lower limb-threatening ischaemia. Br J Surg 1997; 84:207–212.
21. Singh S, Evens L, Datta D, et al. The costs of managing lower limb-threatening ischaemia. Eur J Surg 1996; 12:359–362.
22. Adam DJ, Beard JD, Cleveland T, et al. BASIL trial participants. Bypass versus angioplasty in severe ischaemia of the leg (BASIL): multicentre, randomised controlled trial. Lancet 2005; 366:1925–1934.
23. Cardenas DD, Haselkorn JK, Mcelligott JM, et al. A bibliography of cost-effectiveness practices in physical medicine and rehabilitation: AAPM&R white paper. Arch Phys Med Rehabil 2001; 82:711–719.
24. Whatling PJ, Gibson M, Torrie EP, et al. Iliac occlusions: stenting or crossover grafting? An examination of patency and cost. Eur J Vasc Endovasc Surg 2000; 20: 36–40.
25. Wixon CL, Mills JL, Westerband A, et al. An economic appraisal of lower extremity bypass graft maintenance. J Vasc Surg 2000; 32:1–12.
26. Apelqvist J, Bakker K, van Houtum WH, et al. International consensus and practical guidelines on the management and the prevention of the diabetic foot. International Working Group on the Diabetic Foot. Diabetes Metab Res Rev. 2000; 16 (suppl 1): S84–92.
27. Flores Rivera AR. Risk factors for amputation in diabetic patients: a case-control study. Arch Med Res 1998; 29:179–184.
28. Economic and Health Costs of Diabetes: Hcup Highlight 1. AHRQ Publication No. 05-0034, January 2005. Rockville, MD: Agency for Healthcare Research and Quality. Available at: http://www.ahrq.gov/data/hcup/highlight1/high1.htm.

Kristien Van Acker
Department of Endocrinology, St. Jozef Hospital, Bornem, Belgium

INTRODUCTION

Diabetes is described as a global epidemic of the 21st century. In 2007 over 246 million people were affected by diabetes, and this figure is estimated to rise to a total of 380 million by 2025. As a consequence, complications related to diabetes, including retinopathy, cardiovascular disease, nephropathy, and diabetic foot disease, are also on the rise.

Diabetic foot ulcers and amputations cost both society and individual patients an extremely large amount of money.

In 2005 the International Diabetes Federation (IDF) placed particular emphasis on "diabetic foot," and a special edition of the Lancet journal was dedicated to this specific complication of diabetes. The following statement was the most startling revelation: "Every 30 seconds, a lower limb is lost due to diabetes" (1). Up to 15% of patients with diabetes develop a foot ulcer at some stage, and over one million amputations are carried out each year as a result of diabetes-related complications. In 85% of cases, amputations are preceded by ulcers. Diabetic foot ulcers are examples of "critical limb ischemia" (CLI) disease. As stated in chapter 2, literature shows that at this stage of CLI, there are significant differences between patients with and without diabetes. In the TransAtlantic Inter-Society Consensus (TASC), the former have been recognized and distinguished in a separate subcategory of CLI, "diabetic foot ulcers" (2). The most important difference is the loss of pain perception due to neuropathy in patients with diabetes. As a result of this sensory loss, these patients will have no typical progress of ischemic disease and will rarely suffer from claudication or chronic rest pain in their legs. As the main focus of this chapter, neuropathy influences the time taken for patients to be referred as well as the diagnostic, therapeutic, and preventive approaches used for diabetic patients at risk of losing a foot or developing a foot ulcer.

HISTORICAL ASPECTS

In a recent article by Dr. Henry Connor, we can see why it took so many years before diabetic foot was recognized as an important complication and why it took even longer before diabetologists paid it enough attention, not only in daily practice but also for research purposes (3). An association between gangrene and diabetes was first recognized in 1852 by Marchal de Calvi, who also suggested a causal relationship between diabetes and peripheral nerve damage in 1864 (4,5). Despite these findings, ischemia and infection were seen as the major causes of diabetic foot disease, which led to a neglect of the role of neuropathy with a prolonged period of therapeutic stagnation as a consequence. For many years, disease of the lower limb in diabetic patients was conceptualized as "diabetic gangrene." Until about 1893, no distinction was made between gangrene due to vascular insufficiency and infective gangrene in a limb with a normal or almost normal blood supply. Local thrombosis, resulting in gangrene, because of severe infection is not often recognized by clinicians even today. It was Surgeon Godlee who recognized that the distinction was important because the prognosis in cases of gangrene associated with neuropathy and infection was potentially much better than that in those associated with vascular disease (6). At that time, this knowledge was already significant for considering minor amputation instead of major amputation. For many years, diabetic gangrene was the equivalent of undergoing major amputation and was frequently followed by a hyperglycemic coma and death. The discovery of insulin reduced the risk of surgical intervention, and diabetic foot replaced the hyperglycemic coma as the major cause of diabetes-related mortality. Together with the introduction of aseptic surgery and later on with the discovery of penicillin, the survival rates of diabetic patients with gangrene improved. The risk of infection and gangrene in the stump was diminished, and survival rates improved (7,8). In the same paper, Dr. Henry Connor describes the increasing workload attributable to diabetic foot disease reflected in a fourfold increase in the number of pages that Joslin, an important diabetologist in the early 1990s, devotes to the subject between the second and fourth editions of his textbooks (9). The teaching of diabetic foot care was considered so important that by 1928 the clinic at the Deaconess Hospital in Boston had assigned one graduate nurse and two student nurses to the duty (10). This can be already considered as one of the first multidisciplinary approaches. In the same hospital, the mortality rate following major amputations fell from 11.6% in 1923 to 1943 to 6.6% in 1944 to 1949 (before and after the introduction of penicillin) (11).

History clearly tells us, as well as the conclusion of Dr. Henry Connor, that so long as clinicians continued to think of diabetic foot lesions predominantly in negative terms like gangrene and amputation, it was—*and still is*—almost inevitable that they would—*and will*—do so expressing an attitude of therapeutic nihilism. Only in the 1980s, when more neutral terms were used such as neuropathic ulcer and diabetic foot disease, did diabetologists and surgeons open up to the possibility of therapeutic progress.

Andrew Boulton uses the Chinese proverb "Superior doctors prevent the disease. Mediocre doctors treat the disease before it becomes evident. Inferior doctors treat the full-blown disease" (Huang Dee, China, 2600 BC). He mentions that until recently, doctors entered the inferior category in terms of diabetic foot disease. A search on PubMed for articles published during 2007 on diabetic foot identifies 274 articles, compared with 14 published during 1980 (12), and *The Foot in Diabetes* European textbook is in its fourth edition (13).

EPIDEMIOLOGY, SOCIOECONOMICAL ASPECT, AND ORGANIZATION

The new consensus document of the International Working Group on the Diabetic Foot (IWGDF) includes the following statements (14):

Foot problems are common, very expensive, and life threatening.
Every 30 seconds, a lower limb is lost somewhere in the world as a consequence of diabetes.
Up to 70% of all lower leg amputations are performed on people with diabetes.
Up to 85% of all amputations are preceded by an ulcer.

In developed countries, up to 5% of people with diabetes have a diabetic foot ulcer; 12% to 15% of health care resources are used for diabetes. In developing countries, the latter figure may be as high as 40%.

The prevalence of lower extremity amputations ranges from 0.2% to 4.8%; the annual incidence ranges from 46.1 to 936 per 100,000 people with diabetes. The difference in incidence is in many cases due to differences in study design, demographic factors, and the prevalence of diabetes, as well as variations in registration systems and differences in the reimbursement of various procedures (15).

Singh et al. explains that up to 25% of patients with diabetes will develop a foot ulcer sometime during their lifetime, and even up to 2% of patients may already have undergone amputation (16).

As a consequence of all this data, it is clear that diabetic foot care needs to be improved in all diabetic centers around the world. All health care providers dealing with diabetes, ulcers, and revascularization techniques must be aware of the problem.

General practitioners (GPs) also play a crucial role in reducing amputation rates in diabetic patients. Any contact with a diabetic patient must begin with a foot examination by a member of staff. Mike Edmonds demonstrates that a multidisciplinary approach of diabetic foot ulcers can reduce the rate of amputation (17).

As already stated, the economical impact of amputation is important. Diabetic foot complications result in huge costs for individuals living with diabetes as well as both their families and society in general. Foot problems account for 12% to 15% of health care resources for diabetes. In developing countries, this figure may be as high as 40%. The cost of diabetic foot ulcers not requiring amputation ranges from US$1150 to US$35,758 (2005). The cost of amputation ranges from US$19,052 to US$66,176 (2005) (15,18).

More attention is being paid to the quality of life of patients with diabetic foot ulcers and amputees. Their quality of life has been diminished at the same rate as for patients with cancer or chronic kidney disease undergoing dialysis. The lives of people after amputation are profoundly affected. Many are unable to work, become dependent on others, and cannot pursue an active social life. In developing countries, the situation is even worse because the whole family has no income if the active member is suffering from a chronic ulcer or has undergone amputation.

PHYSIOPATHOLOGY

The physiopathology of the diabetic foot is rather complex. If diabetes is not controlled for several years, complications arise frequently. Vasculopathy and neuropathy are the most important complications leading to diabetic foot problems. Small traumas can have devastating effects. We need to consider three important steps: vasculopathy/neuropathy—trauma will lead to an ulcer—infection increases the risk of amputation, especially if the patient has poor peripheral circulation.

Neuropathy

In literature we can find a prevalence of diabetic neuropathy, ranging from 35% to 60% because of different diagnostic tools used (19–21). Diabetic neuropathy can develop silently and progressively and can have negative symptoms (loss of sensation) or positive symptoms such as paresthesia and allodynia, classified as painful neuropathy (22). *Sensory* neuropathy is characterized by a loss of sensation in terms of pressure, cold/warmth, and pain. This is the reason why patients can suffer injuries while walking barefoot or wearing inappropriate footwear, and because of this phenomenon, they may not even feel their injury or infection. This is also why they do not seek help early on. In more pronounced diabetic neuropathy, *motor deficit* will also arise. The clinical characteristics are atrophy of the intrinsic muscles of the feet. This causes the classic biomechanical changes of the foot with claw toes and prominent metatarsal heads. Here the diabetic patient will have higher pressure and shear stresses, and this will again increase the risk of ulcers. Limited joint mobility can also occur together with this neuropathy. By walking, the propulsion of the foot is disturbed, and these intrinsic changes will put high pressure on the first ray and cause ulcers when unadapted shoes are worn.

Autonomic neuropathy often occurs, and patients will suffer from dry skin and be therefore prone to small ulcers and infections.

Charcot

Charcot foot is a very rare but very typical diabetic foot complication with degenerative changes of the articulations and the subchondrial bone. Incidence ranges from about 0.1% to 0.4% and will occur after a long history of diabetes. Three stages may be recognized (23,24). *The acute stage* appears suddenly as a swollen, warm, and red foot, without any sign of infection or deep thrombosis. Early recognition is mandatory for successful treatment with total contact casting. *The coalescence stage* is the phase without acute edema. *The reconstructive stage* is when damage can be recognized with even subluxation and dislocation of articulations in the foot. Sanders describes the different locations, and we should also mention the prevalence: I, metatarsal phalanges, 18%; II, Lisfranc, 50%; III, Chopart, 20%; IV, ankle, 10%; V, calcaneum, 2% (25).

Vascular Disease

Peripheral arterial disease (PAD) is the most important factor relating to the outcome of a diabetic foot ulcer. The prevalence of PAD in people with diabetes is about four times more frequent than in nondiabetic patients and ranges from 10% to 40% depending on the definition used; approximately 50% of patients with foot ulcers show signs of PAD (15).

Peripheral vascular disease (PVD) in diabetic patients has specific characteristics. PVD will be present in these patients with diabetes at a younger age and is particularly plurisegmental and more often present in distal vessels. Mediasclerosis or Mönckeberg's disease is typical in diabetic patients with neuropathy, leading to more stiffness of the vascular tree and being the cause of more difficult diagnosis of vascular problems using Doppler techniques. Ankle and, occasionally, toe blood pressure readings may be falsely high because of this medial sclerosis. Rest pain due to ischemia may be absent in people with diabetes—probably because of peripheral neuropathy.

In all the multidisciplinary foot clinics in the Western world, a shift has been observed over the last 20 years from neuropathic ulcers to more complex neuroischemic ulcers. It is believed that improved diabetes care of patients and improved prevention strategies play a major role in these changes. On the other hand, we now see more difficult ulcers and gangrene because PVD plays a major role. For this reason, a good knowledge of diagnosis and therapy of PVD is becoming more and more important.

Infections and Osteomyelitis

Infection in a diabetic foot must be seen as a medical emergency. Treatment must be aggressive because such infections increase the risk of amputation, particularly in patients suffering from PVD. This requires prolonged antibiotic therapy, ongoing podiatry input, and one or more surgical procedures. In most cases, infection progresses deeper than expected. Careful diagnosis is essential, and the high risk of osteomyelitis must be recognized. Deep infections are possible without the patient feeling any pain.

Typical clinical signs of infection are not always present: serious infection may occur without fever, elevation of C-reactive protein (CRP), or sedimentation or leucocytosis. Osteomyelitis may occur without redness or other clinical signs such as edema, warmth, etc. Most diabetic foot infections are polymicrobial, and a good microbiological sample is essential. Several studies suggest that osteomyelitis occurs in about 20% of diabetic patients suffering from a foot infection, although in some patients it may also be present with ulcers showing no clinical evidence of inflammation (26). In limb-threatening infections, this figure may rise to over 60% (27).

Risk Classification

With a view toward prevention, work was carried out in the IWGDF on risk classification. This can help us discover further prevention strategies. In Belgium this classification was arranged in five classes. Class 0 for no risk at all and class 3 as a high-risk profile needing intensive follow-up by nurses, podiatrists, general practitioners, patients, and their families. National prevention strategies can be based on this classification. The PEDIS classification or Wagner classification can help health care providers in their daily clinical work involving diagnosis and therapy.

Class 0: No NP or foot deformities
Class 1: Neuropathy (NP) present
Class 2a: NP + orthopedic deformities with acceptable mobility
Class 2b: NP + orthopedic deformities with important rigidity
Class 3: PVD (PEDIS P2-P3, see below)
    Charcot deformations (acute or chronic)
    History of foot ulcer
    History of minor or major amputations

Various systems have been developed to classify diabetic foot ulcers for daily practice. Moreover, no system has been universally accepted for research purposes, which has clearly hampered communication in the field of research. In 2003 the IWDGF introduced, as a progress report, its classification system (PEDIS) for research purposes, which is described in this chapter. This system was developed by experts involved in clinical research from all over the world and was based on the experience gained from using earlier classification systems.

On the basis of scientific literature and expert opinion, five categories were identified, which were considered the most relevant items for research projects in diabetic foot ulcers (15): Perfusion, Extent/size, Depth/tissue loss, Infection, and Sensation. The consensus document should be referred to for further information.

The Wagner-Meggit classification is the oldest classification used. Probe-to-bone test is essential to make a good clinical diagnosis and to recognize the "hidden" osteomyelitis. Another frequently used classification is the TEXAS classification. The vascularization status was integrated in this system.

DIAGNOSIS OF DIABETIC FOOT PROBLEMS
Neuropathy
A good anamnesis is necessary in cases of painful neuropathy. In Europe a simple tool is used, called the DN4 *score*. If four or more items are positive, this test will diagnose neuropathy with a sensitivity of 80% and a specificity of 90% (28).

In daily practice, it is essential to carry out an annual neurological examination of the feet of all patients suffering from diabetes. This examination can include testing of vibratory sense using a 128-Hz tuning fork, discrimination using a pin and deep sensation using a "tendon hammer" (Achilles tendon reflex). In addition to this simple examination, Semmes-Weinstein monofilaments can be used as a semiquantitative test. Prospective studies have shown that the inability to perceive the 10-g monofilament (5.07) on the toes or dorsum of the foot predicts the future occurrence of a diabetic foot ulcer. The advantages of this test are its simplicity and low cost. Nerve conduction studies (NCS) are able to measure the ability of peripheral nerves to conduct electrical signals. The test is abnormal where there are pathological changes in the nerve marrow, the nodes of Ranvier, or the axons. This test is very accurate, but it is not possible to test the small fibers that are frequently involved in painful neuropathy, in superficial pain disturbances, or in the capacity of distinction of warm/cold sensations.

Vasculopathy
Symptoms
When adequate collateral vessels compensate for arterial occlusion, there may be no symptoms at rest, but intermittent claudication may occur when the demand for blood flow increases, for example, during walking. However, <25% of individuals with PAD and diabetes report intermittent claudication, which means that 75% of people with diabetes have so-called "asymptomatic" disease. End-stage symptoms are rest pain—particularly at night—and ulceration/gangrene. Many of these patients also have few symptoms despite extensive tissue loss—probably because of peripheral neuropathy (15,29).

Identifying Peripheral Arterial Disease
Experts from the international consensus of IWGDF recommend that the vascular status of people with diabetes should be examined on an annual basis, paying particular attention to the following (15,29):

1. A history of intermittent claudication or ischemic rest pain is to be distinguished from a history of pain caused by peripheral neuropathy.
2. Palpation of pulses in the posterior tibial and dorsalis pedis arteries is mandatory.

3. Potential signs of critical ischemia are blanching of the feet on elevation, dependent rubor, ulceration, skin necrosis, and gangrene.

Noninvasive Vascular Investigation
Given the uncertainties of history and clinical examination, more objective measurements of skin perfusion are frequently needed. Commonly used techniques include ankle pressure, toe pressure, and (less frequently) transcutaneous oxygen pressure ($TcPO_2$) measurements. These noninvasive vascular tests can be used for

diagnosis and quantification of PAD,
predicting wound healing of a diabetic foot ulcer, and
follow-up and control of treatment.

In a recent study comparing different methods for PAD screening in people with diabetes, the sensitivity of ABI in neuropathic patients was only 53%; significant PVD should always be considered in a patient with a non-healing ulcer—even if no clinical signs of PAD are present and noninvasive testing is not clearly abnormal. In these patients, repeated evaluation may be necessary, and, according to experts, angiography should be considered in a chronic nonhealing ulcer after six weeks of optimal treatment (15).

Osteomyelitis
In the new consensus document of the IWGDF, special attention is paid to the classification of osteomyelitis. A systematic approach is mandatory for every patient with diabetic foot ulceration and infection, as described later on (15).

We consider the following examinations as important for the diagnosis of a possible osteomyelitis.

Probe-to-bone test: After debriding any callus or necrotic material in the wound, a probe-to-bone test should be carried out. A negative result substantially reduces the probability of osteomyelitis, while a positive result makes it more likely. Visible bone or discharging bone fragments also suggest bone infection.

Plain radiographs of the foot: This should be obtained in most cases of suspected osteomyelitis. Bone changes may not become visible until some weeks after the infection. The clinician should always consider the possibility of Charcot neuro-osteoarthropathy.

Isotope bone scanning: This is not really recommended any longer because of its lack of specificity. Noninfectious processes may cause positive scans.

Magnetic resonance imaging (MRI): If available, MRI is useful for proposing the diagnosis, evaluating the extent of bone and soft tissue involvement, and planning surgery or a percutaneous biopsy. White blood cell or antibody scans are alternatives but are inferior in terms of their anatomical resolution and diagnostic value.

Bone biopsy: Bone biopsy for both culture and histopathology, if available, is useful for confirming the diagnosis and for isolating the etiological agent(s) to allow targeted antibiotic therapy. A bone specimen may safely be obtained percutaneously through uninfected skin or as part of an operative procedure. Where possible, antibiotics should be discontinued (for at least

48 hours and preferably up to two weeks) before the biopsy to maximize the yield from cultures; however, the optimal time interval is not known.

The optimal criteria for diagnosing osteomyelitis are not known; however, the IWGDF committee has proposed a scheme for research purposes to assess probability on the basis of various clinical, imaging, and laboratory findings.

Because of a lack of resources and expertise in various locations, many cases currently have to be managed without complex imaging or reliable bone biopsies.

The levels of diagnostic certainty have been arranged into the following four categories:

- *Definite* (posttest probability >90%; "beyond reasonable doubt")
  - Bone sample with positive culture *and* positive histology *OR*
  - Purulence in bone found at surgery *OR*
  - Detached bone fragment removed from ulcer by podiatrist/surgeon *OR*
  - Intraosseous abscess found on MRI *OR*
  - *Any two probable* criteria *OR one* probable *and two* possible criteria *OR any four possible* criteria below

- *Probable* (on the balance of probability, i.e., posttest probability 51% to 90%; "more likely than not")
  - Visible cancellous bone in ulcer *OR*
  - MRI showing bone edema with other signs of osteomyelitis *OR*
  - Bone sample with positive culture but negative or absent histology *OR*
  - Bone sample with positive histology but negative or absent culture *OR*
  - Any two *possible* criteria below

- *Possible* (posttest probability 10–50%; but on balance, less rather than more likely)
  - XR shows cortical destruction *OR*
  - MRI shows bone edema or cloaca *OR*
  - Positive probe-to-bone test or visible cortical bone *OR*
  - ESR >70 mm/hr with no other plausible explanation *OR*
  - Nonhealing wound despite adequate off-loading and perfusion for >6 weeks *OR*
  - Ulcer of >2 weeks duration with clinical evidence of infection

- *Unlikely* (posttest probability <10%)
  - No signs of symptoms of inflammation *AND*
  - Normal X ray *AND*
  - Ulcer present for <2 weeks or absent *AND*
  - If ulcer present, superficial *AND*
  - Normal MRI *AND*
  - Normal bone scan

This scheme also recognizes that the diagnosis of osteomyelitis in diabetic foot problems may not be made or excluded at one point in time but may become increasingly more or less likely as the management of a patient evolves. In likelihood, the diagnostic certainty of osteomyelitis will therefore move up or down as more information is gathered, sometimes over a period of days or even weeks. There are many situations, however, when the diagnosis is either immediately evident or can be excluded with a high degree of confidence. These different degrees of certainty of diagnosis have implications for therapy (15).

THERAPIES
Neuropathy
There are currently no pharmacological treatments with major beneficial effects on the natural history of peripheral diabetic neuropathy, which is a slow but progressive loss of nerve fibers. However, there are pharmacological agents that can relieve symptoms in painful neuropathy. Gabapantines are used more and more nowadays. If diabetic neuropathy is diagnosed, the only treatment option currently available is tight metabolic control to slow the progression of disease, as shown by the DCCT (30) and U.K. Prospective Diabetes Study (UKPDS) trials (31).

Vasculopathy
In patients with foot ulcers, the probability of wound healing should be based on clinical examination and on noninvasive vascular tests. If the probability of healing is deemed to be too low or if the patient has persistent ischemic rest pain, revascularization should always be considered. A second indication for revascularization can be intermittent claudication. Other chapters of this book should be referred to for more details of revascularization since this section contains only general information.

In general, when endovascular revascularization and open repair or bypass of a specific lesion produce equivalent results, endovascular techniques should be used first, given their lower risks and costs (32). A revascularization procedure is technically possible in most patients suffering from critical ischemia. Given that excellent results have been published on distal reconstruction in patients with diabetes, a more aggressive approach to revascularization procedures should be promoted (33). Revascularization should always be considered before a major amputation.

Pharmacological therapy to maintain patency after vascular reconstruction is a controversial topic, although aspirin is used by the majority of vascular surgeons (15). According to recent TASC II guidelines, patients should participate in a clinical surveillance program after bypass surgery, which should be performed in the immediate postoperative period and at regular intervals (usually every 6 months) for at least two years (2).

Risk Factor Modification
Cardiovascular morbidity and mortality are markedly increased in patients with PAD.

Therefore, treatment of neuroischemic ulcers should not be solely focused on the foot but should also aim to reduce the poor survival rate. In patients without diabetes, cessation of smoking has been shown to decrease the risk of developing intermittent claudication and decrease the subsequent risk of amputation. Moreover, if the patient stops smoking, patency rates for vascular reconstruction are higher and the risk of death is lower.

Although there are no studies that demonstrate that treating hypertension and dyslipidemia has any beneficial effect on ischemic foot problems, experts strongly advise that these factors be treated aggressively. In addition, patients with PAD should be treated with low-dose aspirin to reduce vascular comorbidity (15).

Osteomyelitis

Treatment must be aggressive because these infections increase the risk of amputation, especially in patients with PVD. This requires prolonged antibiotic therapy, ongoing podiatry input, and one or more surgical procedures.

The removal of devitalized and infected tissue to control infection and to create an environment favorable to healing, while maximizing the structural and physical integrity of the foot, is regarded as the central goal of surgical intervention in diabetic foot infections. However, inspection of the current data indicates that in the treatment of osteomyelitis, there is little evidence to help choose between medical and surgical therapies, with success rates in the region of 60% to 90% with both approaches. There are no randomized trials or controlled studies directly comparing outcomes with surgery versus medical therapy. Any benefit from surgery in achieving earlier wound healing and arrest of osteomyelitis may be offset by the adverse long-term sequel of foot deformity from bone loss leading to recurrent or transfer ulceration. From the studies assessed in the systematic review, it was not possible to establish whether in patients failing on antibiotic therapy and requiring surgery, the prolonged antibiotic therapy had compromised their subsequent surgical outcome (15,34–36).

None of the studies analyzed demonstrated the superiority of one antibiotic agent over another. Antibiotics with activity predominantly against gram-positive organisms (*Staphylococci* and *Streptococci*) (37) and broad-spectrum antibiotics with additional increased activity against gram-negative organisms and anerobes (38) appear equally efficacious in the management of osteomyelitis. These findings confirm the results of a recent review of the antibiotic management of all types of osteomyelitis (39). While it is not known whether or not the selected antibiotic regimen must be active against all of the isolated organisms from a polymicrobial infection, anti-staphylococcal therapy is almost always warranted. There are no clinical data in diabetic foot osteomyelitis supporting the contention that any particular antibiotic penetrates better into bone. The most appropriate duration of therapy remains elusive. Studies with durations of therapy ranging from two weeks following aggressive surgical debridement (that was most commonly minor amputation) (27) to a mean of 42 weeks (without surgery) (40) have shown comparable results in different studies.

No comparative studies of different durations of antibiotic therapy were found. There are data to support the treatment of patients with intravenous therapy (27), oral antimicrobials (40,41), or step-down therapy from short-duration intravenous therapy to follow on oral therapy (42). No studies could be identified that assessed the efficacy of locally administered antibiotics, for example, in antibiotic-impregnated polymethylmethacrylate or calcium sulfate beads, in diabetic foot osteomyelitis. No particular route of administration has achieved obviously superior results in the studies that were reviewed. We refer to the new classification of the IWGDF on osteomyelitis for therapeutic strategy (see page 282 for diagnosis), which is as follows:

Definite (beyond reasonable doubt) >90%: treat for osteomyelitis

Probable (more likely than not) 51% to 90%: consider treating, but further investigation may be needed

Possible (but on balance, less rather than more likely) 10% to 50%: treatment may be justifiable, but further investigation is usually advised

Unlikely <10%: usually no need for further investigation or treatment

Prevention

Relatively little research has been conducted into the specific effect of education on the incidence of ulcers or amputations. Nevertheless, it is recommended that, as part of a comprehensive foot care program, education should be targeted at high-risk categories of patients, particularly where resources are scarce. Education needs to be directed at professionals as well as patients. Recognition of the at-risk foot and early lesions is the most important responsibility of health care professionals. Unfortunately, foot examination is often neglected despite clear guidelines and recommendations. The objective of education is to change the self-care behavior of the person with diabetes and to enhance adherence to foot care advice (i.e., prescribed shoes). Furthermore, people with diabetes should recognize potential foot problems and then take appropriate action (i.e., seek professional help). Education should be simple, relevant, consistent, and repeated (43). Furthermore, physicians and other health care professionals should receive periodic education and reinforcement of diabetes management skills to improve the care delivered to high-risk individuals (15).

INTERNATIONAL NETWORKS AND ORGANIZATIONS

In the Fifth International Symposium on the Diabetic Foot in the Netherlands, Professor Peter R. Cavanagh from Cleveland, United States was presenting the prestigious Diabetic Foot Award. He tried to give his view on the future for the diabetic foot world. He contacted a lot of experts on the field. Professor Cavanagh divided the experts' prediction into three areas: innovators, policy makers, and implementers (12). Especially, attention was given to the importance of implementation: "several experts suggested that better organization and health care delivery would improve diabetic foot care." He himself reported in 2008 that diabetes-related lower extremity amputations in North England reduced over a five-year period of time during which improvements in the organization of diabetes care were implemented (14). Nowadays, vascular surgeons are more than ever part of the team!

REFERENCES

1. Horton R. Herceptin and early breast cancer: a moment for caution. Lancet 2005; 366:1673–1750.
2. Norgren L, Hiatt WR, Dormandy JA, et al.; for TASC II Working Group. Inter-society consensus for the management of peripheral arterial disease (TASC II). J Vasc Surg 2007; 45(suppl S):S5–S67.
3. Connor H. Some historical aspects of diabetic foot disease. Diabetes Metab Res Rev 2008; 24(suppl 1):S7–S13.
4. Marchal de Calvi A. Des rapports de la gangrene et de la glycosurie. Gazette des Hôpitaux Civils et militaries 1852; 25:178.
5. Marchal de Calvi A. Recherches Sur Les Accidents Diabetiques, Et Essai D'une Theorie Generale Du Diabete. Paris: Asselin, 1864.
6. Godlee RJ. On amputation for diabetic gangrene. Med Chir Trans 1893; 76:37–55.
7. Treves F. A System of Surgery. Vol 1. London: Cassell and Co. Ltd., 1895:268–269.
8. Keen WW, White JW. A Textbook of Surgery for Practitioners and Students. Vol 1. London: WB Saunders and Co., 1903:67.
9. Joslin EP. The Treatment of Diabetes Mellitus. 2nd ed. Philadelphia: Lea and Febiger, 1917:423–427; 4th ed. 1928:785–802.
10. McKittrick LS, Root HF. In: Diabetic Surgery. Philadelphia: Lea and Febiger, 1928: 92–104.

11. McKittrick LS. Recent advances in the care of the surgical complications of diabetes mellitus. N Engl J Med 1946; 235:929–932.
12. Boulton AJM. The diabetic foot: grand overview, epidemiology and pathogenesis. Diabetes Metab Res Rev 2008; 24(suppl 1):S3–S6.
13. Boulton AJM, Cavanagh PR, Rayman G. The Foot in Diabetes. 4th ed. Chichester: John Wiley and Sons, 2006:1–449.
14. Cavanagh RJ, Unwin NC, Connolly VM, et al. Diabetes and non–diabetes related lower extremity amputation incidence before and after the introduction of better organized diabetes foot care. Diabetes Care 2008:31.
15. Bakker K. International Consensus on the Diabetic Foot & Practical Guidelines and Management and Prevention of the Diabetic Foot. Amsterdam, The Netherlands: International Working Group on the Diabetic Foot, 2007.
16. Singh N, Armstrong DG, Lipsky BA. Preventing foot ulcers in patients with diabetes. JAMA 2005; 293:217–228.
17. Edmonds ME, Blundell MP, Morris ME, et al. Improved survival of the diabetic foot: the role of specialised fot clinic. Q J Med 1986; 60:763–771.
18. Boulton AJM, Vileikyte L, Ragnarson Tennvall G, et al. The global burden of diabetic foot disease. Lancet 2005; 366:1719–1724.
19. Boulton AJM, Gries FA, Jervell JA. Guidelines for the outpatient diagnosis and management of diabetic peripheral neuropathy. Diabet Med 1998; 15:508–514.
20. Boulton AJM, Malik RA, Arezzo JC, et al. Diabetic somatic neuropathies: a technical review. Diabetes Care 2004; 27:1458–1486.
21. Boulton AJM, Vinik AI, Arezzo JC, et al. American diabetes association. Diabetic neuropathies: a statement by the American Diabetes Association. Diabetes Care 2005; 28:956–962.
22. Argoff CE, Backonja MM, Belgrade MJ, et al. Consensus guidelines: treatment planning and options. Diabetic peripheral neuropathic pain. Mayo Clin Proc 2006; 81(4 suppl):S12–S25.
23. Armstrong DG, Todd WF, Harkless LB, et al. The natural history of acute Charcot's arthropathy in a diabetic foot specialty clinic. Diabet Med 1997; 14:357–363.
24. Schon LC, Easley ME, Weinfeld SB. Charcot neuroarthropathy of the foot and ankle. Clin Orthop Relat Res 1998; 349:116–131.
25. Sanders LJ, Frykberg RG. Charcot neuroarthropathy of the foot. In: Levin ME, O'Neal LW, Bowker JH, et al., eds. The Diabetic Foot. 6th ed. St Louis: Mosby, 2001:439–465.
26. Newman LG, Waller J, Palestro CJ, et al. Unsuspected osteomyelitis in diabetic foot ulcers. Diagnosis and monitoring by leukocyte scanning with indium in 111 oxy-quinoline. JAMA 1991; 266(9):1246–1251.
27. Grayson ML, Gibbons GW, Habershaw GM, et al. Use of ampicillin/sulbactam versus imipenem/cilastatin in the treatment of limb-threatening foot infections in diabetic patients. Clin Infect Dis 1994; 18(5):683–693.
28. Bouhassira D, Attal N, Alchaar H, et al. Comparison of pain syndromes associated with nervous or somatic lesions and development of a new neuropathic pain diagnostic questionnaire (DN4). Pain 2005; 114:29–36.
29. Williams DT, Harding KG, Price P. An evaluation of the efficacy of methods used in screening for lower-limb arterial disease in diabetes. Diabetes Care 2005; 28:2206–2210.
30. The DCCT Research Group. The effect of intensive treatment of diabetes on the development and progression of long-term complications in insulin-dependent diabetes mellitus. N Engl J Med 1993; 329:977–986.
31. UK Prospective Diabetes Study Group. Intensive blood-glucose control with sulphonylureas or insulin compared with conventional treatment and risk of complications in patients with type 2 diabetes (UKPDS 33). Lancet 1998; 352:837–853.
32. Adam DJ, Beard JD, Cleveland T, et al.; BASIL trial participants. Bypass versus angioplasty in severe ischaemia of the leg (BASIL): multicentre, randomised controlled trial. Lancet 2005; 366:1925–1934.
33. Faglia E, Mantero M, Caminiti M, et al. Extensive use of peripheral angioplasty, particularly infrapopliteal, in the treatment of ischaemic diabetic foot ulcers: clinical

results of a multicentric study of 221 consecutive diabetic subjects. J Intern Med 2002; 252:225–232.

34. Lipsky BA. Osteomyelitis of the foot in diabetic patients. Clin Infect Dis 1997; 25(6):1318–1326.
35. Lipsky BA. A report from the international consensus on diagnosing and treating the infected diabetic foot. Diabetes Metab Res Rev 2004; 20(suppl 1):S68–S77.
36. Lipsky BA, Berendt AR, Deery HG II, et al. IDSA Guidelines: diagnosis and treatment of diabetic foot infections. Clin Infect Dis 2004; 39:885–910.
37. Lipsky BA, Itani K, Norden C. Treating foot infections in diabetic patients: a randomized, multicenter, open-label trial of linezolid versus ampicillin-sulbactam/amoxicillin-clavulanate. Clin Infect Dis 2004; 38(1):17–24.
38. Lipsky BA, Armstrong DG, Citron DM, et al. Ertapenem versus piperacillin/tazobactam for diabetic foot infections (SIDESTEP): prospective, randomised, controlled, double-blinded, multicentre trial. Lancet 2005; 366(9498):1695–1703.
39. Lazzarini L, Lipsky BA, Mader JT. Antibiotic treatment of osteomyelitis: what have we learned from 30 years of clinical trials? Int J Infect Dis 2005; 9(3):127–138.
40. Embil JM, Rose G, Trepman E, et al. Oral antimicrobial therapy for diabetic foot osteomyelitis. Foot Ankle Int 2006; 27(10):771–779.
41. Senneville E, Yazdanpanah Y, Cazaubiel M, et al. Rifampicin-ofloxacin oral regimen for the treatment of mild to moderate diabetic foot osteomyelitis. J Antimicrob Chemother 2001; 48:927–930.
42. Lipsky BA, Baker PD, Landon GC, et al. Antibiotic therapy for diabetic foot infections: comparison of two parenteral-to-oral regimens. Clin Infect Dis 1997; 24(4):643–648.
43. Edmonds ME, Van Acker K, Foster AVM. Education and the diabetic foot. Diabet Med 1996; 13(suppl 1):561–564.

17 Aggressive Wound Healing Strategies

Koen Deloose and Marc Bosiers
Department of Vascular Surgery, AZ St-Blasius, Dendermonde, Belgium

Jürgen Verbist and Patrick Peeters
Department of Cardiovascular and Thoracic Surgery, Imelda Hospital, Bonheiden, Belgium

INTRODUCTION

Chronic wounds are often recalcitrant to healing and often do not follow the expected tract. They are disabling and constitute a significant burden on both the patients' daily life activities and the health care system. It is estimated that lower leg ulcers affect 1% of the adult population and 3.6% of people older than 65 years (1). About 72% of all leg ulcers are associated with venous insufficiency (venous stasis ulcers) (Fig. 1A), 15% with both venous and arterial disorders, and 7% with arterial disorders only (Fig. 1B) (2). One of the most challenging problems in wound care is the diabetic foot pathology. Annually, 2% to 3% of the diabetic population develops a foot ulcer (Fig. 1C), while the lifetime risk to develop a foot ulcer is as high as 25% in diabetics (3). With an expected diabetic boom and an aging society, this problem will rise tremendously.

Over the past few years, the explosion of knowledge related to molecular biology, genetics, and basic science has catapulted wound care and wound healing as a field to the forefront of interest as an exciting but increasingly complex medical speciality.

Also the issue of shorter hospital stays, advocated by patients and families themselves, governments, insurances, and hospital authorities, asks for immediate and efficient solutions for more complex problems.

Holistic patient assessment forms an integral part of wound assessment. A wound can never be treated without the unique physiological and psychological aspects of the human being (4). The history of the patient must be very complete as it guides the practitioner to the proper tests and measurements to determine the underlying cause of the wound and the characteristics that would affect the outcome of different intervention strategies. A thorough anamnesis of the medical and surgical history is obligatory in the screening of disorders that could aggravate the wound, delay healing, or impair efficient wound care. The meticulous documentation of patients' current and chronic medication is an essential step. Medication has a systemic influence on wound healing: some have detrimental effects on the healing process, while others have an important interactive effect on modern wound dressings.

To deal with this challenging problem, the author will incorporate the wound bed preparation model into a practical clinical guide for the treatment of chronic wounds. Central to this paradigm is the importance of treating the underlying cause prior to the local optimization of the wound. The three important components of local wound care that are essential for the optimal wound bed preparation are tissue state (T), infection (I), and moisture balance (M). If the wound bed preparation is optimized and the healing is stalled, the

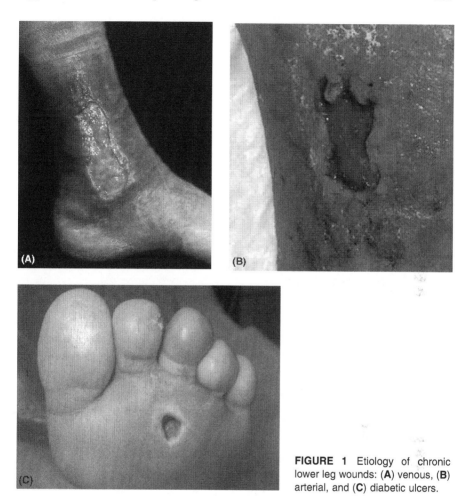

FIGURE 1 Etiology of chronic lower leg wounds: **(A)** venous, **(B)** arterial, and **(C)** diabetic ulcers.

additional edge (E) of slow-healing wounds represents the potential use of advanced active therapies to stimulate healing (TIME).

The key components and relevant questions relating to chronic wound management are the following:

- Causes of the wound; Are these treatable or correctable?
- Local wound factors: T, I, and M
- Other treatments to promote faster woundedge migration after local wound care has been optimized : E

CAUSES OF THE WOUND

It is important to make an accurate diagnosis and correct the cause as a first step. Clinicians must optimize compression therapy in venous disease. Plantar pressure redistribution is obligatory for diabetic neurotrophic foot ulcers. For arterial ulcer management, the plan of care must involve the revascularization and an efficient antithrombotic management.

The healability of a wound is determined by the treatability of its cause, the adequacy of the blood supply, and the coexisting conditions or drugs that may prevent healing (5). The most important requirement for a healable wound is an adequate tissue perfusion. In addition, the presence of decreased vasculature will increase the risk of infection. In case of leg or foot ulcers, the blood supply is usually adequate for the healing process if there is a palpable pulse ($\geq$80 mmHg). If the pulse is not palpable, Doppler examination of the ankle-brachial index (ABI) is necessary to determine healability. An ABI over 0.5 is considered sufficient for adequate blood supply, although calcified vessels can create false elevations. A transcutaneous oxygen tension measurement (>30 mmHg for healing) or a toe pressure measurement (>55 mmHg for healing) is a good alternative determinator.

LOCAL WOUND FACTORS
Tissue State
The wound bed is optimally prepared by aggressive and regular debridements of any firm eschar, necrotic tissue (Fig. 2A), soft fibrin slough (Fig. 2B), and wound fluids. Necrotic tissue serves as a proinflammatory stimulus inhibiting healing while soft yellow fibrin and wound fluids act as culture media for bacterial proliferation. Debridement may also promote healing by removing senescent cells that are deficient in cellular activities and biofilms that shield the

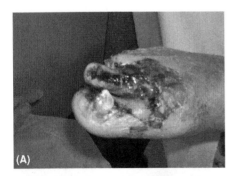

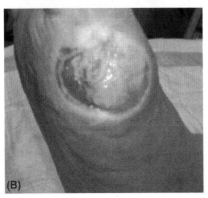

FIGURE 2 Optimal wound bed preparation requires debridement of any (**A**) necrotic tissue and (**B**) soft fibrine slough.

bacterial colonies. Although sharp surgical debridement is the most expeditious, this method may not always be feasible due to pain and bleeding. Alternatively, autolytic debridement can be created by moist wound environments (saline/ ringer/sterile water solutions) to enhance the activities of phagocytic cells and endogenous enzymes on nonviable tissues. However, a regular repeated hydrating of the gauze dressing, even several times a day, or the renewal of the dressing will be required. This is sometimes difficult to maintain in the home-care setting, leading to the selection of more advanced dressings (hydrogels, hydrocolloid dressings, hydropolymer/foam dressings, or alginates) for practical reasons. Enzymatic debridement with dedicated dressings and gels are also well placed for efficient debridements in the homecare setting. Mechanical debridement by wet-to-dry dressings is mostly painful and can create a lot of trauma. Emerging technology using ultrasonic devices and pulse spray cleaners has also been demonstrated to prepare wound beds without painful and traumatic scraping and cutting.

Infection

The presence of microorganisms (wound bioburden), predominantly bacteria but also fungi, can have profound effect on wound healing (6). These organisms, which can be acquired from the surrounding skin, other areas of the body, or the environment, may or may not be pathogens. It is likely that a heavy wound bioburden is the single most important and common factor in the development of pathological wound healing. For the understanding of the events of infection, the difference between contamination, colonization, critical colonization, and infection is important (7). Presence of pathogens in low or moderate numbers (contamination, colonization) is in most cases still kept at a healthy level by the host immune response. Although we know that the colonization by certain bacteria, particularly β-hemolytic streptococci and some anaerobes, of a wound without clinical signs of infection can delay healing (8). This clearly establishes a rationale for control of bioburden as a prophylactic measure to optimize healing. The expression of and evolution to critical colonization and finally infection is individually different and depends on the strength of the hosts' immune response.

As depicted in Table 1, a wide range of important pathogens can be identified in wound infection (9). The number of pathogens (bioburden of

TABLE 1 Range of Important Pathogens in Wound Infection

Escherichia coli
Bacteroides species, e.g., *fragilis*
Enterococcus faecalis
Staphylococcus aureus
Staphylococcus epidermidis
Pseudomonas aeruginosa
Resistant bacterial strains (MRSA, VRE)
Proteus species, e.g., *mirabilis*
Peptostreptococci species, e.g., *asaccharolyticus*
Prevotella species, e.g., *melaninogenica*
β-hemolytic streptococci
Candida albicans

Abbreviations: MRSA, methicillin-resistant *Staphylococcus aureus*; VRE, vancomycin-resistant *Enterococci*.

>10^5 CFU/gm tissue (10)), the type (varying from the so-called commensals or normal skin flora over common infection pathogens to especially virulent and even resistant pathogens), their behavior (creation of biofilms, adhesins, plasmids, and invasins), the specific exo- and endotoxins, the host resistance (uncontrolled edema, smoking, diabetes, poor nutrition, drugs, and so on), the hypoxia in the wound area, and the presence of necrotic tissue will influence the occurrence and course of a wound infection.

Numerous clinical signs and symptoms accompany wound infection. Classic signs are the presence of erythema (local or spreading) and/or pus (abscess formation) (Fig. 3).

Nonhealing of the wound despite appropriate interventions (normally wound size should decrease 30% after four weeks of appropriate treatment and heal by week 12) or an important change in the amount and characteristics (sanguineous, purulent, and so on) of wound exudate can be indicative of bacterial imbalance. A friable, bright red, easily bleeding, and exuberant granulation tissue (granulation tissue should be pink and firm) or the presence of a smell (gram-negative or anaerobe putrid odor or unpleasant sweet odor from pseudomonas) (Fig. 4) reflects bacterial damage.

For treatment indications, it is mainly important to separate superficial from deep infections. The clinician should distinguish superficial wounds with

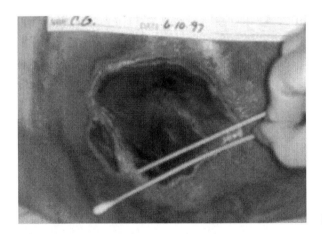

FIGURE 3 Infected wound.

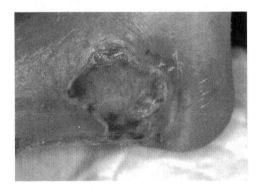

FIGURE 4 Pseudomonas.

increased bacterial burden that may respond to topical antimicrobials from deeper localized infections that usually require the use of systemic antibiotic agents. An increased size from bacterial damage and an increased temperature of the surrounding area are often due to the bacteria spreading from the surface to the surrounding skin and deeper compartments. New satellite areas of skin breakdown that are separated from the main ulcer and exposition of bone (osteomyelitis) are indicative of deep infection. In recent years, studies on chronic wound microbiology have shown that colonizing and/or infecting organisms populate the surface of the wound and deeper tissues beneath the wound bed. Furthermore, synergy and competition between these populations act to control their virulence and growth characteristics (11). Sampling of both superficial and deep wound microflora has to be done by swabbing and deep tissue sampling (especially in complex wounds and diabetic ulcers with complex microbiological environments). Increasingly, more bacterial strains with specific antibiotic resistance are complicating the therapy of infected wounds. For the most important wound infection pathogens, methicillin-resistant *Staphylococcus aureus* (MRSA) has to be named in the first place for clinical significance. Further problematic bacteria with great importance for wound infections are the high degree vancomycin-resistant *Enterococci* (VRE). In the field of wound therapy, only treatment options that avoid topical antibiotic administration and reduce systemic therapy only to where it is necessary should be considered. The use of selected topical antimicrobial agents could be used as a preventive intervention to avoid wound deterioration toward critical colonization and infection. An essential component of preventive treatment is to reduce wound bioburden at an early stage. Wounds may be irrigated with antiseptics, saline, Ringer's solution, or sterile water to remove necrotic tissue and wound fluids.

For the treatment of deep or spreading wounds, appropriate systemic antibiotic therapy has to be selected according to the local practice. This is usually "broad spectrum" in the beginning, but, ideally, it should be according to the identified pathogens after microbiological testing of a deep tissue sample (selective antibiotic therapy) (12). The duration of therapy depends on the improvement in the previously discussed clinical parameters. During systemic therapy, one should consider the development of (multi-) resistant pathogens.

Topical antibiotics, such as antibiotic-containing powders or antibiotic-impregnated gauzes, are generally unsuitable for the elimination of wound infection. Antibiotics administered by this route do not penetrate the different tissue layers, and this can result in resistance development of pathogens, skin sensitizing (hypersensitivity, allergy, and irritation), impaired healing, and sometimes superinfections (13).

Topical antiseptics need a broad-acting spectrum, a low potential for resistance, and inactivation by the wound exudate, low cytotoxic profile, and a low risk of side effects (irritation, allergy, contact dermatitis). Iodine or chlorhexidine compounds and especially silver compounds are dedicated for this application. It is well known from book chapters and review articles that basically all silver salts possess antimicrobial features (14). Especially the silver ions react strongly with membrane-associated and cytoplasm functional bacterial enzymes, create structural damage to the bacterial cell wall, and interact with the bacterial DNA. Silver is not toxic to human tissue as has been demonstrated through centuries of use (15).

Moisture Balance

Appropriate moisture is required to facilitate the action of growth factors, cytokines, and migration of cells including fibroblasts and keratinocytes. Moisture balance is a delicate act: Excessive moisture (Fig. 5A) can potentially cause damage to the surrounding skin by maceration and skin breakdown (16), while inadequate moisture (Fig. 5B) in the wound environment can impede cellular activities and promote eschar formation resulting in poor wound healing.

A suitable modern wound dressing should be able to maintain a moist wound environment over a prolonged period. A period of at least 24 hours is useful to allow sufficient outpatient wound care and prevent drying-out of the wound. Moist gauzes with saline or Ringer solution are the cheapest way to realize moist wound healing. They also cause mechanical autolytic debridement and have antibacterial properties. However, a regular repeated hydrating of the gauze dressing, even several times a day, or renewal of the dressing will be required. This is very unpractical to maintain in the homecare setting, leading to the selection of more advanced dressings for practical reasons. Hydrogels are semipermeable, nonadherent, semitransparent cross-linked hydrophilic polymers used to debride the wound by gentle autolytic action and promote a moist environment for dry or low-exuding wounds. Hydrocolloids are a well-proven method of maintaining a moist wound bed over a prolonged period without frequent dressing changes or the necessity of repeated hydration. The wound exudate binds to the components of the hydrocolloid matrix to form a cohesive gel with endogenous enzymes keeping the wound wet and supporting autolytic debridement. They do not require a secondary dressing. Their impermeability to water sometimes creates overhydration with periwound maceration, and foul odor may be confused with infection. Hydropolymer or foam dressings

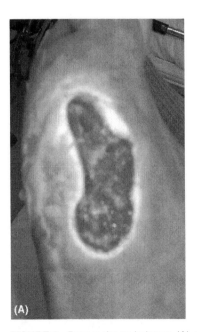 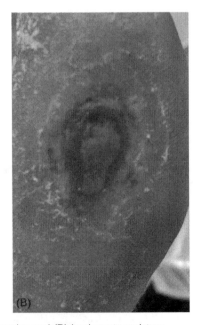

FIGURE 5 Poor moisture balance: (**A**) excessive and (**B**) inadequate moisture.

represent a technical advancement to hydrocolloids. They provide the combined effects of absorption and management of wound exudate to provide a moist wound-healing environment. The exudate management capacity of these dressings and the practical handling (easily cut/shaped to fit difficult wounds) without gel formation (as in hydrocolloids) have been improved. Alginates are derived from seaweed and mostly contain a combination of calcium or sodium alginate. Sodium/calcium ion exchange between exudate and dressing promotes formation of a gel. Alginates are highly absorbent, support wound cleansing by incorporation of autolytic tissue debridement, and stimulate wound healing by the release of ions. They are especially appropriate for the treatment of deep cavernous wounds. Association of all these products with the well-known ant microbial characteristics of silver can increase the efficacy of wound healing, although there are no randomized trials available to prove this statement.

Edge

It is noted that a 20% to 40% reduction in four weeks is likely to be a reliable predictor of healing (17). One measure of beginning healing is the clinical observation of the edge of the wound. A no healing wound may have a cliff-like edge between the upper epithelium and the lower bottom granulation tissue compared with a healing wound with tapered edges like the shore of a sandy beach (Fig. 6) (5).

If the wound edge is not migrating after appropriate wound bed preparation (debridement, bacterial balance, and moisture balance) and healing is stalled, then advanced active wound therapies should be considered. The first step prior to initiating the edge effect therapies is a reassessment of the patient to rule out other causes and cofactors (18). Several active "edge effect" wound therapies support the addition of missing components: growth factors, fibroblasts, epithelial cells, and matrix components. Various growth factors, considered as a subgroup of cytokines, are responsible for the regulation of wound-healing processes. The list of identified growth factors is constantly growing (19). One of the most well known is the platelet-derived growth factor (PDGF), produced by the endothelial cells. This growth factor has hemostatic, proliferate, and antigenic properties. The recombinant PDGF is formulated into a gel, topically applied, and is chemo tactic toward macrophages, neutrophil granulocytes, and fibroblasts, creating a proliferative effect on the number of cells in

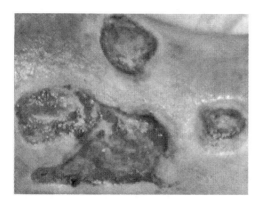

FIGURE 6 Edge of a nonhealing wound.

the wound. Unfortunately, despite the fact that several preclinical studies have shown that the addition of exogenous growth factors can increase tissue synthesis (20,21), the clinical efficacy on wound healing outcome remains speculative (22,23). It has been hypothesized by some authors that the high levels of proteinases in chronic wound exudate degrade the efficacy of the exogenous growth factors (24,25). Chronic wounds can be considered to have an imbalance between tissue deposition stimulated by growth factors and tissue destruction mediated by proteinases. In numerous studies, investigators have shown that the proteinase, and especially the subgroup of matrix metalloproteinases (MMP: Zn-dependent endopeptidases) concentrations are massively increased in the exudate of chronic wounds (compared with acute wound exudate), while their inhibitors are dramatically reduced. The development of collagen plus ORC (oxidized regenerated cellulose) matrices, when applied in a chronic wound absorbing wound exudate and transforming into a soft conformable gel, which bind and inactivate these MMPs and protect the endogenous growth factor binding, looks very promising (26). In the last few years, skin substitutes have been developed. Dermagraft is of human origin and grows as fibroblast culture on a biodegradable mesh. In this way, it becomes a metabolically active tissue that produces collagen, extracellular matrix proteins, and growth hormones. Apligraf is a biosynthetic product, made up of two cell types: epiderma keratinocytes and fibroblasts, and structured in two layers, comparable to human skin. Integra is a collagen-glycosaminoglycan matrix covered by an ultrathin split-skin graft, which stimulates the ingrowth of cells and thus induces a well-ordered regeneration of autolog dermis. Preliminary clinical experiences confirm the efficacy of these skin substitute therapies for chronic ulcers, but more trials are necessary to offer clinical evidence to support their contribution to health economic data.

OTHER THERAPEUTIC APPROACHES

Some randomized trials consider the technique of vacuum wound treatment as a promising approach (Fig. 7A). Here, open cell foam is applied to a suitable wound, adding a seal of adhesive drape, and then subatmospheric pressure is applied to this wound in a controlled way. After application of this negative pressure, an intimate healing-stimulating contact between wound surface and sponge system arises. A direct removal of interstitial fluid volume that increases vascular density and capillary blood flow (27) even as a direct removal of wound effluents (inhibitory cytokines, acute phase proteins, and proteolytic enzymes (28,29) is established, which stimulates the cellular proliferation. The application of negative pressure also leads to bacterial cleansing of the wound and some specific biomechanical effects at cellular level (external application of mechanical stress forces, increase of mitogenic response, and promotion of cell division and angiogenesis) (30). Finally, a mechanical crimp effect leads to a centripetal effect on the wound edges (31). Of course, as mentioned previously, radical debridement must always precede the implementation of vacuum-assisted compression (VAC) therapy. For conditioning of extensive and secreting defects, polyurethane foam should be employed with a continuous suction pressure of 125 mmHg for three to six days (Fig. 8A). When the amount of fluid decreases, intermittent suction can often help to further encourage granulation tissue formation, especially in difficult circulation conditions. Randomized

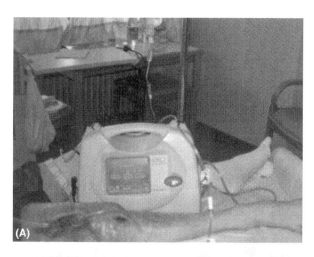

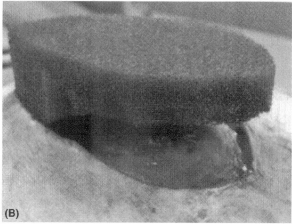

FIGURE 7 Vacuum-assisted compression (VAC) therapy. (**A**) Vacuum therapy unit and (**B**) polyurethane foam application.

well-controlled data are available to show that for complex diabetic foot wounds, VAC therapy seems to be a safe and effective treatment, and could lead to a higher proportion of healed wounds, faster healing rates, and potentially fewer re-amputations than standard care (32,33). Also, for other chronic leg ulcers (venous-arterial cause), VAC therapy should be considered as a therapy of choice owing to its significant advantages in time to complete healing, wound bed preparation time, patient comfort and time involvement, and costs of the nursing staff (an important number of patients can receive treatment on an outpatient basis), compared with the standard moist wound therapy (34). VAC therapy can also be seen as the ideal promoter for wound bed preparation, prior to definitive wound closure with split thickness skin grafts. It can also serve as a postoperative fixation of the split thickness skin grafts (with the interposition of a nonadherent dressing between graft and white polyvinylalcohol foam and a continuous suction of 6 days at 75 mmHg) (Fig. 8) (35).

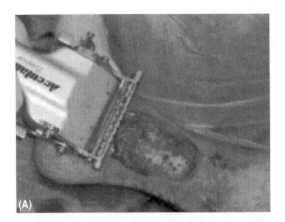

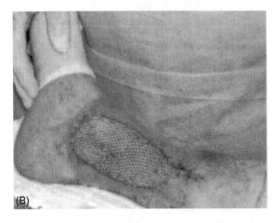

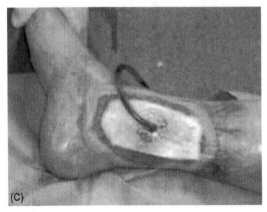

FIGURE 8 Ulcer surgery during a treatment session: (**A**) shaving after repairing the vascular situation with stripping of varicose veins and phlebectomy; (**B**) shaving followed by mesh grafting; (**C**) vacuum therapy to attach the mesh graft transplant; (**D**) Status after five days of continuous vacuum therapy at 75 mmHg.; (**E**) vacuum therapy, cotton padding compression bandage.

(*Continued on next page*)

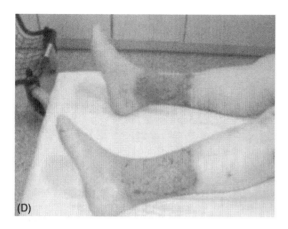

(D)

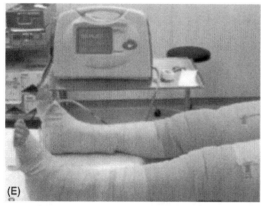

(E)

FIGURE 8 (*Continued*)

Maggot Therapy (Fly Larvae)

Although an ancient remedy, this very successful type of biotherapy for extreme tissue necrosis becomes again more and more "popular." In the case of therapy-resistant chronic wounds, disinfected cultured maggots are applied directly to the wound bed (Fig. 9). They are left on the wound for about four days, covered

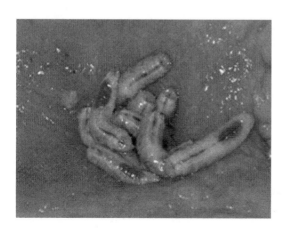

FIGURE 9 Application of disinfected cultured maggots in wound bed.

by a nonadherent woven mesh dressing. Maggots clean wounds, liquefying and ingesting only the dead, devitalized tissues. Dependent on the healing progress, this procedure can be repeated several times.

CONCLUSION
Wound care is definitely not an easy matter to deal with and to coordinate. With correct risk assessment, holistic patient assessment, efficient causal treatment, meticulous wound characteristics analysis, and the use of various modern and high technological dressings, effective wound management is possible. Recognizing red flags that warn of failure to heal and treating the whole patient before the hole in the patient are essential issues to be in the successful and winning team. Clinicians also need to remember that wound healing is not always the primary outcome. Other wound-related outcomes such as reduced pain, reduced bacterial load, reduced dressing changes, or improved quality of life are at least as important.

REFERENCES
1. London NJ, Donnely R. ABC of arterial and venous disease. Ulcerated lower limb. BMJ 2000; 320(7249):1589–1591.
2. Willy C. The Theory and Practice of Vacuum Therapy – Scientific Basis, Indications for Use, Case Reports, Practical Advice. Ulm: Lindqvist Book Publishing, 2006, p. 431.
3. Brem H, Sheehan P, Rosenberg H, et al. Evidence-based protocol for diabetic foot ulcers. Plast Reconstr Surg 2006; 117:193S–209S.
4. Naudé L. Wound assessment incorporating the WHASA wound assessment form. Wound Healing Southern Africa 2008; 1(1):16–21.
5. Sibbald RG, Woo KY, Ayello E. Wound bed preparation: DIM before DIME. Wound Healing Southern Africa 2008; 1(1):29–34.
6. Bowler PG. The 10^3 bacterial growth guideline: reassessing its clinical relevance in wound healing. Ostomy Wound Manage 2003; 49(1):44–53.
7. Kingsley A. A proactive approach to wound infection. Nurs Stand 2002; 15(30):50–59.
8. Halbert AR, Stacey MC, Rohr JB. The effect of bacterial colonization on venous ulcer healing. Australas J Dermatol 1992; 33(2):75–80.
9. Bowler PG. Duerden BI, Armstrong DG. Wound microbiology and approaches to wound management. Clin Microbiol Rev 2001; 14:244–269.
10. Cooper R, Kingsley A, White RJ. Wound Infection & Microbiology. Whitstone, Holsworthy: Medical Communications UK Ltd, 2002.
11. Velicer GJ. Social strife in the microbial world. Trends Microbiol 2003; 11(7):330–337.
12. Lanis S, Ryan S, Woo K, et al. Infections in chronic wounds. In: Krasner D, Sibbald G, Rodeheaver GT, et al. Chronic Wound Care: A Clinical Source Book for Healthcare Professionals. 4th ed. HMP communications, 2007:299–321.
13. Cutting KF. A dedicated follower of fashion? In White RJ ed. Topical Medications and Wounds. Br J Nurs 2001; 10:S9–S16.
14. Russell AD, Hugo WB. Antimicrobial activity and action of silver. In: Ellis GP, Luscombe DK, eds. Progress in Medicinal Chemistry. Vol 31. Amsterdam: Elsevier Science, 1994:351–370.
15. Demling RH, De Santi L. The role of silver technology in wound healing. Wounds 2001; 13(1):A5–A15.
16. Okan D, Woo K, Ayello EA, et al. The role of moisture balance in wound healing. Adv Skin Wound Care 2007; 20(1):39–52.
17. Margolis DJ, Allen-Taylor L, Hoffstad O, et al. The accuracy of venous leg ulcer prognostic models in wound care systems. Wound Repair Regen 2004; 12:163–168.

18. Woo K, Ayello EA, Sibbald RG. The edge effect: current therapeutic options to advance the wound edge. Adv Skin Wound Care 2007; 20(2):99–117.
19. Vogt PM, Peter FW, Topsakal E, et al. Zum einsatz von wachstumsfaktoren in der therapie chronischer wunden. Experimentelle, klinische und finanzielle aspekte. Chirurg 1998; 69(11):1197–1206.
20. Greenhalgh DG, Hummel RP, Albertson S. Synergistic actions of platelet derived growth factor and the insulin-like growth factors in vivo. Wound Repair Regen 1993; 1:69–81.
21. Mellin TN, Cashen DE, Ronan JJ. Acidic fibroblast growth factor accelerates dermal wound healing in diabetic mice. J Invest Dermatol 1995; 104(5):850–855.
22. Robson MC. The role of growth factors in the healing of chronic wounds. Wound Repair Regen 1997; 5:12–17.
23. Brantigan CO. The history of the understanding of the role of growth factors in wound healing. Wounds 1996; 8:78–90.
24. Falanga V. Growth factors and chronic wounds: the need to understand the micro-environment. J Dermatol 1992; 19(11):667–672.
25. Yager DR, Chen SM, Ward SI. Ability of chronic wound fluids to degrade peptide growth factors is associated with increased levels of elastase activity and diminished levels of proteinase inhibitors. Wound Repair Regen 1997; 5:23–32.
26. Veves A, Sheehan P, Pham H. A randomised controlled trial of a collagen/oxidised regenerated cellulose dressing vs. standard therapy in the management of diabetic foot ulcers. Arch Surg 2002; 137(7):822–827.
27. Chen SZ. Effects of vacuum-assisted closure on wound microcirculation: an experimental study. Asian J Surg 2005; 28(3):211–217.
28. Plikaitis CM, Molnar JA. Subatmospheric pressure wound therapy and the vacuum-assisted closure device: basic science and current clinical successes. Expert Rev Med Devices 2006; 3(2):175–846.
29. Tang SY. Influence of vacuum-assisted closure technique on expression of Bcl2 and NGF/NGFmRNA during wound healing. Zonghua Zheng Xing Wai Ke Za Zhi 2004; 20(2):139–142.
30. Saxena V, Hwang CW, Huang S, et al. Vacuum-assisted closure: microdeformations of wounds and cell proliferation. Plast Reconstr Surg 2004; 114(5):1086–1096 (discussion 1097–1098).
31. Morykwas MJ, Argenta LC, Shelton-Brown EI, et al. Vacuum-assisted closure: a new method for wound control and treatment: animal studies and basic foundation. Ann Plast Surg 1997; 38(6):553–562.
32. Armstrong DG, Lavery LA. Negative pressure wound therapy after partial diabetic foot amputation: a multicentre, randomised controlled trial. Lancet 2005; 366(9498): 1704–1710.
33. Blume PA. North American Center of Limb preservation, New Haven, Connecticut, United States; 2007; Annual Scientific Meeting of the American Podiatric Medicine. Randomised controlled trial.
34. Vuerstaek JDD, Veraart JC, Wuite J, et al. A new concept in active healing of mixed or resistant venous ulcers: vacuum assisted closure: a 3 year experience. Phlebologie 2002; 55(1):15–19.
35. Gesslein M, Horch RE. Interdisciplinary management of complex chronic ulcers using vacuum assisted closure therapy and "buried chip skin grafts." Zentralbl Chir 2006; 131(S1):170–173.

18 Growth Factor and Cell Therapy in Patients with Critical Limb Ischemia

Ralf W. Sprengers
Departments of Vascular Surgery and Nefrology and Hypertension, University Medical Center Utrecht, Utrecht, The Netherlands

Marianne C. Verhaar
Departments of Nefrology and Hypertension, University Medical Center Utrecht, Utrecht, The Netherlands

Frans L. Moll
Department of Vascular Surgery, University Medical Center Utrecht, Utrecht, The Netherlands

KEY POINTS

- Exploring new treatment strategies for patients with no other options than amputation is of major importance.
- Growth factor therapy and progenitor cell–mediated therapy for the stimulation of postnatal neovascularization have been identified as potential new treatment alternatives.
- Growth factor therapy and progenitor cell–mediated therapy have been shown to effectively restore blood flow to the ischemic target tissue in animal models.
- Small uncontrolled clinical trials have demonstrated the safety and suggest efficacy of growth factor therapy and cell-mediated therapy in patients with CLI.
- Well-designed, larger, randomized and placebo-controlled clinical trials are warranted to confirm the initial promising results.
- Further development and optimization of both strategies might offer a novel treatment option for CLI patients in the coming years.
- Cardiovascular risk management might further enhance the success of growth factor and progenitor cell–mediated neovascularization.

INTRODUCTION

Recent advances in surgical and radiological revascularization techniques have led to better treatment options for patients with critical limb ischemia (CLI) (1). However, in approximately 40% of these patients, surgical or radiological revascularization is still not possible because of the anatomical location of the atherosclerotic lesions, the extent of the disease, or extensive comorbidity (2,3). With no effective pharmacological therapy available (4), new experimental strategies, such as growth factor and cell therapy to enhance neovascularization, are currently being explored.

Blood vessel growth or neovascularization in the adult involves several processes: angiogenesis, vasculogenesis, and arteriogenesis. Angiogenesis involves the sprouting of new capillaries from the preexisting vasculature. In addition to this migratory and proliferative process of mature endothelial cells, sprouting may also occur through a process referred to as postnatal vasculo-genesis. During embryonic development, vasculogenesis comprises the in situ formation of blood vessels from angioblasts. Recent evidence suggests that also in the adult, neovascularization may occur through migration and differentia-tion of bone marrow–derived endothelial progenitor cells (EPCs) (5). Hypoxia and the key transcriptional system hypoxia-inducible factor (HIF) are major triggers for both angiogenesis and vasculogenesis (6,7), enhancing the synthesis of proangiogenic factors like vascular endothelial growth factor (VEGF), angiopoietin, and inducible nitric oxide synthase (iNOS) (6,8,9).

Arteriogenesis, or collateral vessel formation, denotes the enlargement of preexisting vasculature and, unlike vasculogenesis and angiogenesis, does not depend on local tissue hypoxia, but rather on activation of the endothelial cell layer by changes in shear stress (8,9). In this process, the activated endothelium releases several chemoattractants, like monocyte chemoattractant protein 1 (MCP-1) and intercellular adhesion molecule 1 (ICAM-1), which recruit a variety of inflammatory cells. These cells, in turn, produce several proangiogenic factors such as VEGF, fibroblast growth factor (FGF), and platelet-derived growth factor (PDGF) that ultimately lead to the remodeling of a small arteriole into a larger conducting collateral (10,11).

In the adult, all three processes of neovascularization may occur. How-ever, in patients with peripheral arterial occlusive disease they are insufficient to overcome the loss of blood flow as a result of occluded arteries (8,12). Thera-peutic neovascularization focuses on the augmentation of new vessel formation to improve tissue perfusion through all three mechanisms: vasculogenesis and/ or angiogenesis in the ischemic tissue as well as collateral vessel formation via arteriogenesis.

This chapter will provide an overview of the strategies, currently being investigated in the clinic, that aim to augment postnatal neovascularization, as well as the future perspectives for these therapies for CLI.

GROWTH FACTOR THERAPY

One potential strategy to augment neovascularization in ischemic tissue is the supply of proangiogenic growth factors, either in the form of a recombinant protein or by use of gene therapy for the introduction of genes coding for a proangiogenic factor. The proangiogenic factors VEGF and basic fibroblast growth factor (FGF) are the most widely studied factors for therapeutic neo-vascularization (13,14) and will therefore be discussed in more detail below. Other growth factors that have been studied clinically for their potential to stimulate neovascularization include hepatocyte growth factor (HGF) and granulocyte macrophage colony-stimulating factor (GM-CSF) (15,16). Further-more, the therapeutic effects of the induction of key transcription factors, such as HIF-1α, are currently being explored (17).

ANGIOGENIC FACTORS

VEGF can be induced by hypoxia, hypoglycemia, and inflammation (13,18). To date, six growth factors have been identified that belong to the VEGF family: VEGF-A (also named VEGF or VEGF-1), VEGF-B (VEGF-3), VEGF-C (VEGF-2), VEGF-D, VEGF-E, and placental growth factor (PLGF). VEGF-A was the first cloned member of the VEGF family and is still the most extensively studied member (18,19). It is expressed in several different isoforms, as a result of alternative splicing of mRNA from an eight-exon gene. All isoforms have comparable angiogenic potential, but differ in their extracellular matrix–binding properties. The smaller isoforms can diffuse more easily into tissues, whereas the larger isoforms have longer-lasting effects (13,18,19).

Receptors for VEGF are expressed on mature EC, monocytes, and hematopoietic stem cells and EPCs. Four VEGF receptors (VEGFR) have been identified: VEGFR-1 (also called Flt-1), VEGFR-2 [kinase insert domain receptor (KDR) or Flk-1], VEGFR-3 (Flt-4), and neuropilin 1. Binding of a VEGF member to VEGFR-2 stimulates proliferation and migration, while binding to VEGFR-1 mediates tube formation (13,18,20).

The FGF family consists of 22 different members, which can generally be divided into seven subfamilies (21). FGF-1 (acidic FGF) and FGF-2 (FGF) are widely studied for their pronounced angiogenic activity (13). Whereas most other FGFs have a signal sequence that allows them to be secreted, FGF-1 and FGF-2 bind to the cell membrane and the extracellular matrix and are released upon tissue damage. Most other FGF members are proliferation or differentiation factors involved in developmental processes, and have very low expression levels in adult tissues (13,18,21).

Receptors for FGF are expressed on a wide variety of cells, including smooth muscle cells and endothelial cells. Four separate genes that code for FGF receptors (FGFR) have been identified, of which three can lead to two different isoforms via the alternative splicing of mRNA. Thus, seven receptors can be distinguished in total, named FGFR-1 (B and C), FGFR-2 (B and C), FGFR-3 (B and C), and FGFR-4. In contrast to VEGF, FGF activity is mainly regulated by the expression of FGF receptors in the target tissue and not by the level of expression of the growth factors itself (18,21).

GROWTH FACTOR ADMINISTRATION METHODS AND DELIVERY ROUTES

Two methods for the delivery of proangiogenic factors are the administration of a recombinant protein form of the proangiogenic factor and the delivery of genes encoding for a proangiogenic factor either by viral or nonviral methods. The use of recombinant proteins allows for the precise control of the administered dose (18). However, a relatively high dose of the recombinant protein is usually required to induce a therapeutic effect, which may result in an increase in the occurrence and intensity of adverse events (13,18,22). Moreover, repeated administration of the proangiogenic recombinant protein is often required as recombinant proteins have a short half-life in vivo due to rapid degradation by circulating proteases (13,18).

The most commonly used nonviral approach to deliver genes coding for a proangiogenic factor is the direct injection of unmodified (naked) plasmid DNA, coding for the desired proangiogenic factor (20). This approach is relatively simple and well tolerated with respect to toxicity and immune response initiation properties, but the transfection efficacy is low and, because of metabolism by nucleases, it has a short-lasting effect (13,14,18,20). To improve the transfection efficiency, DNA plasmids can be coupled to a nonviral lipophylic vector (e.g., cationic phospholipids) that facilitates the transportation of DNA across the cell membrane. In addition, the use of lipophylic vectors allows transportation of large DNA molecules (14,20,23). Furthermore, membrane permeabilization of the target cell to enhance the uptake of the vector can be achieved by using ultrasound exposure to microbubble echocontrast agents (acoustic cavitation) (14,20,24,25) or by means of electropermeabilization (26,27).

Human adenoviruses are most widely used as viral vectors for gene transfer (18,20). In viral vectors, the sequences necessary for replication are replaced by the DNA sequence encoding the proangiogenic factor, thus rendering the virus replication deficient (18). Viral gene transfer is markedly more efficient than nonviral gene delivery, because viral vectors can transduce both dividing as well as nondividing cells (20), and because these vectors can easily be produced in large quantities (18). An important limitation of viral vectors, however, is the potential induction of inflammatory and immune responses (18,20).

Gene transfer can be performed either ex vivo, where target cells are removed from the patient and transfected in vitro before reintroducing them into the patient or can be performed in vivo using systemic, local intravascular, perivascular, or intramuscular delivery techniques (13,20,23). Local intravascular delivery can be performed surgically or in catheter-mediated manner by temporarily isolating the vascular segment (by clamping or balloon dilatation) and incubating the segment with the desired vector solution. The perivascular delivery method comprises the placement of a biodegradable adventitial collar or gel around a vascular segment to target the segment from the outside. In addition, perivascular delivery can also be performed by injection of a vector directly into the adventitia. Percutaneous intramuscular injection can be performed to obtain a local, sustained paracrine effect on the target tissue (23). To date, only balloon catheter–mediated local intravascular delivery and percutaneous intramuscular delivery have been used in clinical studies on CLI.

Pre-clinical and Clinical Studies

In the 1990s, several animal studies demonstrated beneficial effects of the administration of proangiogenic factors on myocardial and hind limb neovascularization. In dog myocardial ischemia models, it was shown that intracoronary VEGF and FGF administration enhanced collateral artery development and increased blood flow delivery after coronary artery occlusion (28,29). In rabbit models of hind limb ischemia, both intramuscular injection as well as intraarterial administration of VEGF resulted in earlier distal arterial reconstitution and enhanced neovascularization (30,31). These animal studies established proof of principle that growth factor administration enhances neovascularization and led to several small clinical trials in patients with myocardial ischemia, intermittent claudication (IC), and limb ischemia. Here, the clinical studies in patients with CLI will be discussed (Table 1).

The first study on the clinical application of gene transfer for the treatment of CLI was published in 1996 by Isner et al. (32). In this case report, a DNA plasmid coding for VEGF was attached to a hydrogel polymer coating on angioplasty balloon and delivered intra-arterially in a 70-year-old patient with CLI (gangrene). A total dose of 2000-µg VEGF was delivered. Up to 12 weeks after gene transfer, an increase in collateral vessels formation was observed in the ischemic limb at knee, mid-tibial, and ankle level as well as an increase in rest and maximum blood flow velocity of 82% and 72%, respectively. In reaction to the treatment, transient peripheral edema developed seven days after administration,

TABLE 1 Overview of Clinical Studies on Growth Factor Therapy in CLI Patients

Author, year (reference number)	Study type	Patient characteristics (number of patients)	Delivery method	Intervention Vector	Intervention Dose	Results
Isner et al., 1996 (32)	CR	CLI (1)	Intra-arterial with hydrogel-coated balloon	VEGF$_{165}$ plasmid	2,000 µg	Improvement in collateral vessels (angiography), resting and maximum flow
Isner et al., 1995 and Isner, 1998 (33, 34)	PS	CLI (8)[a]	Intra-arterial with hydrogel-coated balloon	VEGF$_{165}$ plasmid	100–2,000 µg	No improvement in ABI. Improvement in flow (MRA, intravascular Doppler) in high-dose patients. Collateral vessel formation (angiography) in one high-dose patient.
Baumgartner et al., 1998 (35)	PS	CLI (9)	Intramuscular	VEGF$_{165}$ plasmid	4,000 µg	Significant improvement in ABI. Improved distal flow (MRA). Newly visible collateral blood vessels (angiography). Ulcer healing
Rajagopalan et al., 2001 (36)	PS	IC (4), CLI (2)	Intramuscular	VEGF$_{121}$ adenovirus	$4 \times 10^{8.5}$– 4×10^{10} units	Significant improvement in endothelium function (endothelium-dependent vasodilatation)
Comerota et al., 2002 (37)	PS	CLI (51)	Intramuscular	FGF-1 plasmid	500–16,000 µg	Significant improvement in rest pain, TcPO$_2$, ABI, and ulcer healing
Mäkinen et al., 2002 (38)	RCT	IC (40), CLI (14)	Intra-arterial with balloon catheter	VEGF$_{165}$ plasmid vs. VEGF$_{165}$ adenovirus vs. control	2,000 µg vs. 2×10^{10} units vs. control	Significant improvement in vascularity (angiography) for VEGF-treated groups. Significant improvement of ABI and Rutherford class in all groups. No differences in major amputation, ulcer healing or resolution of rest pain
Shyu et al., 2003 (39)	PS	CLI (21)	Intramuscular	VEGF$_{165}$ plasmid	400–2,000 µg	Significant improvement in ABI. Improved distal flow (MRA). Improvement in rest pain. Ulcer healing

Study	Design	Condition (n)	Route	Agent	Dose	Results
Kim et al., 2004 (40)	PS	TAO (7), ASO (2)	Intramuscular	VEGF$_{165}$ plasmid	2,000–8,000 µg	Significant improvement in rest pain, ABI, and collateral vessel formation (angiography). Ulcer healing
Morishita et al., 2004 (15)	PS	TAO (3), ASO (3)	Intramuscular	HGF plasmid	4,000 µg	Significant improvement in ABI, TcPO$_2$ after O$_2$, ulcer size, and rest pain
Kusumanto et al., 2006 (41)	RCT	CLI with DM (54)	Intramuscular	VEGF$_{165}$ plasmid vs. placebo	2,000 µg	No difference in number of amputations. Significant hemodynamic improvement and ulcer healing. Improvement in rest pain
TALISMAN 201[b]	RCT	CLI (125)	Intramuscular	FGF-1 plasmid vs. placebo	16,000 µg vs. control	No difference in wound healing. Significant reduction in the number of amputations
HGF-STAT[b]	RCT	CLI (104)		HGF plasmid vs. HGF plasmid vs. HGF plasmid vs. placebo	12,000 µg vs. 8,000 µg vs. 1,200 µg vs. control	Significant increase in TcPO$_2$ between highest dose and placebo only. No difference in ulcer status

Papers are sorted by date of publication.

[a]Includes the patient reported in the CR from 1996 by the same author.

[b]Preliminary data.

Abbreviations: VEGF, vascular endothelial growth factor; MRA, magnetic resonance angiography; FGF, fibroblast growth factor; HGF, hepatocyte growth factor; RCT, randomized controlled trial; PS, patient series; CR, case report; CLI, critical limb ischemia; IC, intermittent claudication; ASO, arteriosclerosis obliterans; TAO, thromboangitis obliterans; ABI, ankle-brachial index; TcPO$_2$, transcutaneous oxygen pressure; DM, diabetes mellitus.

together with spider angiomas over the ankle and forefoot, which resolved after four and eight weeks, respectively. In 1998, the Isner group described the interim results of the first eight patients participating in a dose-escalating clinical trial in 22 CLI patients. In this study, no increase in collateral vessel formation was observed in patients receiving lower VEGF dosages (<1000 μg) and increased blood flow was only seen on magnetic resonance angiography (MRA) in three out of five patients receiving 1000-μg VEGF. No improvements in ankle-brachial index (ABI) were observed. In all but one patient, which is also the patient described in the above-mentioned case report and the first patient to receive 2000-μg VEGF in this trial, no adverse events attributable to VEGF administration were observed (33). Similar results were reported by Shyu et al. in 2003, who treated 21 patients in a dose-escalating manner with similar VEGF doses and found a minimal effective dose of 2400-μg VEGF, on the basis of the ankle-brachial index improvements (39). Kim et al. reported no VEGF dose-response effects (with a minimal administered dose of 2000 μg) (40).

To date, two small, randomized trials comparing VEGF gene transfer with placebo treatment in CLI patients and one larger randomized trial in patients with IC [Regional Angiogenesis with Vascular Endothelial growth factor (RAVE) study] have been published (38,41,42). Mäkinen et al. compared local catheter-mediated intra-arterial VEGF delivery, either via an adenovirus vector (in 14 IC and 4 CLI patients) or via a VEGF DNA plasmid (in 11 IC and 6 CLI patients), with placebo treatment with Ringer's lactate. Although both VEGF delivery strategies significantly improved vascularity on digital subtraction angiography when compared with the placebo group, no significant differences in amputation rate, clinical status (ulcer healing, rest pain), or ABI were found among the three groups (38). The RAVE study, a double-blinded, placebo-controlled study in 105 IC patients comparing the efficacy of a single low- or high-dose intramuscular injection of $VEGF_{121}$ with that of placebo treatment also found no differences in exercise performance or quality of life between the groups (42). In contrast, Kusumanto et al., who compared intramuscular delivery of a VEGF plasmid with placebo treatment in 54 diabetic CLI patients, showed significantly improved wound healing and significant hemodynamic improvement, defined by an absolute increase in ABI >15% in the VEGF-treated group (41). Clinical improvement was observed in over 50% of patients treated with the DNA plasmid, which is comparable to earlier success rates reported by Baumgartner et al., Shyu et al., and Kim et al. (35,39,40). Although no reports have been published comparing intramuscular and intra-arterial delivery strategies for gene therapy, the negative results of the trial by Mäkinen and the RAVE study were suggested to be related to the use of an intra-arterial delivery route instead of the intramuscular route used by the other trials (41).

Other proangiogenic factors have clinically been studied. Comerota et al. treated 51 patients with CLI with a naked plasmid DNA coding for FGF in a dose-escalating manner and demonstrated a significant reduction in pain and ulcer size, together with a significant increase in transcutaneous oxygen pressure ($TcPO_2$) and ABI (37). Although administration of the plasmid DNA was reported to be well tolerated, a relatively high number of adverse events (66 in 51 patients) were seen in this trial (37). A randomized trial on the effects of a single or double intra-arterial dose of FGF in 190 CI patients [the Therapeutic Angiogenesis with Recombinant Fibroblast Growth Factor-2 for Intermittent Claudication (TRAFFIC) study] reported a significant difference in the peak walking time change from baseline at 90 days between the placebo-treated group and the single-dose FGF group, but placebo treatment did not differ from the double dose–treated group. Moreover, the difference between the placebo group and the single-dose FGF group was no longer observed at 180 days (43). Preliminary data from the TALISMAN 201 trial in patients with CLI show no difference in would healing between intramuscular FGF treatment and placebo, but do show a significantly reduced risk of amputation in the FGF-treated group.

Intramuscular injection of HGF plasmid DNA in three patients with arteriosclerosis obliterans and three patients with Buerger disease (all staged Fontaine III or IV) showed a significant increase in ABI and $TcPO_2$ at 12 weeks after the start of the treatment and a significant decrease in ulcer size and pain indicated on a visual analog scale (15). Preliminary data from the HGF-STAT trial in 104 CLI patients demonstrated a significant increase in $TcPO_2$ between the highest administered dose (12,000 µg) and placebo treatment without differences in ulcer status. No significant differences were observed between the other groups (44).

Recently, a phase 1 clinical trial demonstrated the safety of gene transfer of the key transcription factor HIF-1α, which is able to induce the production of multiple proangiogenic factors, in patients with CLI (17). A phase 2 clinical trial on HIF-1α gene transfer is currently being conducted in 300 patients with IC.

Overall, the initial uncontrolled studies using VEGF, as well as FGF and HGF, in patients with CLI showed promising results. However, subsequent large placebo-controlled trials in myocardial ischemia and IC patients were mainly disappointing (42,43,45–47) and reported only a limited success (48). Several factors may have negatively influenced the results of these trials, such as the administered dose, the achieved duration of gene expression, heterogeneity between patients included in the trials, and poor end point selection (48). Moreover, all clinical studies published so far have investigated the effects of a single proangiogenic factor. Larger randomized placebo-controlled trials currently being conducted on the effects of gene transfer of key transcription factors, such as the phase 2 trial on HIF-1α, might be able to provide additional answers.

Cell Therapy

The observation in the 1990s that peripheral blood contains EPCs which can contribute to neovascularization by differentiating into functional endothelial cells, but also by paracrine effects on the resident endothelium (5,7,49–55), has led to new strategies aimed at therapeutic neovascularization that involve bone marrow or peripheral blood progenitor cell administration.

Cell Populations

In response to mobilizing stimuli (e.g., tissue ischemia), EPCs are released from the bone marrow into the peripheral blood (7) and subsequently home to sites where new vessel formation is required (7,50,54). Importantly, when these progenitor cells are taken from the bone marrow and implanted in animal models of myocardial or limb ischemia, neovascularization of the ischemic tissue is augmented (12,56–60). The (endothelial) progenitor cells involved in postnatal neovascularization are generally believed to originate from the

CD34$^+$ hematopoietic precursor cell population within the mononuclear cell (MNC) fraction of the bone marrow, analogous to the common hemangioblast precursor during embryonic development (50,52). On the other hand, other studies have shown that also CD34$^-$ hematopoietic precursor cells (5,61), as well as non-hematopoietic mesenchymal precursor cells and myeloid/monocyte lineage cells (CD14$^+$), can transdifferentiate into cells with EPC characteristics (62–65) and play an important role in postnatal neovascularization, probably through the paracrine effects of secreted angiogenic factors (66,67). Most likely, the beneficial effects of cell-based neovascularization therapy are the results of an interplay between different cell populations within the MNC fraction of the bone marrow, and may act via direct incorporation and differentiation into the vessel's endothelial layer, via the production of angiogenic factors, or via a combination of both.

Most clinical trials thus far use the whole MNC fraction to augment neovascularization in CLI. Whether selective administration of isolated cell populations is more effective remains to be elucidated.

DELIVERY ROUTES

Three delivery routes may be used for the administration of cells for treatment of patients with limb ischemia: intra-arterial infusion, intramuscular injection, or a combination of both. With intra-arterial infusion, the cells are injected into the common femoral artery of the ischemic leg and travel with the blood flow to the border zone of the ischemic tissue (68–70). There, the cells migrate from the lumen to the vessel wall and into the ischemic tissue to exert their effect via angiogenesis and vasculogenesis mechanisms described above. Intramuscular injection comprises the injection of cells directly into the ischemic muscle, often at multiple sites along a grid. These local depots of cells then augment neovascularization through vasculogenesis and paracrine mechanisms (8).

Both delivery techniques have advantages and disadvantages. With intra-arterial infusion, the injected cells travel in a nutrient- and oxygen-rich environment (the circulation), but the ischemic tissue might be targeted less efficiently, because the cells need to migrate into the vessel wall and surrounding tissue. Although this is not the case for the intramuscular approach, it has been suggested that for this approach the survival of cells is decreased, because they are injected into a nutrient- and oxygen-depleted environment (68,71,72).

To date, no study has reported on a comparison between the two approaches or between a single and combined approach for therapeutic neovascularization in CLI patients. In an animal ischemic hind limb model, similar angiogenic effects were observed after intramuscular and intra-arterial injection of cells (58).

Clinical Studies

The promising results of cell-mediated neovascularization in animal models of tissue ischemia were soon followed by several small clinical trials in patients with CLI and myocardial ischemia. Here we will provide an overview of the clinical trials on bone marrow–derived (BM) or peripheral blood–derived (PB) progenitor cells for CLI thus far (Table 2).

In 2002, the Therapeutic Angiogenesis using Cell Transplantation (TACT) study was the first to report on the use of BM-MNC for therapeutic

TABLE 2 Overview of Clinical Studies on Therapeutic Angiogenesis with Autologous BM-Derived Progenitor Cells for CLI

Author, year (Ref)	Study type	Patient characteristics (number of patients)	Intervention	Mean implanted cell number (SD)	Results
Tateishi-Yuyama, et al., TACT Study Investigators, 2002 (73)	Pilot	Unilateral CLI (25)	Intramuscular BM-MNC	$1.6\ (0.6) \times 10^9$	Significant improvement in ABI, $TcPO_2$, rest pain, and pain-free walking time at 4 and 24 wk.
	RCT	Bilateral CLI (20)	Intramuscular BM-MNC Intramuscular PB-MNC	$1.5\ (0.6) \times 10^9$	Significant improvement in ABI, $TcPO_2$, rest pain, and pain-free walking time at 4 and 24 wk.
Esato et al., 2002 (74)	PS	TAO (4), ASO (4)	Intramuscular BM-MNC	$6.1^{a,b} \times 10^9$	Improvement in rest pain. Improvement in subjective symptoms at 4 wk. Increase in local skin temperature. Ulcer healing.
Higashi et al., 2004 (75)	PS	CLI (7)	Intramuscular BM-MNC	$1.6\ (0.3) \times 10^9$	Improvement in ABI, $TcPO_2$, rest pain, and pain-free walking time at 4 and 24 wk.
Miyamoto et al., 2004 (76)	PS	CLI (12)	Intramuscular BM-MNC	$4.0\ (0.3) \times 10^9$	Significant improvement in pain-free walking time. Improved ABI, reduction in pain (visual analog score), and improved perfusion.
Saigawa et al., 2004 (77)	PS	ASO (8)	Intramuscular BM-MNC	$6.0\ (1.6) \times 10^7/kg$	Significant improvement in ABI at 4 wk and significant improvement in $TcPO_2$ at 2 and 4 wk.
Bartsch et al., 2006 (78)	PS	PAD (10)	Intra-arterial/ intramuscular BM-MNC	$0.1^a \times 10^9$	Significant improvement in walking distance, ABI, and oxygen saturation at 2 mo.
Durdu et al., 2006 (79)	PS	TAO (28)	Intramuscular BM-MNC	$101^{a,b} \times 10^9$	Improved ABI and significant improvement in rest pain, peak walking time, and quality of life at 6 mo. Newly visible collateral blood vessels (angiography). Ulcer healing.
Miyamoto et al., 2006 (80)	PS	TAO (8)	Intramuscular BM-MNC	$3.5\ (0.8) \times 10^9$	Improvement in limb status (pain and skin ulcers) at 4 wk. Adverse events during long-term follow-up.
Kajiguchi et al., 2007 (81)	PS	TAO (3), ASO (4)	Intramuscular BM-MNC Intramuscular PB-MNC	$4.7^{a,b} \times 10^9$	Improvement in subjective symptoms (VAS) and objective findings (extent of ulcer, ABI, $TcPO_2$, thermography, and angiography) for TAO patients only.
Sugihara et al., 2005 (82)	CR	CLI (1)	Intramuscular PB-MNC	9.5×10^9	Improvement in $TcPO_2$ and skin temperature. Ulcer healing.

(Continued)

TABLE 2 Overview of Clinical Studies on Therapeutic Angiogenesis with Autologous BM-Derived Progenitor Cells for CLI (*Continued*)

Author, year (Ref)	Study type	Patient characteristics (number of patients)	Intervention	Mean implanted cell number (SD)	Results
Huang et al., 2004 (83)	PS	ASO (5)	Intramuscular G-CSF mobilized PB-MNC	$3.0^a \times 10^9$	Significant improvement in clinical manifestations, ABI, blood flow, and laser Doppler blood perfusion at 12 wk.
Kawamura et al., 2005 (84)	PS	CLI (30)	Intramuscular G-CSF mobilized PB-MNC	$19^{a,b} \times 10^9$	Prevention of limb amputation in 73%. Improvement of symptoms.
Lenk et al., 2005 (85)	PS	CLI (7)	Intra-arterial G-CSF mobilized PB-MNC after ex vivo culturing	^{a}	Significant improvement in ABI, TcPO₂, pain-free walking time, and endothelium-dependent vasodilatation at 12 wk.
Huang et al., 2005 (86)	RCT	Diabetic patients with CLI (28)	Intramuscular G-CSF mobilized PB-MNC	$3^a \times 10^9$	Significant improvement in ulcer healing, lower limb pain, limb blood perfusion, and ABI at 12 wk. Significantly less amputations in transplant group.
Ishida et al., 2005 (87)	PS	TAO (5), ASO (1)	Intramuscular G-CSF mobilized PB-MNC	$39.9\ (19.6) \times 10^9$	Improvement in ABI and ischemic ulcers, mean maximal walking distance, and physiological functioning subscale (SF-36)
Kawamura et al., 2006 (88)	PS	All stage of PAD (92) of which 75 with CLI	Intramuscular G-CSF mobilized PB-MNC	$19^{a,b} \times 10^9$	Improvement of subjective symptoms, temperature on thermograms, and arterial detection on CT. Prevention of limb amputation in 91%.
Kudo et al., 2003 (89)	CR	CLI (2)	Intramuscular G-CSF mobilized CD34⁺ cells		Improvement in TcPO₂, and clinical symptoms. Newly visible collateral blood vessels (angiography).
Cañizo et al., 2007 (90)	CR	ASO (1)	Intramuscular G-CSF mobilized CD133⁺ cells		Limb salvage after 17 mo. Improved walking distance and blood flow on magnetic resonance angiography.

Papers are sorted by cell source and date of publication.
^{a}Not reported.
^{b}Calculated from published data.
Abbreviations: MNC, mononuclear cell; G-CSF, granulocyte colony-stimulating factor; RCT, randomized controlled trial; PS, patient series; CR, case report; CLI, critical limb ischemia; ASO, arteriosclerosis obliterans; TAO, thromboangitis obliterans; PAD, peripheral arterial disease; ABI, ankle-brachial index; TcPO₂, transcutaneous oxygen pressure; VAS, Visual Analogue Scale.
Source: Adapted from Ref. 91.

neovascularization in patients with CLI (73). In the first part of this study, 25 patients with unilateral limb ischemia received an intramuscular injection of BM-MNC, which resulted in a significant improved ABI, TcPO$_2$ and pain score for the treated leg, as well as a significant increase in pain-free walking distance up to six months after treatment. A subsequent controlled trial in 22 patients with bilateral limb ischemia, who received intramuscular BM-MNC injections in one limb and the same number of PB-MNC in the other, again showed improvements in ABI and TcPO$_2$ for both legs, but more so in the BM-MNC-treated than in the PB-MNC-treated legs. Because the CD34$^+$ cell fraction is a 500-fold larger in the bone marrow than in the peripheral blood, these data supported the concept that the progenitor cells involved in postnatal neovascularization originate from a common CD34$^+$ precursor cell.

Since the TACT study, 17 clinical studies have been reported on progenitor cell therapy in patients with CLI (74–90). These studies differ in study design, patient populations, cell populations, and cell numbers. Eight of the studies also used BM-MNC, whereas nine used PB-mobilized cells, mostly after granulocyte colony-stimulating factor (G-CSF) to mobilization. One study used non-mobilized PB-MNC (82), one used G-CSF mobilized CD34$^+$ cells (89) and one other G-CSF mobilized CD133$^+$ cells (90). The majority of studies using PB-MNC used apheresis to harvest the cells; one drew 400 mL of blood (85). In the studies using BM-derived progenitor cells, the amount of aspirated bone marrow varies from 80 to 1000 mL and an approximately 125-fold difference in the number of isolated MNC/mL has been reported (Table 2).

Despite these differences, all studies thus far have shown similar results with respect to improvements in rest pain, pain-free walking distance, ABI, and/or TcPO$_2$. However, most of the studies have been small and uncontrolled. The results of larger randomized placebo-controlled trials are urgently awaited. Several of such studies are currently recruiting (Table 3).

Perspectives

Both growth factor and cell therapy are promising new strategies to augment neovascularization in CLI patients. However, many questions will have to be answered to develop optimal strategies for therapeutic neovascularization. For growth factor, therapy questions regard the administered dose, the duration of the expression of the gene coding for the desired proangiogenic factor, and patient selection (48). The discrepancies between the first studies on growth factor therapy and the subsequent larger trials may in part have been related to these issues. On the other hand, induction of a single proangiogenic factor may be inferior to the induction of multiple proangiogenic factors by augmenting key transcription factors (17). For cell-based therapy, important questions involve the optimal cell population, the optimal route of administration, the optimal dose, the need for repeated administration, and the impact of progenitor cell dysfunction (91).

Simultaneous administration of growth factor and cell-based therapies may be beneficial, for example, intramuscular gene therapy in the calf muscles as pretreatment of the target tissue to augment homing, combined with intra-arterial administration of progenitor cells into the femoral artery of the affect limb. Indeed, in a hind limb ischemia animal model combined administration of growth factors (VEGF and angiopoietin-1 via a viral vector) and EPC resulted in a higher blood flow recovery, cellularity, and capillary density than administration of either treatment strategy alone (92). Gene therapy could also be

314

Sprengers et al.

TABLE 3 Overview of Ongoing Clinical Studies on Therapeutic Angiogenesis with Autologous BM-Derived Progenitor Cells for CLI

NCT number[a]	Country	Sponsor	Number of patients	Start date	Randomized	Placebo controlled	Double blinded	Intervention
NCT00145262	Japan	Investigator	b	August 2003	No	No	No	BM-MNC, route unknown
NCT00411840	Germany	Investigator	100	July 2004	No	No	No	BM-MNC via combined intra-arterial and intramuscular approach
NCT00113243	United States	Investigator	20	December 2004	No	No	No	Intramuscular BM-derived stem cells
NCT00306085	Italy	Investigator	20	April 2005	No	No	No	BM-MNC, route unknown
NCT00311805	United States	Investigator	24	April 2006	Yes	Yes	Yes	Intramuscular PB CD34+
NCT00488020	Brazil	Investigator	10	April 2006	No	No	No	Intramuscular BM-MNC + albumin
NCT00371371	Netherlands	Investigator	109–160[c]	September 2006	Yes	Yes	Yes	Intra-arterial BM-MNC
NCT00392509	United States	Industry	20	October 2006	Yes	Active control	Yes	Intramuscular ALDH-br BM-MNC
NCT00442143	Denmark	Investigator	10	January 2007	No	No	No	Intramuscular BM-MNC
NCT00468000	United States	Industry	120	April 2007	Yes	Yes	Yes	Intramuscular TRC BM-MNC
NCT00434616	Germany	Investigator	90	April 2007	Yes	Yes	Yes	Intramuscular BM-MNC
NCT00518401	United States	Industry	10	June 2007	No	No	No	Intramuscular stem cells
NCT00539266	Netherlands	Investigator	108	October 2007	Yes	Yes	Yes	Intramuscular BM-MNC
NCT00498069	United States	Industry	48	b	Yes	Yes	Yes	Intramuscular BM aspirate concentrate

Overview consists of all relevant trials registered in the ISRCTN register (controlled-trials.com), U.S. National Institutes of Health trial register (clinictrials.gov), Dutch trial register (trialregister.nl), and the meta-register of controlled trials (mRCT).
Studies are sorted by date of initiation of the study.
[a]Study identification number in the clinical trial register of the U.S. National Institutes of Health (ClinicalTrials.gov).
[b]Unknown.
[c]Variable number of patients to be included because of applied group sequential interim analysis.
Abbreviations: MNC, mononuclear cell; ALDH-br, Aldehyde Dehydrogenase-Bright.

applied to the progenitor cells ex vivo, to enhance their homing, migration, incorporation, and/or (trans)differentiation capacities. For example, VEGF-transfected EPC have improved proliferation and adhesion capacities in vitro, and enhance neovascularization by VEGF supply to the target tissue in animal models (93). Transduction of EPC with telomerase reverse transcriptase, which increases telomerase length and thereby delays senescence of the cells, was shown to significantly improve survival and proliferation of EPC in vitro and to enhance neovascularization with improved limb salvage in a mouse hind limb ischemia model (94). Moreover, in vitro and in vivo EPC function was demonstrated to improve with the upregulation of protein kinase Akt activity (95,96). Akt is considered an appealing therapeutic target for its role in apoptosis blocking, proliferation, and angiogenesis augmentation (97).

It is important to realize that patients in need of therapeutic neovascularization often have cardiovascular risk factors, which may influence the effect of therapy. Patients with cardiovascular risk factors have reduced numbers of EPC with impaired function with respect to clonogenic and adhesion capacities (98,99). These functional impairments extend to the whole bone marrow–derived MNC fraction and may limit the potential of cell-mediated therapy (100). Optimizing cardiovascular risk factors is therefore of crucial importance. Ex vivo pretreatment of progenitor cells with several drugs that target cardiovascular risk factors (statins, certain antihypertensive drugs) have been shown to improve progenitor cell function in vitro and neovascularization capacity in vivo in animal models (101–108).

For CLI patients without other treatment options than amputation, postnatal revascularization via growth factor therapy or progenitor cell–mediated therapy seems to provide an ultimate relief. Both preclinical studies to further elucidate underlying mechanisms of (therapeutic) neovascularization as well as large randomized controlled clinical trials with well-defined endpoints are needed for further optimization of strategies aimed at therapeutic neovascularization. Hopefully, this will lead to crucial advances in the treatment of CLI in the near future and ultimately to better options for prevention of progression to CLI by interventions in earlier stages.

REFERENCES

1. Norgren L, Hiatt WR, Dormandy JA, et al. Inter-society consensus for the management of peripheral arterial disease (TASC II). Eur J Vasc Endovasc Surg 2007; 33(suppl 1):S1–S75.
2. Guidelines for percutaneous transluminal angioplasty. Standards of practice committee of the society of cardiovascular and interventional radiology. Radiology 1990; 177:619–626.
3. Valentine RJ, Myers SI, Inman MH, et al. Late outcome of amputees with premature atherosclerosis. Surgery 1996; 119:487–493.
4. Hiatt WR. Medical treatment of peripheral arterial disease and claudication. N Engl J Med 2001; 344:1608–1621.
5. Asahara T, Murohara T, Sullivan A, et al. Isolation of putative progenitor endothelial cells for angiogenesis. Science 1997; 275:964–967.
6. Pugh CW, Ratcliffe PJ. Regulation of angiogenesis by hypoxia: role of the HIF system. Nat Med 2003; 9:677–684.
7. Takahashi T, Kalka C, Masuda H, et al. Ischemia- and cytokine-induced mobilization of bone marrow-derived endothelial progenitor cells for neovascularization. Nat Med 1999; 5:434–438.

8. Zhou B, Poon MC, Pu WT, et al. Therapeutic neovascularization for peripheral arterial diseases: advances and perspectives. Histol Histopathol 2007; 22:677–686.
9. Simons M. Angiogenesis: where do we stand now? Circulation 2005; 111:1556–1566.
10. Schaper W, Scholz D. Factors regulating arteriogenesis. Arterioscler Thromb Vasc Biol 2003; 23:1143–1151.
11. Hoefer IE, van RN, Rectenwald JE, et al. Arteriogenesis proceeds via ICAM-1/Mac-1-mediated mechanisms. Circ Res 2004; 94:1179–1185.
12. Kalka C, Masuda H, Takahashi T, et al. Transplantation of ex vivo expanded endothelial progenitor cells for therapeutic neovascularization. Proc Natl Acad Sci U S A 2000; 97:3422–3427.
13. Shah PB, Losordo DW. Non-viral vectors for gene therapy: clinical trials in cardiovascular disease. Adv Genet 2005; 54:339–361.
14. Khan TA, Sellke FW, Laham RJ. Gene therapy progress and prospects: therapeutic angiogenesis for limb and myocardial ischemia. Gene Ther 2003; 10:285–291.
15. Morishita R, Aoki M, Hashiya N, et al. Safety evaluation of clinical gene therapy using hepatocyte growth factor to treat peripheral arterial disease. Hypertension 2004; 44:203–209.
16. van RN, Schirmer SH, Atasever B, et al. START Trial: a pilot study on STimulation of ARTeriogenesis using subcutaneous application of granulocyte-macrophage colony-stimulating factor as a new treatment for peripheral vascular disease. Circulation 2005; 112:1040–1046.
17. Rajagopalan S, Olin J, Deitcher S, et al. Use of a constitutively active hypoxia-inducible factor-1alpha transgene as a therapeutic strategy in no-option critical limb ischemia patients: phase I dose-escalation experience. Circulation 2007; 115:1234–1243.
18. Rissanen TT, Vajanto I, Yla-Herttuala S. Gene therapy for therapeutic angiogenesis in critically ischaemic lower limb—on the way to the clinic. Eur J Clin Invest 2001; 31:651–666.
19. Yla-Herttuala S, Rissanen TT, Vajanto I, et al. Vascular endothelial growth factors: biology and current status of clinical applications in cardiovascular medicine. J Am Coll Cardiol 2007; 49:1015–1026.
20. Bobek V, Taltynov O, Pinterova D, et al. Gene therapy of the ischemic lower limb—Therapeutic angiogenesis. Vascul Pharmacol 2006; 44:395–405.
21. Itoh N. The Fgf families in humans, mice, and zebrafish: their evolutionary processes and roles in development, metabolism, and disease. Biol Pharm Bull 2007; 30:1819–1825.
22. Hariawala MD, Horowitz JR, Esakof D, et al. VEGF improves myocardial blood flow but produces EDRF-mediated hypotension in porcine hearts. J Surg Res 1996; 63:77–82.
23. Manninen HI, Makinen K. Gene therapy techniques for peripheral arterial disease. Cardiovasc Intervent Radiol 2002; 25:98–108.
24. Tsutsui JM, Xie F, Porter RT. The use of microbubbles to target drug delivery. Cardiovasc Ultrasound 2004; 2:23.
25. Lawrie A, Brisken AF, Francis SE, et al. Microbubble-enhanced ultrasound for vascular gene delivery. Gene Ther 2000; 7:2023–2027.
26. McMahon JM, Wells DJ. Electroporation for gene transfer to skeletal muscles: current status. BioDrugs 2004; 18:155–165.
27. Andre F, Mir LM. DNA electrotransfer: its principles and an updated review of its therapeutic applications. Gene Ther 2004; 11(suppl 1):S33–S42.
28. Banai S, Jaklitsch MT, Shou M, et al. Angiogenic-induced enhancement of collateral blood flow to ischemic myocardium by vascular endothelial growth factor in dogs. Circulation 1994; 89:2183–2189.
29. Yanagisawa-Miwa A, Uchida Y, Nakamura F, et al. Salvage of infarcted myocardium by angiogenic action of basic fibroblast growth factor. Science 1992; 257:1401–1403.
30. Pu LQ, Sniderman AD, Brassard R, et al. Enhanced revascularization of the ischemic limb by angiogenic therapy. Circulation 1993; 88:208–215.
31. Takeshita S, Zheng LP, Brogi E, et al. Therapeutic angiogenesis. A single intraarterial bolus of vascular endothelial growth factor augments revascularization in a rabbit ischemic hind limb model. J Clin Invest 1994; 93:662–670.

32. Isner JM, Pieczek A, Schainfeld R, et al. Clinical evidence of angiogenesis after arterial gene transfer of phVEGF165 in patient with ischaemic limb. Lancet 1996; 348:370–374.
33. Isner JM. Arterial gene transfer of naked DNA for therapeutic angiogenesis: early clinical results. Adv Drug Deliv Rev 1998; 30:185–197.
34. Isner JM, Walsh K, Symes J, et al. Arterial gene therapy for therapeutic angiogenesis in patients with peripheral artery disease. Circulation 1995; 91:2687–2692.
35. Baumgartner I, Pieczek A, Manor O, et al. Constitutive expression of phVEGF165 after intramuscular gene transfer promotes collateral vessel development in patients with critical limb ischemia. Circulation 1998; 97:1114–1123.
36. Rajagopalan S, Shah M, Luciano A, et al. Adenovirus-mediated gene transfer of VEGF(121) improves lower-extremity endothelial function and flow reserve. Circulation 2001; 104:753–755.
37. Comerota AJ, Throm RC, Miller KA, et al. Naked plasmid DNA encoding fibroblast growth factor type 1 for the treatment of end-stage unreconstructible lower extremity ischemia: preliminary results of a phase I trial. J Vasc Surg 2002; 35:930–936.
38. Mäkinen K, Manninen H, Hedman M, et al. Increased vascularity detected by digital subtraction angiography after VEGF gene transfer to human lower limb artery: a randomized, placebo-controlled, double-blinded phase II study. Mol Ther 2002; 6:127–133.
39. Shyu KG, Chang H, Wang BW, et al. Intramuscular vascular endothelial growth factor gene therapy in patients with chronic critical leg ischemia. Am J Med 2003; 114:85–92.
40. Kim HJ, Jang SY, Park JI, et al. Vascular endothelial growth factor-induced angiogenic gene therapy in patients with peripheral artery disease. Exp Mol Med 2004; 36:336–344.
41. Kusumanto YH, van Weel V, Mulder NH, et al. Treatment with intramuscular vascular endothelial growth factor gene compared with placebo for patients with diabetes mellitus and critical limb ischemia: a double-blind randomized trial. Hum Gene Ther 2006; 17:683–691.
42. Rajagopalan S, Mohler ER III, Lederman RJ, et al. Regional angiogenesis with vascular endothelial growth factor in peripheral arterial disease: a phase II randomized, double-blind, controlled study of adenoviral delivery of vascular endothelial growth factor 121 in patients with disabling intermittent claudication. Circulation 2003; 108:1933–1938.
43. Lederman RJ, Mendelsohn FO, Anderson RD, et al. Therapeutic angiogenesis with recombinant fibroblast growth factor-2 for intermittent claudication (the TRAFFIC study): a randomised trial. Lancet 2002; 359:2053–2058.
44. Powell RJ, Dormandy J, Simons M, et al. Therapeutic angiogenesis for critical limb ischemia: design of the hepatocyte growth factor therapeutic angiogenesis clinical trial. Vasc Med 2004; 9:193–198.
45. Simons M, Annex BH, Laham RJ, et al. Pharmacological treatment of coronary artery disease with recombinant fibroblast growth factor-2: double-blind, randomized, controlled clinical trial. Circulation 2002; 105:788–793.
46. Henry TD, Annex BH, McKendall GR, et al. The VIVA trial: vascular endothelial growth factor in ischemia for vascular angiogenesis. Circulation 2003; 107:1359–1365.
47. Grines CL, Watkins MW, Mahmarian JJ, et al. A randomized, double-blind, placebo-controlled trial of Ad5FGF-4 gene therapy and its effect on myocardial perfusion in patients with stable angina. J Am Coll Cardiol 2003; 42:1339–1347.
48. Simons M, Ware JA. Therapeutic angiogenesis in cardiovascular disease. Nat Rev Drug Discov 2003; 2:863–871.
49. Crosby JR, Kaminski WE, Schatteman G, et al. Endothelial cells of hematopoietic origin make a significant contribution to adult blood vessel formation. Circ Res 2000; 87:728–730.
50. Asahara T, Masuda H, Takahashi T, et al. Bone marrow origin of endothelial progenitor cells responsible for postnatal vasculogenesis in physiological and pathological neovascularization. Circ Res 1999; 85:221–228.

51. Capla JM, Ceradini DJ, Tepper OM, et al. Skin graft vascularization involves precisely regulated regression and replacement of endothelial cells through both angiogenesis and vasculogenesis. Plast Reconstr Surg 2006; 117:836–844.

52. Shi Q, Rafii S, Wu MH, et al. Evidence for circulating bone marrow-derived endothelial cells. Blood 1998; 92:362–367.

53. Shintani S, Murohara T, Ikeda H, et al. Mobilization of endothelial progenitor cells in patients with acute myocardial infarction. Circulation 2001; 103:2776–2779.

54. Shintani S, Murohara T, Ikeda H, et al. Augmentation of postnatal neovascularization with autologous bone marrow transplantation. Circulation 2001; 103:897–903.

55. Kamihata H, Matsubara H, Nishiue T, et al. Implantation of bone marrow mononuclear cells into ischemic myocardium enhances collateral perfusion and regional function via side supply of angioblasts, angiogenic ligands, and cytokines. Circulation 2001; 104:1046–1052.

56. Murohara T, Ikeda H, Duan J, et al. Transplanted cord blood-derived endothelial precursor cells augment postnatal neovascularization. J Clin Invest 2000; 105:1527–1536.

57. Finney MR, Greco NJ, Haynesworth SE, et al. Direct comparison of umbilical cord blood versus bone marrow-derived endothelial precursor cells in mediating neovascularization in response to vascular ischemia. Biol Blood Marrow Transplant 2006; 12:585–593.

58. Yoshida M, Horimoto H, Mieno S, et al. Intra-arterial bone marrow cell transplantation induces angiogenesis in rat hindlimb ischemia. Eur Surg Res 2003; 35:86–91.

59. Kocher AA, Schuster MD, Szabolcs MJ, et al. Neovascularization of ischemic myocardium by human bone-marrow-derived angioblasts prevents cardiomyocyte apoptosis, reduces remodeling and improves cardiac function. Nat Med 2001; 7:430–436.

60. Kawamoto A, Gwon HC, Iwaguro H, et al. Therapeutic potential of ex vivo expanded endothelial progenitor cells for myocardial ischemia. Circulation 2001; 103:634–637.

61. Rookmaaker MB, Verhaar MC, Loomans CJ, et al. CD34+ cells home, proliferate, and participate in capillary formation, and in combination with. Arterioscler Thromb Vasc Biol 2005; 25:1843–1850.

62. Harraz M, Jiao C, Hanlon HD, et al. CD34—blood-derived human endothelial cell progenitors. Stem Cells 2001; 19:304–312.

63. Fernandez PB, Lucibello FC, Gehling UM, et al. Endothelial-like cells derived from human CD14 positive monocytes. Differentiation 2000; 65:287–300.

64. Rehman J, Li J, Orschell CM, et al. Peripheral blood "endothelial progenitor cells" are derived from monocyte/macrophages and secrete angiogenic growth factors. Circulation 2003; 107:1164–1169.

65. Urbich C, Heeschen C, Aicher A, et al. Relevance of monocytic features for neovascularization capacity of circulating endothelial progenitor cells. Circulation 2003; 108:2511–2516.

66. Ziegelhoeffer T, Fernandez B, Kostin S, et al. Bone marrow-derived cells do not incorporate into the adult growing vasculature. Circ Res 2004; 94:230–238.

67. Heil M, Ziegelhoeffer T, Mees B, et al. A different outlook on the role of bone marrow stem cells in vascular growth: bone marrow delivers software not hardware. Circ Res 2004; 94:573–574.

68. Dimmeler S, Zeiher AM, Schneider MD. Unchain my heart: the scientific foundations of cardiac repair. J Clin Invest 2005; 115:572–583.

69. Bartsch T, Brehm M, Zeus T, et al. Autologous mononuclear stem cell transplantation in patients with peripheral occlusive arterial disease. J Cardiovasc Nurs 2006; 21:430–432.

70. Strauer BE, Brehm M, Zeus T, et al. Repair of infarcted myocardium by autologous intracoronary mononuclear bone marrow cell transplantation in humans. Circulation 2002; 106:1913–1918.

71. Zhang M, Methot D, Poppa V, et al. Cardiomyocyte grafting for cardiac repair: graft cell death and anti-death strategies. J Mol Cell Cardiol 2001; 33:907–921.

72. Toma C, Pittenger MF, Cahill KS, et al. Human mesenchymal stem cells differentiate to a cardiomyocyte phenotype in the adult murine heart. Circulation 2002; 105:93–98.
73. Tateishi-Yuyama E, Matsubara H, Murohara T, et al. Therapeutic angiogenesis for patients with limb ischaemia by autologous transplantation of bone-marrow cells: a pilot study and a randomised controlled trial. Lancet 2002; 360:427–435.
74. Esato K, Hamano K, Li TS, et al. Neovascularization induced by autologous bone marrow cell implantation in peripheral arterial disease. Cell Transplant 2002; 11:747–752.
75. Higashi Y, Kimura M, Hara K, et al. Autologous bone-marrow mononuclear cell implantation improves endothelium-dependent vasodilation in patients with limb ischemia. Circulation 2004; 109:1215–1218.
76. Miyamoto M, Yasutake M, Takano H, et al. Therapeutic angiogenesis by autologous bone marrow cell implantation for refractory chronic peripheral arterial disease using assessment of neovascularization by 99mTc-tetrofosmin (TF) perfusion scintigraphy. Cell Transplant 2004; 13:429–437.
77. Saigawa T, Kato K, Ozawa T, et al. Clinical application of bone marrow implantation in patients with arteriosclerosis obliterans, and the association between efficacy and the number of implanted bone marrow cells. Circ J 2004; 68:1189–1193.
78. Bartsch T, Falke T, Brehm M, et al. [Transplantation of autologous adult bone marrow stem cells in patients with severe peripheral arterial occlusion disease.] Med Klin (Munich) 2006; 101(suppl 1):195–197.
79. Durdu S, Akar AR, Arat M, et al. Autologous bone-marrow mononuclear cell implantation for patients with Rutherford grade II-III thromboangiitis obliterans. J Vasc Surg 2006; 44:732–739.
80. Miyamoto K, Nishigami K, Nagaya N, et al. Unblinded pilot study of autologous transplantation of bone marrow mononuclear cells in patients with thromboangiitis obliterans. Circulation 2006; 114:2679–2684.
81. Kajiguchi M, Kondo T, Izawa H, et al. Safety and efficacy of autologous progenitor cell transplantation for therapeutic angiogenesis in patients with critical limb ischemia. Circ J 2007; 71:196–201.
82. Sugihara S, Yamamoto Y, Matsubara K, et al. Autoperipheral blood mononuclear cell transplantation improved giant ulcers due to chronic arteriosclerosis obliterans. Heart Vessels 2006; 21:258–262.
83. Huang PP, Li SZ, Han MZ, et al. Autologous transplantation of peripheral blood stem cells as an effective therapeutic approach for severe arteriosclerosis obliterans of lower extremities. Thromb Haemost 2004; 91:606–609.
84. Kawamura A, Horie T, Tsuda I, et al. Prevention of limb amputation in patients with limbs ulcers by autologous peripheral blood mononuclear cell implantation. Ther Apher Dial 2005; 9:59–63.
85. Lenk K, Adams V, Lurz P, et al. Therapeutical potential of blood-derived progenitor cells in patients with peripheral arterial occlusive disease and critical limb ischaemia. Eur Heart J 2005; 26:1903–1909.
86. Huang P, Li S, Han M, et al. Autologous transplantation of granulocyte colony-stimulating factor-mobilized peripheral blood mononuclear cells improves critical limb ischemia in diabetes. Diabetes Care 2005; 28:2155–2160.
87. Ishida A, Ohya Y, Sakuda H, et al. Autologous peripheral blood mononuclear cell implantation for patients with peripheral arterial disease improves limb ischemia. Circ J 2005; 69:1260–1265.
88. Kawamura A, Horie T, Tsuda I, et al. Clinical study of therapeutic angiogenesis by autologous peripheral blood stem cell (PBSC) transplantation in 92 patients with critically ischemic limbs. J Artif Organs 2006; 9:226–233.
89. Kudo FA, Nishibe T, Nishibe M, et al. Autologous transplantation of peripheral blood endothelial progenitor cells (CD34+) for therapeutic angiogenesis in patients with critical limb ischemia. Int Angiol 2003; 22:344–348.
90. Cañizo MC, Lozano F, Gonzalez-Porras JR, et al. Peripheral endothelial progenitor cells (CD133 +) for therapeutic vasculogenesis in a patient with critical limb ischemia. One year follow-up. Cytotherapy 2007; 9:99–102.

91. Sprengers RW, Lips DJ, Moll FL, et al. Progenitor cell therapy in patients with critical limb ischemia without surigcal options. Ann Surg 2008; 247(3):411–420.

92. Chen F, Tan Z, Dong CY, et al. Combination of VEGF(165)/Angiopoietin-1 gene and endothelial progenitor cells for therapeutic neovascularization. Eur J Pharmacol 2007; 568:222–230.

93. Iwaguro H, Yamaguchi J, Kalka C, et al. Endothelial progenitor cell vascular endothelial growth factor gene transfer for vascular regeneration. Circulation 2002; 105:732–738.

94. Murasawa S, Llevadot J, Silver M, et al. Constitutive human telomerase reverse transcriptase expression enhances regenerative properties of endothelial progenitor cells. Circulation 2002; 106:1133–1139.

95. Cho HJ, Youn SW, Cheon SI, et al. Regulation of endothelial cell and endothelial progenitor cell survival and vasculogenesis by integrin-linked kinase. Arterioscler Thromb Vasc Biol 2005; 25:1154–1160.

96. Choi JH, Hur J, Yoon CH, et al. Augmentation of therapeutic angiogenesis using genetically modified human endothelial progenitor cells with altered glycogen synthase kinase-3beta activity. J Biol Chem 2004; 279:49430–49438.

97. Seeger FH, Zeiher AM, Dimmeler S. Cell-enhancement strategies for the treatment of ischemic heart disease. Nat Clin Pract Cardiovasc Med 2007; 4(suppl 1):S110–S113.

98. Vasa M, Fichtlscherer S, Aicher A, et al. Number and migratory activity of circulating endothelial progenitor cells inversely correlate with risk factors for coronary artery disease. Circ Res 2001; 89:E1–E7.

99. Fadini GP, Sartore S, Albiero M, et al. Number and function of endothelial progenitor cells as a marker of severity for diabetic vasculopathy. Arterioscler Thromb Vasc Biol 2006; 26:2140–2146.

100. Heeschen C, Lehmann R, Honold J, et al. Profoundly reduced neovascularization capacity of bone marrow mononuclear cells derived from patients with chronic ischemic heart disease. Circulation 2004; 109:1615–1622.

101. Dimmeler S, Aicher A, Vasa M, et al. HMG-CoA reductase inhibitors (statins) increase endothelial progenitor cells via the PI 3-kinase/Akt pathway. J Clin Invest 2001; 108:391–397.

102. Llevadot J, Murasawa S, Kureishi Y, et al. HMG-CoA reductase inhibitor mobilizes bone marrow—derived endothelial progenitor cells. J Clin Invest 2001; 108:399–405.

103. Vasa M, Fichtlscherer S, Adler K, et al. Increase in circulating endothelial progenitor cells by statin therapy in patients with stable coronary artery disease. Circulation 2001; 103:2885–2890.

104. Assmus B, Urbich C, Aicher A, et al. HMG-CoA reductase inhibitors reduce senescence and increase proliferation of endothelial progenitor cells via regulation of cell cycle regulatory genes. Circ Res 2003; 92:1049–1055.

105. Shantsila E, Watson T, Lip GY. Endothelial progenitor cells in cardiovascular disorders. J Am Coll Cardiol 2007; 49:741–752.

106. Pistrosch F, Herbrig K, Oelschlaegel U, et al. PPARgamma-agonist rosiglitazone increases number and migratory activity of cultured endothelial progenitor cells. Atherosclerosis 2005; 183:163–167.

107. Wang CH, Ting MK, Verma S, et al. Pioglitazone increases the numbers and improves the functional capacity of endothelial progenitor cells in patients with diabetes mellitus. Am Heart J 2006; 152:1051–1058.

108. Sasaki K, Heeschen C, Aicher A, et al. Ex vivo pretreatment of bone marrow mononuclear cells with endothelial NO synthase enhancer AVE9488 enhances their functional activity for cell therapy. Proc Natl Acad Sci U S A 2006; 103:14537–14541.

Index